Mental Health in Historical Perspective

Series Editors
Catharine Coleborne
School of Humanities and Social Science
University of Newcastle
Callaghan, NSW, Australia

Matthew Smith
Centre for the Social History of Health and Healthcare
University of Strathclyde
Glasgow, UK

Covering all historical periods and geographical contexts, the series explores how mental illness has been understood, experienced, diagnosed, treated and contested. It will publish works that engage actively with contemporary debates related to mental health and, as such, will be of interest not only to historians, but also mental health professionals, patients and policy makers. With its focus on mental health, rather than just psychiatry, the series will endeavour to provide more patient-centred histories. Although this has long been an aim of health historians, it has not been realised, and this series aims to change that.

The scope of the series is kept as broad as possible to attract good quality proposals about all aspects of the history of mental health from all periods. The series emphasises interdisciplinary approaches to the field of study, and encourages short titles, longer works, collections, and titles which stretch the boundaries of academic publishing in new ways.

More information about this series at
http://www.palgrave.com/gp/series/14806

David Freis

Psycho-Politics between the World Wars

Psychiatry and Society in Germany, Austria, and Switzerland

palgrave
macmillan

David Freis
Institute of Ethics, History
and Theory of Medicine
University of Münster
Münster, Germany

Mental Health in Historical Perspective
ISBN 978-3-030-32701-9 ISBN 978-3-030-32702-6 (eBook)
https://doi.org/10.1007/978-3-030-32702-6

Cover credit: Balfore Archive Images/Alamy Stock Photo

This Palgrave Macmillan imprint is published by the registered company Springer Nature Switzerland AG
The registered company address is: Gewerbestrasse 11, 6330 Cham, Switzerland

Acknowledgements

This book has been long in the making and over the years has crossed the paths of many people. Most of what is good about this book is due to their suggestions, their feedback, advice, encouragement, and support. Everything else is, of course, entirely to blame on me. What follows is only an incomplete list of those who helped me to see this project through to the end.

My interest in the history of psychiatry was sparked by Regina Schulte, whose seminars and excursions introduced me to the archives and to historical thinking. Martin Kohlrausch supported this project from the very beginning and went on to serve as an external supervisor when I relocated from the Ruhr University's béton brut to the Tuscan hills. At the European University Institute in Florence, Dirk Moses's rigorous supervision greatly helped me to turn my research into a readable text and initiated me to the art of the topic sentence. Pavel Kolář provided feedback and encouragement. Alexander Etkind as second reader and Mitchell Ash, who kindly joined the examination board, supplied their vast expertise. My thanks also go out to all the people, researchers, academic and non-academic staff, too many to name here, who made and make the EUI the unique institution and community that it is, to the EUI library for providing a great environment to work, to their incredible interlibrary loan service, and to the German Academic Exchange Service for offering me this wonderful possibility. Research for this project would not have been possible without the friendly and helpful staff in many libraries and archives, and writing it would have been a lot less pleasant without the grumpy waiters in many coffee houses in Vienna and elsewhere. Regina Schulte, Lucian Hölscher, Martin Kohlrausch, Mitchell Ash, Friedrich Stadler, John Zilcosky, Wolf Kittler, and Thomas Beddies offered me the possibility to present and discuss aspects of this research in their seminars. The Deutsche Gesellschaft für Geschichte der Nervenheilkunde, the journal *Medical History*, and the Fachverband Medizingeschichte kindly awarded prizes for this project and its offshoots. I also thank Volker Roelcke, Heiner Fangerau, Elizabeth Danto, and, in particular, Hans-Georg Hofer for their advice and support.

That my research eventually took the form of this book is thanks to Molly Beck and Maeve Sinnott at Palgrave Macmillan, who kindly and patiently guided me through the publication process. Many thanks to Matt Smith and Cathy Colborne for adding this book to an increasingly long list of great titles in their series. I would also like to thank the anonymous reviewer for their kind and constructive feedback.

Finally, all of this would never have been possible without Elisabeth and her tireless encouragement and unbelievable patience.

Contents

About the Author

David Freis is a research associate in the Institute for the Ethics, History, and Theory of Medicine at the University of Münster. He received his Ph.D. in history and civilisation from the European University Institute and is the author of numerous articles and chapters in the history of psychiatry and psychotherapy.

CHAPTER 1

Introduction

After the First World War, psychiatrists captured the imagination of the public. Two of the eponymous villains of early Weimar cinema's most successful and iconic films were mad doctors as much as mad-doctors. In the 1920 movie, a nameless alienist-turned-lunatic styles himself as the early-modern showman Caligari and uses his suggestive abilities to force a patient into becoming his tool for murder. Soon after, the demonic Dr. Mabuse, a physician and psychoanalyst, appeared as the main figure in the film adaption of the recent best-seller. Amidst the post-war commotion, he employs his hypnotic powers to subtly influence his surroundings, to gamble, spy, and to manipulate the stock market. The mastermind behind an enormous criminal conspiracy, his aim is to create and rule a utopian community in the South American jungles. Both films mark the beginning of a cinematic occupation with an uncanny image of the psychiatrist that continued through the twentieth century.[1]

In his influential analysis of Weimar cinema, Siegfried Kracauer argued that the figure of the hypnotic psychiatrist symbolically foreshadowed transformations in the exercise of political power that Germany would experience with the rise of Nazism.[2] However, as film historian Anton Kaes has more recently shown, the doctors Caligari and Mabuse also related to the actual history of psychiatry during and after the war.[3] On first sight, the real psychiatrists of 1918 had little in common with these caricatures of malevolent quacks—although, about two decades later, a number of them would

D. Freis, *Psycho-Politics between the World Wars*,
Mental Health in Historical Perspective,
https://doi.org/10.1007/978-3-030-32702-6_1

turn into more gruesome murderers than early Weimar film-makers would have been able to imagine. But there was more to psychiatrists' depiction in these films than only the evocative narrative of madness affecting those who promised to cure it. Older tales of patient abuse and fears of wrongful confinement in madhouses merged with more recent reports of the brutal treatment of 'hysterical' soldiers and mass starvation in psychiatric asylums during the war.

Like other 'mad scientists' in popular culture, post-war cinema's psychiatrists reflected an ambivalence about the threats and promises of modern science. The fascination with progress was mixed with fears that representatives of a discipline claiming a privileged insight into the deepest layers of the functioning of the human mind could use this knowledge to manipulate individuals and collectives.[4] And in fact, while psychiatrists in 1918 were neither delusional killers nor megalomaniac criminals, many of them firmly believed in shifting the boundaries of their professional authority further into society and politics, targeting not only the insane but also the apparently normal, and in restructuring society on the basis of their scientific insights. Often these calls for socio-medical interventions translated directly into visions of psychiatrists transcending their traditional role as physicians and becoming guides and leaders of the nation on the way towards 'mental reconstruction'.[5]

The shrillest of these voices faded into silence during the political and economic consolidation of the early 1920s. Nonetheless, in the following decades psychiatrists' attempts to bring diagnosis and treatment outside the asylum and the clinic continued in different shapes. Many of the ideas discussed in this context were not entirely new. Throughout the nineteenth century, psychiatrists had drawn political conclusions from clinical observations and had framed their diagnoses of perceived social and political problems in medical terms.[6] After all, psychiatry both as a science and as a practice was, from the onset, concerned with social norms and the maintenance of social order and thus always had one foot in the political sphere. Only after the First World War, however, did psychiatrists' socio-political ideas grow into systematic programmes and became institutionalised as associations and societies.

This book examines the radical reformulation of psychiatrists' role in society in the period between the First World War and the Second World War. Out of a vast range of possible stories that could be told, I focus on three attempts to redefine psychiatry's relation to society and politics: the psycho-political diagnoses of the defeat and the revolution in 1918/1919, 'applied psychiatry', and mental hygiene. While the larger trend of an increasing presence of experts from the psy-ences in all fields of political, social, and cultural life beginning in the inter-war period has been noted by scholars from different perspectives, we know less about the specific historical configurations shaping this process. As I show, psychiatry's 'need for expansion', which was already observed by contemporaries, was far from monolithic.[7] It sprung from very different motives and circumstances and happened at the intersection of the larger lines of political history with intra-psychiatric and intra-medical developments and against the background of growing competition with other actors in the differentiating field of the psy-ences. My main goal is to examine psychiatry's move out of the asylum and the clinic and into society and politics in both detail and context. I ask about continuities and discontinuities to pre-war psycho-political thinking, and how the experience of the First World War and the political turmoil that followed it accelerated and shaped the redefinition of psychiatrists' self-understanding in the inter-war period. Furthermore, I also take a close look at the interplay, competition, and conflict between different actors in the scientific field, both inside the psychiatric discipline, in the wider realm of the psy-ences, and beyond.

My point of departure is the end of the First World War. Like for many other areas of politics, culture, and science, the first global and industrial war marked a significant caesura in the history of psychiatry as a medical speciality. The need to treat hundreds of thousands of 'war neurotics' had given psychiatry an important role in the conduct of war and brought the discipline into even closer proximity to the state.[8] Following a rationale of efficiency and rationalisation, the mass treatment of war neuroses through a range of newly invented or re-discovered methods promised a therapeutic breakthrough. It presented psychiatry with the prospect of finally overcoming an era of 'therapeutic nihilism', in which important scientific advances had changed little about psychiatry's notorious inability to heal its patients. For psychiatry as a 'belated science',[9] this recently gained prestige and treatment success promised an opportunity to close up to more successful medical specialties such as bacteriology and surgery, which had experienced a most impressive development in the previous decades. With the military defeat of the Central Powers and the post-war turmoil, however, these war gains were threatening to unravel quickly. Public and patient protests and the dissolution of military hierarchies profoundly altered the relation between doctors and their patients and effectively abolished the foundations of psychiatry's therapeutic success, which often had been based on the almost unconditional subordination of soldier-patients under their military physicians.[10]

Medical debates about the treatment of the war neurotics and the impact of the war on individual patients were accompanied and mirrored by a discourse transposing the issue from the individual to the level of the collective. Drawing on nineteenth-century psychologies of the collective such as French *psychologie des foules* and German *Völkerpsychologie*, prominent psychiatrists discussed how the war had created, affected, jolted, or united a 'national soul' (*Volksseele*) and how collective psychology and psychopathology could explain the behaviour of the enemy. Oscillating between analogy, metaphor, and actual diagnosis, the concept of the *Volksseele* complemented the ubiquitous wartime talk of an organic body politic and allowed to discuss politics from a psychological and psychiatric perspective. In the wake of defeat and revolution, the concept of the *Volksseele* helped reframe the political, cultural, and medical crisis of the immediate post-war period as a crisis of a collective psyche. Against this backdrop, prominent right-wing psychiatrists radicalised their views of their role in society, shifting the focus from the mental health of the individual patient to that of the nation as a whole. They combined alarmist psycho-political diagnoses about collective mental 'shocks' and 'nervous breakdowns' with calls for far-reaching socio-medial programs, which only they themselves, invested with privileged insights into the medical and spiritual needs of the people, would be legitimised to lead.

The most ambitious and aggressive of these programmes was 'applied psychiatry', for which the Viennese psychiatrist Erwin Stransky (1877–1962) untiringly and stubbornly campaigned throughout the interwar period. Introduced in 1918 as an expansive vision of 'medical imperialism' of the psychiatric profession by the right-wing nationalist Stransky, and radicalised politically after the end of the war, its history took a surprising turn during the 1920s. Conflicted between cooperation and competition with the Vienna psychoanalysts and individual psychologists, applied psychiatry became a uniquely interdisciplinary forum, bringing together scholars from very different backgrounds using psychopathology to examine culture, society, and politics. It reached its zenith with a first international conference, when some of the greatest minds in psychiatry and its border areas gathered in Vienna in the summer of 1930. A projected second conference never took place, as the rise of Nazism and Austro-fascism severed the networks and forced key actors into exile for both 'racial' and political reasons. In the end, applied psychiatry yielded few palpable results, but its grandiose claims and the peculiar concurrence of aggressive disciplinary expansionism and interdisciplinary cooperation *avant la lettre* make it one of the most fascinating forgotten episodes in the history of the psy-ences.

As a movement, mental hygiene originally was a product of American pre-war philanthropism that entered the European stage in the mid-1920s. The founding of mental hygiene associations in Europe was the result of lobbying by protagonists of the vastly more successful movement in the United States. But the Europe associations directly built upon various pre-existing local reform programmes in psychiatry. Mental hygiene brought together different approaches to psychiatric reform and prophylaxis in common national frameworks and engaged them in the international 'politics of comparison'.[11] Simultaneously, reform-minded psychiatrists used the prestige of being part of an up-and-coming international movement to bolster their own position at home. Mental hygiene introduced an unprecedented degree of internationalism to the professional networks of reform-minded psychiatrists and—in the same year as applied psychiatry—reached its apogee in 1930 with a large international meeting in Washington, DC. In the following decade, and against the backdrop of rising political tensions, meetings of European mental hygienists continued. During this time, mental hygiene's internationalism became increasingly charged with political notions of mutual understanding among nations and the prevention of war. These notions, however, could also be instrumentalised by the foreign policy propaganda of the 'Third Reich'.

From the very beginning, there were considerable discrepancies between what mental hygiene actually meant on both sides of the Atlantic. In the wake of the world economic crisis, the different national branches of the international movement drifted even further apart. US mental hygienists believed in the importance of the environment and used Freudian notions to propagate early adjustment in childhood as well as social and political reform. By contrast, German mental hygienists subscribed to the social-Darwinist view that the most effective way to prevent mental illness was to prevent the mentally ill from reproducing. Although the initial agenda of the German Association for Mental Hygiene was broad, its activities increasingly narrowed down to the propagation of racial hygiene and eugenics. In Switzerland, mental hygiene was on yet another intellectual trajectory. Strongly influenced by pre-war psycho-utopianism and psychoanalysis, leading representatives of the Swiss movement envisioned mental hygiene as far more than a medical speciality and even as the pedagogical and philosophical foundation of a future society.

The introduction of catchy brand names such as 'applied psychiatry' and 'mental hygiene' was in itself telling. After the First World War, scientific expertise increasingly became an actively traded commodity. Experts from all fields entered a booming market, in which different resources—such as research money and equipment, influence, power, prestige, legitimacy, and recognition—were traded, not only between scientists and political actors, but also inside disciplines, among them, and in the public sphere.[12] Hence, these names reflect the need to situate and advertise different approaches in a competitive environment and to strategically distinguish them from similar ideas.[13]

Evidently, the examples discussed here were not the only reason for and not the only expression of the shift into the social sphere that psychiatry and psychiatric knowledge experienced during this period. This process should be seen as the outcome of a complex conjuncture of scientific, political, social, economic, and cultural factors. The programmes mentioned above were, in some way or another, influenced by the expansion of the welfare state and the debates about pensions for mentally wounded soldiers, which created an increasing demand for psychiatric expertise in welfare legislation and bureaucracy.[14] Advances in heredity research, which added to the scientific prestige of this field of psychiatry and brought the discipline as a whole closer to the already well-established movement for eugenics and 'racial hygiene', also stimulated visions of psychiatric prophylaxis.[15] Other important impulses came from the professionalisation and expansion of psychotherapy and from the increasing circulation of psychoanalytic ideas among scholars, intellectuals, artists, and the public.

This book wants to offer a new perspective on the history of psychiatry in the years between the world wars and psychiatry's shift into the social sphere. It focuses not only on psychiatrists' most explicit attempts to move the boundaries of their discipline beyond the clinic and the asylum, but distinguishes three different layers of this process: *diagnosis*, *expansion*, and *prophylaxis*. The clearest example for the first is the psycho-political writings in the aftermath of the 1918/1919 revolution. They relied on a double extension of the range of psychiatry's diagnoses, both on a group of 'psychopathic' individuals who were rarely found in the asylum and the clinic and on the entire nation, which was described as showing the same symptoms as an hysteric individual. Many of these tracts moved from diagnosis to therapy and proposed socio-medical interventions that went far beyond the usual boundaries of psychiatry. This expansion is the topic of the second case study. Visions of an expansion of psychiatry's sphere of authority were nowhere articulated as clearly and radically as in the case of applied psychiatry. Erwin Stransky was less interested in solving specific social and medical problems and more with psychiatry's aggressive expansion on all fronts. The third aspect, prophylaxis, became the pivotal idea of the movement for mental hygiene. The notion of a prevention of mental illness was directly connected to foundational research into its causation, but it also involved a redefinition of the boundaries of psychiatrists' activities. In all three of these interconnected case studies, I ask the same question: How did the conjuncture of national politics, professional politics inside the psy-ences, and medical and psychiatric ideas shape and redefine psychiatrists' self-understanding in the inter-war period?

Throughout this book, the focus is not only on visions, ideas, and institutions, but also on the individuals who conceived them. I situate their views on psycho-political diagnoses, disciplinary expansion, and mental prophylaxis in the context of their careers and professional trajectories and the actors themselves in their broader historical context. The goal is of course not to return to a narrative of great men and their deeds and ideas that has long dominated the historiography of medicine. Even if one were to endorse this approach, many of the protagonists introduced in this study would hardly qualify. Instead, the aim is to use the biographies of a number of protagonists as a method among others in order to gain an additional layer of analysis. While a top-down view on larger discourses and macro-structures would perhaps produce a neater account, a perspective moving more freely between individual biographies and broader contexts has the potential to overcome the temptation of all too linear stories and an homogenising view of modern psychiatry. Following individual scholars through their historical contexts offers a way to avoid some of the pitfalls of the teleological narrative of an ever-increasing permeation of society by the psy-ences, instead highlighting individual agency, contingency, and historicity, allowing for a more complex understanding of continuities and discontinuities through the political caesuras and crises of the early twentieth century.

'Following the actors' may lead to unexpected places.[16] The boundaries of scientific and medical disciplines were far more porous than commonly assumed, and the networks around these protagonists included surprising connections between diverse scholars and their respective approaches, likely and less-likely alliances and long-standing enmities. At the same time, a more long-term perspective on the careers of these scholars can contribute to a more comprehensive analysis of the development of their ideas, continuities and discontinuities, and the impact of individual and collective experiences. Finally, a closer look at the protagonists allows to relate the expansion of scientific expertise in the early twentieth century to the changes in political, medical, and academic self-perceptions that animated, accompanied, and legitimised this process.

Escaping the Straitjacket of Confinement: The History of Twentieth-Century Psychiatry

Although this study takes its inspirations and perspectives from a variety of different historiographical fields, it is clearly situated in the history of psychiatry. Over the last decades, the historiography of psychiatry has developed into a vibrant and highly diverse historical sub-discipline. Recently, historians in the field have again broadened their perspective, increasingly situating the history of psychiatry in the broader context of society, culture, science, and technology.[17] Nevertheless, despite its expansion and diversification, the field is still conspicuously shaped by the impulses that vaulted it out of a narrowly defined, Whig history of medicine in the 1960s. The historiography of twentieth-century psychiatry faces two challenges: finding suitable narratives and concepts capable of describing the specifics of psychiatry in the twentieth century and taking into account both the internal complexities of psychiatry as a discipline and its location in a wider field of sciences and practices targeting the human mind.

Since the last third of the twentieth century, the historiography of psychiatry was closely intertwined with attempts to change psychiatry. The symbiotic relationship between sociological and historical research on psychiatry and the international movement for its reform was particularly clear in the case of two seminal books: Michel Foucault's *Folie et déraison* and Erving Goffman's *Asylums*, both published in 1961. Among others, these two studies placed psychiatry in the mid of historical, sociological, and philosophical debates, while at the same time defining and politicising the outlook of the so-called anti-psychiatric movement. Despite considerable differences in their scope and intellectual approach, Foucault and Goffman shared an understanding of psychiatry as an institution of social control and of the asylum as the space in which this control was exerted. Goffman in particular stressed how the asylum as a 'total institution' could itself shape its inmates and their behaviour, showing how mental illness could be examined as the result of a process of social construction. But he also prepared the more trenchant charge that psychiatry itself might be pathogenic, manufacturing categories of mental illness in order to uphold and expand its role in a system of social control.[18]

'Anti-psychiatry' and the radical politics associated with it have since largely faded into obscurity (partly to re-emerge as objects of historical research more recently).[19] And yet, the debates of the 1960s and 1970s decisively shaped the field of the history of psychiatry and continue to have some influence on present-day debates. In Germany, reform psychiatrist Klaus Dörner and social historian Dirk Blasius were among the first to examine the history of psychiatry in a broader social and political context.[20] Taking their cues from Foucault and Goffman, they described the emergence of psychiatry as a profession and as a tool of social control during the nineteenth century, stressing the close relation between bourgeois demands for the preservation of social order and the exclusion of unproductive individuals in an emerging capitalist society. At the centre of this narrative was the asylum, and psychiatry's pendulum-like swings between reform on the one hand, and confinement, neglect, and coercion on the other.

Over the following decades, the history of psychiatry received important impulses from general and medical history that could still be accommodated into the broader narrative focused on confinement and the asylum. The history of everyday life, microhistory, and 'history from below' gave more weight to the perspective of the inmates and patients, examining their everyday experiences and their agency, while also tapping patient files as a rich source for historical inquiry.[21] Around the same time, scholars from women's and gender history made a crucial contribution to the field when they pointed out that neither medical practice nor diagnostic categories such as hysteria were independent from gender norms and hierarchies.[22] In the first decade of the twenty-first century, these perspectives experienced a considerable boom in the German-language historiography of psychiatry, when numerous scholars began unearthing the archives of former and existing asylums to examine everyday life, material cultures of psychiatric institutions, patient narratives, and experiences 'from below'.[23]

But despite its undeniable merits, a historiography of psychiatry centred on the asylum, confinement, and social control may have considerable limitations. As Volker Hess and Benoît Majerus argued in 2011, this is especially pertinent when historians write the history of twentieth-century psychiatry.[24] The grand narrative of confinement inspired by Foucault's works, they argue, provided an authoritative framework for the history of psychiatry in the eighteenth and nineteenth century. The attempt, however, to extend its range into the twentieth century would necessarily fail to describe what happened to psychiatry in the twentieth century. Hess and Majerus took little notice of the heated debates revolving around Foucault's works about the history of psychiatry since the 1970s and therefore overstate the degree of consensus reached in the history of psychiatry in the 'long' nineteenth century and before.[25] Even so, they accurately describe an important and overlooked issue in the historiography of psychiatry. Hess and Majerus have in mind mostly the mutations that psychiatry underwent after the Second World War that brought about the end of traditional institutional treatment—the rise of social psychiatry, psychopharmacology, and neurophysiological aetiologies.[26] Nevertheless, their interjection is equally relevant for the history of psychiatry in the inter-war period, which cannot be told as a linear continuation of nineteenth-century asylum psychiatry, but was shaped by parallel, conflicting, complementary, and sometimes contradictory trends such as the introduction of social psychiatry, the rise of the eugenic paradigm, the development of 'heroic' somatic therapies, and the increasing competition with other psy-ences.

The same also holds true for Greg Eghigian's call for a 'deinstitutionalisation' of the history of contemporary psychiatry.[27] Again, the focus of his research is on the last third of the twentieth century, and it is to this period that the specific notion of deinstitutionalisation is linked. Nevertheless, the process that Eghigian examines—psychiatry leaving the clinic and the hospital and becoming 'a technoscience that operates in numerous settings'—began decades earlier. This is the shift that this book is about, when I examine psychiatrists' early attempts to reach out of the clinic and into society. The movement for mental hygiene is a particularly clear and early example for an effort to 'deinstitutionalise' psychiatry, and the movement was a direct precursor of approaches that only came to fruition after the Second World War under the new umbrella of 'mental health'. Even eugenics and racial hygiene, advocated by many protagonists of this study, are today rightly considered as appalling abuses of medical power but followed a rationale of 'deinstitutionalisation' rather than one of confinement.

When understood in these very broad terms, the 'deinstitutionalisation' of psychiatry was no linear process, and it did not happen overnight. Institutional and non-institutional approaches coexisted, overlapped, and completed each other for much of the twentieth century, and shifts from one to the other were not only driven by internal debates in psychiatry, but also by changing aetiologies of mental illness, new treatment methods, by political actors, broader changes in the welfare system, and economic concerns. In this perspective, the aftermath of the First World War was a time when a gradual shift from a paradigm of institutional care and confinement to one of 'deinstitutionalisation', open care, and (eugenic and non-eugenic) prophylaxis reached a tipping point.

Historians of psychiatry may not yet have found authoritative narratives to describe the larger trends of the twentieth century. Nevertheless, there is ample research in the field. While studies in eighteenth- and nineteenth-century psychiatry still make up the bigger part of publications, interest in the twentieth century has been steadily growing for some time now.[28] As far as the history of psychiatry in the German-speaking countries is concerned, scholars' interest has very much focused on two particular, momentous episodes, between which the topic of this book is wedged: the treatment of mentally traumatised soldiers during the First World War and the mass sterilisation and mass killing of patients committed by psychiatrists under Nazi rule. As these two are at the beginning and the end of my narrative respectively, it will be useful to comment briefly on some of the more relevant trends in this research.

During the last two decades, the military psychiatry of the First World War has become one of the most densely researched topics in the field. Apart from the recently rekindled interest in all aspects of the 1914–1918 war in the context of its centenary, this is to no small degree due to the emergence of new perspectives on wartime psychological injuries around the turn of the millennium. These were in turn part of a much broader, cross-disciplinary debate about concepts of trauma taking place during this time. The most important impulses for the remarkable currency of trauma were formulated outside historiography in the second half of the 1990s before being picked up by historians of psychiatry.[29] While scholars from different disciplines used a broadly defined, psychoanalytically inspired notion of 'cultural trauma' to understand how the catastrophes and cataclysms of the twentieth century could have been experienced and narrated, cultural historians discovered that 'shell shock', the iconic diagnosis of the First World War, was in fact a 'social disease'.[30] More than just a result of individual traumatisation due to the somatic and psychological impacts of the war, the symptoms, aetiologies, treatment methods, and narratives of 'shell shock' conveyed cultural and political meanings accessible to historical hermeneutics. Since then, 'shell shock' has moved out of the clinical context and has become a catchphrase encapsulating the individual and collective ordeal of the war—as it had already been during and immediately after the war.[31]

In Germany, the psychiatric experience of the First World War was long seen in the light of the second.[32] The drastic and painful methods of 'active treatment' were decried as torture and coercive abuses of medical power by sadist, right-wing militarist psychiatrists, foreshadowing the crimes of Nazi psychiatry. However, even if there are some grains of truth to this narrative, simplistic assumptions about a *Sonderweg* of German psychiatry obscured more than they actually revealed, leaving little space for contingencies, complexities, and discontinuities, while at the same time reducing the period between the world wars to a mere interlude.

Paul Lerner's monograph *Hysterical Men* marked an important shift in the historiography on German First World War psychiatry around the turn of the twenty-first century.[33] It offered a differentiated account beyond the juxtaposition of authoritarian neuropsychiatrists and sympathetic psychoanalysts and connected the topic to ongoing debates about trauma, masculinity, and modernity. In the first decade of the twenty-first century, the First World War became one of the single best-researched topics in the history of German and Austrian psychiatry.[34] The proliferation of research about military psychiatry also opened up new perspectives on the previously understudied history of psychiatry in the years between the world wars, even if mostly as a postlude to the First World War.[35] In the last ten years, numerous studies have examined how mentally wounded veterans' pension claims became the issue of a heated and politicised debate in inter-war Germany and how they affected welfare legislation. Moreover, historians' new interest in the psychiatric dimension of the First World War coincided with a time when the history of psychiatry received fresh impulses from adjacent fields. In discussing the embattled nerves of the trench warriors as a medium through which the experience of the war and the state of the nation could be understood, these studies shifted the focus from psychiatry as a discipline to the wider political and cultural implications of its diagnoses, a perspective that drew on research on the role of 'nerves' in modern German history.

It was at a time when more forward-thinking scholars like Friedrich Kittler prophesied the imminent end of the 'age of the nerves' that historians discovered the topic.[36] Joachim Radkau's study about the 'age of nervousness' could not live up to some of its all too encompassing claims, but it introduced the elusive diagnosis of nervousness as a contemporary catch-phrase for the experiences and mental strains of an accelerating and crisis-ridden modernity to a broader historical audience.[37] At the same time, by situating the nerves (and with them, the human body and subjectivity) between Wilhelmine, Weimar, and Nazi politics on the one side, and the rapid development of electrical and communication technologies on the other, Radkau's study opened up the history of psychiatry towards both a cultural history of politics and the history of science and technology. Since then, other scholars have taken up neurasthenia from various perspectives and used it to contribute to a broadly conceived history of pre-war and inter-war psychiatry as part of a history of German modernity.[38]

Any book about inter-war psychiatry in the German-speaking countries inevitably has to consider the history of German psychiatry after 1933. This is especially true when it comes to understanding the prophylactic and socio-medical approaches of inter-war psychiatry, as they were connected to the crimes of Nazi psychiatry not only through a shared set of medical and political ideas, but also through protagonists whose career led them from being key actors in Weimar reform programme to being actively engaged in Nazi 'euthanasia'. This is hardly surprising. Right-wing nationalist views were common among German physicians long before the First World War, and the nexus between turn-of-the-century social Darwinism, eugenics, and Nazi psychiatry has been thoroughly researched since the second half of the 1980s.[39] The First World War and its aftermath became an important caesura, pushing forward the institutionalisation of eugenics and radicalising the medico-political outlook of its protagonists. It was in 1920 that jurist Karl Binding and psychiatrist Alfred Hoche introduced the now-infamous notion of 'life unworthy of life' and initiated a debate that would eventually culminate in the mass murder of psychiatric inmates committed by German psychiatrists after 1939.[40]

The issue of eugenics and Nazi psychiatry presents the historiography of inter-war psychiatry in the German-speaking countries with a methodological challenge. Many studies about the eugenics movements in other parts of the world, as well as research with a comparative perspective or a focus on international networks, have shown that eugenics were not a German *Sonderweg*, but a global trend in the first half of the twentieth century.[41] In addition, eugenics were not necessarily linked to right-wing politics, but could also be part of more progressive and left-wing varieties of 'social engineering'. The link between Nazi medicine and eugenics, one might say, works better in one direction than in the other: while Nazi psychiatry after

1933 narrowed itself down to eugenics and 'racial hygiene', the history of eugenics cannot be narrowed down to that of Nazi psychiatry.

This has two important implications. First, when dealing with eugenic ideas in the inter-war period, even when focusing on the German-speaking countries, one should avoid teleological perspectives leading straight to Nazi medicine. While it may be easy and plausible to retrospectively describe the eugenic ideas in inter-war Germany as direct precursors, the actual developments and debates were more open and left considerable room for contingency. Second, the eugenics movement was far from homogeneous, calling for a complex understanding that sees eugenics in multiplicity. There was not one single approach to eugenics, but many varieties, depending on different national contexts as well as political and scientific allegiances. German racial hygiene after 1933 stands out due to the sheer scale and brutality of its implementation and its close connection to Nazi ideology and politics. The more productive question, however, is not 'what is National Socialist about eugenics?' but rather what was specific about German 'racial hygiene' in a much wider history of global eugenics?[42]

The issue of eugenics not only raises the question of international comparison and contextualisation, but also helps problematising the role of established disciplines in newly emerging fields of scientific theory and practice. While psychiatry can serve as a vantage point to examine the development of eugenics, one must also take into account that psychiatrists were far from being the only ones who pushed eugenic ideas. Instead, eugenics emerged in a crowded field, where psychiatry was merely one discipline among others and where biologists, social hygienists, geneticists, criminologists, jurists, and anthropologists were also staking out their claims. The involvement of politicians and welfare bureaucrats further complicates the picture, as does the fact that intellectuals, philosophers, and writers also took part in debates about degeneration and the selective breeding of human beings. Hence, eugenics could be described as an emerging discipline, an interdisciplinary project, a political movement, a discourse, or—most accurately—all of the above.

Similar issues are also at stake when writing the history of psychiatry in the twentieth century and of psychiatry beyond the asylum in particular. The first third of the century saw the simultaneous emergence and professionalisation of a number of related psy-ences with similar and overlapping claims of explaining the human mind as well as understanding, diagnosing, and treating mental illness. Applied psychology and *Psychotechnik* promised to put to practical use the findings of experimental psychology. Different approaches for the treatment of psychic disorders through psychic methods became known under the label of psychotherapy. And the most successful of these, Freudian psychoanalysis, established itself as an autonomous discipline, developed an elaborate social and cultural theory, and eventually became one of the most influential intellectual movements of the twentieth century, while at the same time spawning dissident schools such as Adlerian 'individual psychology' and Jungian 'analytic psychology'. The exploration of the human psyche attracted a multitude of different disciplines and actors, who interacted in different ways that ranged from cooperation, mutual or unilateral influence, and overlaps on the one hand, to open competition, ignorance, enmity, and fierce demarcation disputes on the other. To make things more complicated, none of these disciplines should be considered as a black box. Psychiatry, for example, was anything but monolithic. Apart from being members of various schools and local traditions, different psychiatrists worked under different circumstances, some conducting cutting-edge research in relatively well-equipped urban university clinics, while others administered run-down and overcrowded asylums in the countryside.[43]

Although this book mainly focuses on psychiatry and psychiatrists, psychoanalysis may serve to concisely illustrate how the relation between different approaches and disciplines in the broader field of the psy-ences reappears in every single chapter. Like many of the protagonists of this study, psychoanalysts shared the idea that concepts of mental illness and psychopathology could be used to understand and change society. The eminent psychoanalysts Otto Fenichel, Siegfried Bernfeld, and Paul Federn, among many others, extensively discussed the social role of their discipline. And when right-wing psychiatrists diagnosed the revolution and the revolutionaries in 1918/1919, psychoanalysts and Adlerian individual psychologists did the same, mostly from a moderate left-wing perspective. Erwin Stransky's applied psychiatry emerged and developed in inter-war Vienna both in cooperation with local psychoanalysts and in a fierce competition with them. And while the mental hygiene movement in Europe was dominated by reform-minded psychiatrists who had little interest in psychoanalysis, in the United States, it strongly relied on a specific reading of Freud to legitimise its ideology of adaptation. At the same time, Paul Federn and Heinrich Meng tried to popularise psychoanalysis, advertising its potentials for everyday prophylaxis and mental hygiene.[44] While psychoanalysis remained separate from the mental hygiene movement in Germany, it became an integral part of more encompassing notion of mental hygiene in Switzerland before the Second World War.

What these examples show is that even while focusing on psychiatry, one cannot ignore the permeability of its boundaries and the influence of neighbouring and related disciplines. What is required is a broader perspective, capable of describing the assemblage of disciplines, discourses, and techniques that began to clutter around the problem of the human mind from the eighteenth century on. British sociologist Nikolas Rose's notion of the 'psychological complex' points in this direction, describing the emerging science of psychology as 'a complex of discourses, practices, agents and techniques' deployed in a range of different social and institutional settings.[45] It helps to see these disciplines not as monolithic, but as complex and multi-layered. More recently, neologism such as the 'psy-ences' or the 'psy-disciplines' has been used to speak about psychiatry, psychology, psychoanalysis, psychotherapy, neurology, and related fields as different parts of a large array of sciences gathered around the human psyche. These concepts are both catchy and useful, as they help to elucidate the complex relations of various scientific disciplines. They are, however, still descriptive rather than analytical, and it is up to historical (as well as sociological and ethnological) studies to fill them with concrete content.

A Few Thoughts About Psychiatry, Society, and Politics

One argument that I propose in this book is that psychiatric attempts to diagnose and treat society can shed light on the political history of the inter-war period. This is not only because psychiatrists directly discussed and diagnosed events that were evidently political—such as the First World War or the 1918/1919 German revolution—or because some of their approaches were supported and implemented by the state. It is also the case because the programmes discussed in this study—despite frequent affirmations of a non-political, non-partisan, and objective stance—were clearly political. By framing political and social phenomena as medical in nature, their protagonists followed and radicalised Rudolf Virchow's 1848 dictum that 'politics are medicine on a large scale'.[46] They amalgamated political and medical concepts and rhetoric; they blurred and redrew the boundaries between science and politics.

Declaring oneself non-political can in fact be highly political. Thomas Mann's 'observations of a non-political man' (*Betrachtungen eines Unpolitischen*), penned during the war and published in 1918, are a case in point and rank among the most important testimonials of German conservative thought in the twentieth century.[47] More importantly, being emphatically non-political was not just a way for conservative novelists to come to terms with current events (and, in Mann's case, his older brother), but also a crucial part of the self-understanding of physicians and scientists since the nineteenth century.

By affirming their non-political stance, they did not relinquish their say about how society should be organised and administered. On the contrary, a non-partisan and objective scientific and technological rationality was presented as a viable alternative to the alleged myopia, emotionality, and self-interestedness of party politics. While utopian imaginations of large-scale scientific and technological solutions for social problems already gained momentum early in the nineteenth century, the years between the world wars became the heyday of utopian ideas of 'social engineering' and saw the rise and fall of technocracy—the term itself introduced in 1919—as a movement. The belief that society had to be reshaped and its problems solved rationally, objectively, and by techno-scientific means united experts from different disciplines behind a vision of anti-political politics. As an influential 'background ideology', technocratic ideas cut across the boundaries between established political camps and across the boundaries of a traditional definition of politics as well.[48]

When it came to non-political politics, medicine did not stand apart.[49] Throughout the nineteenth century, physicians had forcibly distanced themselves from the political sphere and insisted on the non-partisanship and autonomy of their discipline. Towards the end of the century, the emphatic rejection and denigration of anything political increasingly accompanied calls for an appropriation of political responsibilities by medical experts. As Tobias Weidner has shown, these two strands of the medical discourse about politics were two sides of the same coin, as the medical repudiation of politics became the lynchpin of an anti-political agenda that rejected traditional party politics in favour of scientocratic ideas.[50]

Physicians' aspirations to partake in the solving of societal problems were part of a broader process of a 'scientisation of the social' (*Verwissenschaftlichung des Sozialen*).[51] Introduced in 1996 by historian Lutz Raphael, this concept describes developments in the human sciences that accompanied Max Weber's much-quoted 'disenchantment of the world'.[52]

In Raphael's words, scientisation was one of the 'basic processes' of modernity, characterised by 'the continuing presence of experts from the human sciences, their arguments and their findings, in administrations and corporations, in political parties and parliaments, and even in the everyday world of meaning (*Sinnwelt*) of social groups, classes, and milieus'.[53] Raphael's concept describes a process that was, and remains, a formative part of modernity. It is, however, almost too generalising. As the many examples in his programmatic article show, scientisation left almost no facet of modern life untouched and little escapes his notion of 'the social'. A monograph about the scientisation of the social in the twentieth century would hardly be possible; instead, the concept has shown its value in numerous case studies, where it has served as a framework to relate different contemporaneous developments to each other and to understand underlying dynamics.[54]

The scientisation of the social was, however, no linear development.[55] With the concept—and *telos*—of scientisation in mind, it is tempting to describe the history of modern societies as an undeviating development towards an ever-increasing role of the human sciences in all fields of society. In the case of the psy-ences, this narrative connects seamlessly to polemical warnings against the gradual colonisation of society by psychiatrists, psychologists, and psychoanalysts and the emergence of a 'therapeutic culture' or a 'therapeutic state'.[56] Tellingly, Raphael has recently used a similar terminology to describe the most recent configuration of the scientisation of the social, beginning in the 1970s, as an 'age of therapy'.[57] Nikolas Rose has repeatedly made a similar argument for modern Britain. Drawing on a Foucauldian notion of governmentality, he describes an increasing permeation of British society by psychological knowledge and institutions from the late nineteenth century onwards.[58]

On first sight, the sources discussed in this book seem to support a similar interpretation for the German-speaking countries. The protagonists themselves routinely and explicitly voiced the idea of expanding psychiatry's authority into the social sphere: Erwin Stransky's applied psychiatry was nothing less than a call for a psychiatric expertocracy, and some of the prophylactic measures proposed by mental hygienists read like battle plans for a psychiatric invasion of society. Psychiatrists' visions of the future were the fears of others. In 1919, simultaneously to the publication of the most radical psycho-political tracts, the journal of the German 'anti-psychiatric' movement—anticipating the rhetoric of its indirect successors in the 1960s—cautioned against a 'psychiatric need for expansion' that would lead to the 'psychiatrisation' (*Verpsychiatrisierung*) of society.[59]

Yet, aspirations and apprehensions should not be confused with realities. The fact that none of the programmes discussed here came even close to being fully implemented is a reminder that there are good reasons to be cautious about such a linear, and teleological, story. The influence of the human sciences in many fields of society manifestly increased in the twentieth century, and the psy-ences had a significant role to play in this process. Nevertheless, this development should neither be taken for granted, nor as automatic and unavoidable. What I propose instead is a more probing stance. To avoid the pitfalls of teleology, this story should include the failures and contingencies, the competition between different disciplines, the unintended outcomes of attempts to extend the social range of human sciences and of experiments of social engineering, and also—to use a notion that is both political and psychological—the resistances that these projects met and provoked.

That the psy-ences could be used politically is not a recent idea. In the nineteenth century already, scholars used concepts derived from psychiatry and psychology to describe socio-political dynamics as well as cultural developments.[60] These approaches were, however, usually diagnostic rather than therapeutic. With the odd exception of the renegade psychoanalyst Otto Gross, few believed that the psy-ences had the ability and authority to remake society. It was during and immediately after the cataclysm of the First World War that visions of a more active political role of the psy-ences rapidly gained traction among professionals and the public. In a much-noticed article in 1919, German psychiatrist Hugo Marx claimed that 'the Anglo-American psychologist' had won the war.[61] To save and rebuild the nation, psycho-knowledge and its applications had to become an integral part of modern statecraft. This idea neither limited by partisan divides, nor by divides inside the psy-ences. In 1918 already, psychoanalyst Sándor Ferenczi mocked the Bolsheviks for their psychological ignorance. Their problems to maintain and use their newly gained political power, he argued, were their obsession with politics and economy had led them to forget about the dynamics of the human soul.[62] The idea that the knowledge and the methods of the psy-ences could improve present society or create a new and better one became one of the grand utopian narratives of the inter-war period. It was the Soviet avant-garde artist Kazimir Malevich who stated that 'the state is an apparatus by which the nervous systems of its inhabitants are regulated'.[63]

In these few examples, psychiatric and psychological concepts were directly conflated with politics. The overall scope of this book is broader and encompasses other, subtler ways in which psychiatry tried to leave the asylum and the clinic, but the encounter and entanglement of psychiatric and political thought are a recurring theme. To describe these ideas and approaches, I use the notion 'psycho-politics' and, more often, the adjective 'psycho-political'.

As a combination of the ubiquitous prefix 'psycho-' with 'politics', the concept may at first seem self-explanatory, but comes with a history of its own. The German term *Psychopolitik* first appeared in the second half of the 1920s and was already elusive then. It was independently introduced by two scholars, Heinrich Rogge and Siegfried Bernfeld, who each endowed it with a different meaning. Together, these two historical uses of the term psycho-politics stake out the scope of this study, ranging from the direct application of psychiatric and psychological concepts to the political sphere on the one hand, to ideas of large-scale prophylaxis and public health on the other. Visions of psycho-politics appealed to scholars on the left and right, but could entail very different ideas about how society should be.

When the jurist Heinrich Rogge (1886–1966) discussed 'psycho-politics and the problem of the leader' in 1925, it was in direct continuation of the psychiatric debates of the immediate post-war period.[64] Rogge asked how the collective psychology of a 'mass soul' influenced politics and how these dynamics unfolded in the relation between masses and leader. As he saw it, 'politics and psychology are identical: both should be the science of the soul of the community'.[65] This science, which he alternatingly called 'psychological politics', 'political psychology', or 'psycho-politics', was not only descriptive and analytical, it was also about reshaping politics: 'The final and highest form of psycho-politics is that psychology [...] tackles the education and self-education of the political leaders'. With its longing for a new kind of psychologically proficient leader, Rogge's article reflected the political imaginary of its time[66] and shows how ideas that had been formulated in psychological and psychiatric debates were appropriated by members of other disciplines. Rogge's concept of psycho-politics revolved around a recurring utopian theme of the contemporary debate about psycho-knowledge and politics, the idea that knowledge about the human mind would allow to overcome current social and political struggles through a rational and scientific form of politics.

The second time the notion of psycho-politics appeared in the interwar period was in a 1930 essay about 'psychology and the labour movement' by the Austrian left-wing psychoanalyst and educationalist Siegfried Bernfeld.[67] For Bernfeld, the synthesis of psychology and politics meant a synthesis of Freudian and Marxian thought. He argued that the disciplines concerned with mental disorders, namely psychiatry, psychotherapy, psychoanalysis, and neurology, had to acknowledge that many of these widespread ills were not individual, but had societal causes. Hence, they would have to consider 'the mass character of mental ills to search for methods that go beyond the therapeutic treatment of individuals and aim at overcoming the *mass problem*'. Other medical specialties, Bernfeld wrote in 'Red Vienna', had already made this step from individual treatment to social reform and prophylaxis, but the psy-ences lagged behind: 'Health policy measures are placed over the prescription of drugs. Of such a development of psychology towards "psycho-politics", the first, vague rudiments are barely recognisable'.[68] Unmentioned by Bernfeld, the movement for mental hygiene at the same time proposed similar transformations of psychiatry into a form of social medicine. However, what set apart Bernfeld's notion of psychiatric prophylaxis as distinctly psycho-political was that for him, mental prophylaxis was part of a broader appropriation of psychology by the political left that would equip the labour movement with 'a *new weapon* in its intellectual and economic class struggles'.[69]

Between 1930 and the present day, the concept of psycho-politics reappeared several times. A particularly ambitious but futile attempt to reintroduce the concept was made by the philosopher Paul Feldkeller (1889–1972), who published a 'dictionary of psycho-politics' in 1967.[70] What Feldkeller, who claimed to have invented the term in 1947, called psycho-politics was a new kind of politics that would overcome the struggles of present-day politics through science and humanist ethics: 'Thus, the term "psycho-politics" means a psychologically-oriented politics that until now has not existed [...]. With these politics-made-science a cultural and moralizing moment is added to the non-scientific and non-moral scuffle (since the days of Younger Stone Age)'.[71] Feldkeller's psycho-politics were an eclectic and vaguely defined project drawing on many different sources,[72] but despite the evident differences, the psycho-politics of Heinrich Rogge, Siegfried Bernfeld, and Paul Feldkeller had something in common. For all three scholars, psycho-politics had yet to become reality and only then would change the world for the better. In one way or another, uniting the psy-ences and politics was something positive, and even utopian.

In the next decades, this discourse changed direction. After the experiences of the Second World War and against the backdrop of the Cold War, psycho-politics turned dystopian. The connection of psychology and politics became increasingly associated with propaganda and manipulation, with brain-washing and psychological warfare. In 1967, Paul Feldkeller stressed that his psycho-politics had nothing to do with the political abuses of psychology for 'the continuation of old wars and the preparation of new ones'.[73] Since then, however, the term has mainly been used in a more critical vein, most prominently in Peter Sedgwick's (1934–1983) left-wing critique of the shortcomings of 1960s 'anti-psychiatry', and subsequently by scholars and activists affiliated with 'anti-psychiatry', critical theory, and post-colonial studies, or combinations thereof, to describe the psychology of political power relations and pillory the political instrumentalisation of psycho-knowledge.[74] Many of these studies have been influenced by Michel Foucault—not only by following his view the psy-ences as agents of social normalisation and control, but also by alluding to Foucauldian notions of 'bio-politics'.

The most recent, and hitherto most successful, use of the notion of psycho-politics builds directly on this reference to Foucault. In his best-selling 2014 essay *Psychopolitik*, German philosopher Byung-Chul Han used the term psycho-politics to criticise what he saw as a particularly perfidious form of power in present-day, neo-liberal society.[75] Foucault's notion of bio-politics, Han (inaccurately) claimed, was limited to the external discipline of bodies and populations. It describes the governmental rationale of earlier societies, but is 'inadequate for the neo-liberal regime, which mainly exploits the *psyche*'.[76] To describe the neo-liberal techniques to exploit and deform the mind, Han proposed the notion of psycho-politics. Like all earlier uses of the concept, Han's psycho-politics are symptomatic of the intellectual trends of their time. His essay, however, tells less about the actual problems of neo-liberal capitalism and more about the pitfalls of a specific sort of its critique. The underlying a-historical concept of neo-liberalism is as homogenising as it is totalising, turning it into a catch-all phrase for the real and imagined discontents of the early twenty-first century. Somewhat like in a conspiracy theory without conspirators, Han attributes neo-liberalism with agency and intentionality that seems almost consciously intent on destroying anything good and authentic that is left in the world. This is old-fashioned cultural conservatism thinly disguised as progressive thinking.

These different uses of a notion of psycho-politics can serve as a point of departure for thinking about a concept better attuned to historical analysis. As I argue, to tackle the historical material, at least two problems are to be avoided. First and most obviously, a category for historical analysis should not be primarily normative. All of the concepts of psycho-politics mentioned above have one thing in common. Regardless of whether psycho-politics were thought as being utopian or dystopian, the term was used to make normative claims about the relation between the psy-ences, psycho-knowledge, and politics. As an historical concept, by contrast, it will have to be able to describe these specific constellations in a given historical context. The normative dimension is not absent, but it is the historical actors themselves who fill it with content.

Second, while the allusion to Foucauldian bio-politics is tempting and may help to situate psycho-politics in a broader historiographical and conceptual framework, the link should not be overstressed. One reason is that the concept of bio-politics was already quite broad and elusive when introduced by Michel Foucault in the mid-1970s. Since then, and in the last decade in particular, the concept has proliferated and inflationary use has added to the confusion, so that bio-politics today can apparently describe almost any kind of public health or population policy and much beyond that.[77] Introducing a concept of psycho-politics with a similar range would be neither useful nor necessary. Moreover, when doing so, as Byung-Chul Han has done, one risks reproducing a body–mind dualism by implying that bio-politics target only bodies, whereas psycho-politics pertain to the mind.[78] This is not only an idealist and simplistic conception of the body—mind relation, but in an historical study, it would also mean ignoring the historical actors' own understanding of this relation. As other scholars have done, the notion of psycho-politics should not be defined by its assumed target, but also by the specific disciplines and the bodies of knowledge that were involved. Psycho-politics then describes bio-political public health interventions conducted by members of the psy-ences or in the name of mental health. Psychiatric eugenics or campaigns against alcoholism, for example, were propagated by psychiatrists; they have, however, little to do with a clear-cut distinction between body and mind. This definition would also be able to accommodate Siegfried Bernfeld's notion of psycho-politics as the psy-ences' prospective contribution to social medicine, and it covers the greater part of the agenda of the movement for mental hygiene.

To complicate things further, some of the historical uses of the term psycho-politics, as well as many of the writings, programmes, visions, and ideas discussed in this study, evade a definition directly derived from bio-politics. To some extent, this is a matter of translation. The Foucauldian notion of bio-politics is concerned with governmental techniques and practices that are policy rather than politics—a distinction that the French *biopolitique* does not convey. But not everything that happened at the intersection of the psy-ences and politics was situated on this level. Moreover, even those programmes, schemes, and utopian ideas that could most accurately be described in terms of large-scale public health policies emerged from the messier, local contexts of everyday politics.

A concept of politics that is probably more useful for the analytic needs of this book can be derived from recent research in the cultural history of politics. Instead of relying on a preconceived definition, scholars in the field have tried to historicise the concept of politics and the political itself and have argued for a 'dynamic and constructivist understanding of the political' that problematises the historical uses of the concept. In this perspective, the boundaries between what is political and what is not and between the political, the public, and the private are constantly redrawn and renegotiated.[79] When the 'politics' in psycho-politics are understood in this historicised and multi-layered perspective, the concept and the perspective move closer to the actual motivations and self-understandings of the historical actors. This notion of psycho-politics, which moves more freely between the micro- and macro-dimensions of the interactions between the psy-ences and politics, runs through this book as a common thread. In all three case studies and in all five chapters, from the diagnoses of the nation in the wake of defeat and revolution, to applied psychiatry and mental hygiene, the psychiatrists who conceived, wrote, and organised these programs shared the same idea: that they, as professionals concerned with the pathologies of the human mind, had the knowledge, the authority, and the responsibility to change society for the better. And in one way or another, these doctors and their ideas all became deeply entangled in the political history of their age.

Notes

1. Stefan Andriopoulos, *Possessed: Hypnotic Crimes, Corporate Fiction, and the Invention of Cinema*, trans. Peter Jansen and Stefan Andriopoulos (Chicago: University of Chicago Press, 2008); Anton Kaes, *Shell Shock Cinema: Weimar Culture and the Wounds of War* (Princeton and Oxford: Princeton University Press, 2009); Andrew Scull, 'Some Reflections on Madness and Culture in the Post-war World', *History of Psychiatry* 25 (2014): 395–403.
2. Siegfried Kracauer, *Von Caligari zu Hitler: Ein Beitrag zur Geschichte des deutschen Films* (Reinbek bei Hamburg: Rowohlt, 1958).
3. Kaes, *Shell Shock Cinema*.

4. Philipp Sarasin, 'Das obszöne Genießen der Wissenschaft: Über Populärwissenschaft und mad scientists', in *Geschichtswissenschaft und Diskursanalyse* (Frankfurt am Main: Suhrkamp, 2003), 231–57.
5. Erwin Stransky, 'Der seelische Wiederaufbau des deutschen Volkes und die Aufgaben der Psychiatrie: Erweiterter Vortrag, gehalten auf der Deutschen Psychiaterversammlung in Hamburg, am 27./28. Mai 1920', *Zeitschrift für die gesamte Neurologie und Psychiatrie* 60, no. 1 (1920): 271–80; Robert Gaupp, *Die zukünftige Stellung des Arztes im Volke: Ansprache an die Studierenden der Medizin der Universität Tübingen (23. X. 1919)* (Tübingen: H. Laupp, 1919).
6. Volker Roelcke, *Krankheit und Kulturkritik: Psychiatrische Gesellschaftsdeutungen im bürgerlichen Zeitalter (1790–1914)* (Frankfurt am Main: Campus, 1999); Daniel Pick, *Faces of Degeneration: A European Disorder, c. 1848–c. 1918* (Cambridge: Cambridge University Press, 1989); Jaap van Ginneken, *Crowds, Psychology and Politics, 1871–1899* (Cambridge: Cambridge University Press, 1992).
7. Anonymous, 'Psychiatrisches Ausbreitungsbedürfnis', *Die Irrenrechts-Reform* 11 (1919): 197–99.
8. Volker Roelcke, 'Die Entwicklung der Psychiatrie zwischen 1880 und 1932: Theoriebildung, Institutionen, Interaktionen mit zeitgenössischer Wissenschafts- und Sozialpolitik', in *Wissenschaften und Wissenschaftspolitik: Bestandsaufnahmen zu Formationen, Brüchen und Kontinuitäten im Deutschland des 20. Jahrhunderts*, ed. Rüdiger vom Bruch and Brigitte Kaderas (Stuttgart: Franz Steiner, 2002), 119–20.
9. Dirk Blasius, *Einfache Seelenstörung: Geschichte der deutschen Psychiatrie 1800–1945* (Frankfurt am Main: Fischer, 1994), 117.
10. Paul Lerner, *Hysterical Men: War, Psychiatry, and the Politics of Trauma in Germany, 1890–1930* (Ithaca: Cornell University Press, 2003).
11. Martin Kohlrausch and Helmuth Trischler, *Building Europe on Expertise: Innovators, Organizers, Networkers* (Houndmills, Basingstoke: Palgrave Macmillan, 2014), 1.
12. Mitchell G. Ash, 'Wissenschaft und Politik als Ressourcen für einander', in *Wissenschaften und Wissenschaftspolitik: Bestandsaufnahmen zu Formationen, Brüchen und Kontinuitäten im Deutschland des 20. Jahrhunderts*, ed. Rüdiger vom Bruch and Brigitte Kaderas (Stuttgart: Franz Steiner, 2002), 32–51; Mitchell G. Ash, 'Wissenschaft(en) und Öffentlichkeit(en) als Ressourcen füreinander: Weiterführende Bemerkungen zur Beziehungsgeschichte', in *Wissenschaft und Öffentlichkeit als Ressourcen füreinander: Studien zur Wissenschaftsgeschichte im 20. Jahrhundert*, ed. Sybilla Nikolow and Arne Schirrmacher (Frankfurt am Main and New York: Campus, 2007), 349–64.
13. Sonu Shamdasani, 'Psychotherapy: The Invention of a Word', *History of the Human Sciences* 18, no. 1 (2005): 1–22.

14. Stephanie Neuner, *Politik und Psychiatrie: Die staatliche Versorgung psychisch Kriegsbeschädigter in Deutschland 1920–1939* (Göttingen: Vandenhoeck & Ruprecht, 2011); Jason Crouthamel, *The Great War and German Memory: Society, Politics and Psychological Trauma, 1914–1945* (Exeter: University of Exeter Press, 2009); Jason Crouthamel and Peter Leese, eds., *Psychological Trauma and the Legacies of the First World War* (Basingstoke: Palgrave Macmillan, 2017).
15. Volker Roelcke, 'Psychiatrische Wissenschaft im Kontext nationalsozialistischer Politik und Euthanasie: Zur Rolle Ernst Rüdins und der Deutschen Forschungsanstalt für Psychiatrie/Kaiser-Wilhelm-Institut', in *Geschichte der Kaiser-Wilhelm-Gesellschaft im Nationalsozialismus: Bestandsaufnahme und Perspektiven der Forschung*, ed. Doris Kaufmann, vol. 1 (Göttingen: Wallstein, 2000), 112–50; Matthias M. Weber, 'Rassenhygienische und genetische Forschungen an der Deutschen Forschungsanstalt für Psychiatrie/Kaiser-Wilhelm-Institut in München vor und nach 1933', in *Geschichte der Kaiser-Wilhelm-Gesellschaft im Nationalsozialismus: Bestandsaufnahme und Perspektiven der Forschung*, ed. Doris Kaufmann, vol. 1 (Göttingen: Wallstein, 2000), 95–111.
16. Bruno Latour, *Science in Action: How to Follow Scientists and Engineers Through Society* (Cambridge, MA: Harvard University Press, 1987).
17. Volker Hess and Heinz-Peter Schmiedebach, *Am Rande des Wahnsinns: Schwellräume einer urbanen Moderne* (Vienna, Cologne, and Weimar: Böhlau, 2012); Hans-Walter Schmuhl and Volker Roelcke, *'Heroische Therapien': Die deutsche Psychiatrie im internationalen Vergleich 1918–1945* (Göttingen: Wallstein, 2013); Christine Wolters, Christof Beyer, and Brigitte Lohff, *Abweichung und Normalität: Psychiatrie in Deutschland vom Kaiserreich bis zur Deutschen Einheit* (Bielefeld: transcript, 2013); Heinz-Peter Schmiedebach, ed., *Entgrenzungen des Wahnsinns: Psychopathie und Psychopathologisierungen um 1900* (Berlin and Boston: Walter de Gruyter, 2016).
18. Thomas Szasz, *The Myth of Mental Illness: Foundations of a Theory of Personal Conduct* (New York: Harper & Row, 1961).
19. Gerald N. Grob, 'The Attack on Psychiatric Legitimacy in the 1960s: Rhetoric and Reality', *Journal of the History of the Behavioral Sciences* 47, no. 4 (2011): 398–416; Cornelia Brink, 'Keine Angst vor dem Psychiater: Psychiatrie, Psychiatriekritik und Öffentlichkeit in der Bundesrepublik Deutschland (1960–1980)', in *'Moderne' Anstaltspsychiatrie im 19. und 20. Jahrhundert: Legitimation und Kritik*, ed. Heiner Fangerau and Karen Nolte (Stuttgart: Steiner, 2006), 341–60.
20. Klaus Dörner, *Bürger und Irre: Zur Sozialgeschichte und Wissenschaftssoziologie der Psychiatrie* (Frankfurt am Main: Fischer, 1975); Blasius, *Einfache Seelenstörung*.

21. Roy Porter, 'The Patient's View: Doing Medical History from Below', *Theory and Society* 14, no. 2 (1985): 175–98.
22. Esther Fischer-Homberger, *Krankheit Frau: Zur Geschichte der Einbildungen* (Darmstadt: Luchterhand, 1984); Elaine Showalter, *The Female Malady: Women, Madness and English Culture, 1830–1980* (New York: Pantheon Books, 1985).
23. Roy Porter and David Wright, *The Confinement of the Insane: International Perspectives 1800–1965* (Cambridge: Cambridge University Press, 2003); Karen Nolte, *Gelebte Hysterie: Erfahrung, Eigensinn und psychiatrische Diskurse im Anstaltsalltag um 1900* (Frankfurt am Main: Campus, 2003); Cornelia Brink, *Grenzen der Anstalt: Psychiatrie und Gesellschaft in Deutschland 1860–1980* (Göttingen: Wallstein, 2010).
24. Volker Hess and Benoît Majerus, 'Writing the History of Psychiatry in the 20th Century', *History of Psychiatry* 22, no. 2 (2011): 139–45.
25. Arthur Still and Irving Velody, *Rewriting the History of Madness: Studies in Foucault's Histoire de La Folie* (London: Routledge, 1992); Andrew Scull, 'A Failure to Communicate? On the Reception of Foucault's Histoire de La Folie by Anglo-American Historians', in *The Insanity of Place/The Place of Insanity: Essays on the History of Psychiatry* (London and New York: Routledge, 2006), 30–37.
26. Mark S. Micale, 'The Ten Most Important Changes in Psychiatry Since World War II', *History of Psychiatry* 25, no. 4 (2014): 485–91.
27. Greg Eghigian, 'Deinstitutionalizing the History of Contemporary Psychiatry', *History of Psychiatry* 22, no. 2 (2011): 201–14.
28. Ibid., 202.
29. Cathy Caruth, *Unclaimed Experience: Trauma, Narrative, and History* (Baltimore: Johns Hopkins University Press, 1996); Mark S. Micale and Paul Lerner, eds., *Traumatic Pasts: History, Psychiatry, and Trauma in the Modern Age, 1870–1930* (Cambridge: Cambridge University Press, 2001); Jeffrey C. Alexander, *Trauma: A Social Theory* (Cambridge and Malden: Polity, 2012).
30. George L. Mosse, 'Shell-Shock as a Social Disease', *Journal of Contemporary History* 35, no. 1 (2000): 101–8.
31. Jay Winter, 'Shell-Shock and the Cultural History of the Great War', *Journal of Contemporary History* 35, no. 1 (2000): 7–11.
32. Peter Riedesser and Axel Verderber, *Maschinengewehre hinter der Front: Zur Geschichte der deutschen Militärpsychiatrie* (Frankfurt am Main: Fischer, 1996).
33. Lerner, *Hysterical Men.*
34. Julia Barbara Köhne, *Kriegshysteriker: Strategische Bilder und mediale Techniken militärpsychiatrischen Wissens (1914–1920)* (Husum: Matthiessen, 2009); Hans-Georg Hofer, *Nervenschwäche und Krieg: Modernitätskritik und Krisenbewältigung in der österreichischen Psychiatrie (1880–1920)*

(Vienna, Cologne, and Weimar: Böhlau, 2004); Crouthamel, *The Great War and German Memory.*
35. Lerner, *Hysterical Men*, 193–248; Neuner, *Politik und Psychiatrie.*
36. Friedrich Kittler, *Short Cuts* (Frankfurt am Main: Zweitausendeins, 2002), 142.
37. Joachim Radkau, *Das Zeitalter der Nervosität: Deutschland zwischen Bismarck und Hitler* (Munich: Hanser, 1998).
38. Andreas Killen, *Berlin Electropolis: Shock, Nerves, and German Modernity* (Berkeley, Los Angeles, and London: University of California Press, 2006); Michael Cowan, *Cult of the Will: Nervousness and German Modernity* (University Park, PA: The Pennsylvania State University Press, 2008); Hofer, *Nervenschwäche und Krieg*; Marijke Gijswijt-Hofstra and Roy Porter, eds., *Cultures of Neurasthenia from Beard to the First World War* (Amsterdam: Rodopi, 2001).
39. Hans-Walter Schmuhl, *Rassenhygiene, Nationalsozialismus, Euthanasie: Von der Verhütung zur Vernichtung 'lebensunwerten Lebens,' 1890–1945* (Göttingen: Vandenhoeck & Ruprecht, 1987); Paul Weindling, *Health, Race and German Politics Between National Unification and Nazism, 1870–1945* (Cambridge: Cambridge University Press, 1989); Peter Weingart, Jürgen Kroll, and Kurt Bayertz, *Rasse, Blut und Gene: Geschichte der Eugenik und Rassenhygiene in Deutschland* (Frankfurt am Main: Suhrkamp, 1992).
40. Karl Binding and Alfred Hoche, *Die Freigabe der Vernichtung lebensunwerten Lebens: Ihr Maß und ihre Form* (Leipzig: F. Meiner, 1920).
41. Mark B. Adams, *The Wellborn Science: Eugenics in Germany, France, Brazil, and Russia* (New York: Oxford University Press, 1990); Stefan Kühl, *Die Internationale der Rassisten: Aufstieg und Niedergang der internationalen Bewegung für Eugenik und Rassenhygiene im 20. Jahrhundert* (Frankfurt am Main and New York: Campus, 1997).
42. Paul Weindling, 'The Sonderweg of German Eugenics: Nationalism and Scientific Internationalism', *The British Journal for the History of Science* 22, no. 3 (1989): 321–33.
43. Volker Roelcke, 'Continuities or Ruptures? Concepts, Institutions and Contexts of Twentieth-Century German Psychiatry and Mental Health Care', in *Psychiatric Cultures Compared: Psychiatry and Mental Health Care in the Twentieth Century: Comparisons and Approaches*, ed. Marijke Gijswijt-Hofstra et al. (Amsterdam: Amsterdam University Press, 2005), 162–83.
44. Paul Federn and Heinrich Meng, eds., *Das psychoanalytische Volksbuch* (Stuttgart: Hippokrates, 1926).
45. Nikolas Rose, *The Psychological Complex: Psychology, Politics, and Society in England, 1869–1939* (London and Boston: Routledge & Kegan Paul, 1985), 9.
46. Rudolf Virchow, 'Der Armenarzt', *Die medicinische Reform*, no. 18 (1848): 125; Constantin Goschler, 'Wahrheit zwischen Seziersaal und Parlament:

Rudolf Virchow und der kulturelle Deutungsanspruch der Naturwissenschaften', *Geschichte und Gesellschaft* 30, no. 2 (2004): 219–49; Tobias Weidner, *Die unpolitische Profession: Deutsche Mediziner im langen 19. Jahrhundert* (Frankfurt am Main: Campus, 2012), 112–29.

47. Thomas Mann, *Betrachtungen eines Unpolitischen* (Berlin: S. Fischer, 1918); Willibald Steinmetz and Heinz-Gerhard Haupt, 'The Political as Communicative Space in History: The Bielefeld Approach', in *Writing Political History Today*, ed. Willibald Steinmetz, Ingrid Gilcher-Holtey, and Heinz-Gerhard Haupt (Frankfurt am Main and New York: Campus, 2013), 25–26.
48. Dirk van Laak, 'Technokratie im Europa des 20. Jahrhunderts - eine einflussreiche Hintergrundideologie', in *Theorien und Experimente der Moderne: Europas Gesellschaften im 20. Jahrhundert*, ed. Lutz Raphael (Cologne, Vienna and Weimar: Böhlau, 2012), 101–28; Thomas Etzemüller, *Die Ordnung der Moderne: Social Engineering im 20. Jahrhundert* (Bielefeld: transcript, 2009).
49. van Laak, 'Technokratie', 124.
50. Weidner, *Die unpolitische Profession.*
51. Ibid., 16, 28.
52. Lutz Raphael, 'Die Verwissenschaftlichung des Sozialen als methodische und konzeptionelle Herausforderung für eine Sozialgeschichte des 20. Jahrhunderts', *Geschichte und Gesellschaft* 22, no. 2 (1996): 165–93.
53. Ibid., 166.
54. Kerstin Brückweh et al., eds., *Engineering Society: The Role of the Human and Social Sciences in Modern Societies, 1880–1980* (London: Palgrave Macmillan, 2012).
55. Mathew Thomson, 'The Psychological Sciences and the Scientization and Engineering of Society in Twentieth-Century Britain', in *Engineering Society: The Role of the Human and Social Sciences in Modern Societies, 1880–1980*, ed. Kerstin Brückweh et al. (London: Palgrave Macmillan, 2012), 141–44.
56. Philip Rieff, *The Triumph of the Therapeutic* (New York: Harper & Row, 1966); Thomas Szasz, *The Therapeutic State: Psychiatry in the Mirror of Current Events* (Buffalo, NY: Prometheus Books, 1984); James L. Nolan, *The Therapeutic State: Justifying Government at Century's End* (New York: New York University Press, 1998); Timothy Aubry and Trysh Travis, *Rethinking Therapeutic Culture* (Chicago: Chicago University Press, 2015); Pascal Eitler et al., *Das beratene Selbst: Zur Genealogie der Therapeutisierung in den 'langen' Siebzigern* (Bielefeld: transcript, 2011).
57. Lutz Raphael, 'Embedding the Human and Social Sciences in Western Societies, 1880–1980: Reflections on Trends and Methods of Current Research', in *Engineering Society: The Role of the Human and Social Sciences in Modern Societies, 1880–1980*, ed. Kerstin Brückweh et al. (London: Palgrave Macmillan, 2012), 53–54.

58. Rose, *The Psychological Complex*; Nikolas Rose, *Inventing Our Selves: Psychology, Power, and Personhood* (Cambridge: Cambridge University Press, 1996).
59. Anonymous, 'Psychiatrisches Ausbreitungsbedürfnis', 197.
60. van Ginneken, *Crowds*; Pick, *Faces*; Roelcke, *Krankheit.*
61. Hugo Marx, 'Aerztliche Gedanken Zur Revolution', *Berliner Klinische Wochenschrift* 12 (1919): 279.
62. Sándor Ferenczi, 'Die Psychoanalyse der Kriegsneurosen', in *Zur Psychoanalyse der Kriegsneurosen: Diskussion gehalten auf dem V. Internationalen Psychoanalytischen Kongress in Budapest, 28. und 29. September 1918* (Leipzig and Vienna: Internationaler psychoanalytischer Verlag, 1919), 9–10.
63. Boris Groys, *The Total Art of Stalinism: Avant-Garde, Aesthetic, Dictatorship, and Beyond*, trans. Charles Rougle (Princeton, NJ: Princeton University Press, 1992), 17.
64. Heinrich Rogge, 'Psychopolitik und Führerproblem', *Zeitschrift für Menschenkunde* 1, no. 1 (1925): 18–24.
65. Ibid., 23.
66. Thomas Mergel, 'Führer, Volksgemeinschaft und Maschine: Politische Erwartungsstrukturen in der Weimarer Republik und dem Nationalsozialismus 1918–1936', in *Politische Kulturgeschichte der Zwischenkriegszeit 1918–1939*, ed. Wolfgang Hardtwig (Göttingen: Vandenhoeck & Ruprecht, 2005), 91–128; Yves Cohen, *Le siècle des chefs: Une histoire transnationale du commandement et de l'autorité (1890–1940)* (Paris: Éditions Amsterdam, 2013).
67. Siegfried Bernfeld, 'Die Psychologie in der Arbeiterbewegung', in *Antiautoritäre Erziehung und Psychoanalyse: Ausgewählte Schriften*, ed. Lutz von Werder and Reinhart Wolff, 3rd ed., vol. 2 (Frankfurt am Main: März, 1970), 497–506.
68. Ibid., 503.
69. Ibid., 506.
70. Paul Feldkeller, *Wörterbuch der Psychopolitik* (Berne and Munich: A. Francke, 1967).
71. Ibid., 1.
72. Ibid., 106–10.
73. Ibid., 107.
74. Peter Sedgwick, *Psychopolitics: Laing, Foucault, Goffman, Szasz, and the Future of Mass Psychiatry* (New York: Harper & Row, 1982); Hannah Proctor, 'Lost Minds: Sedgwick, Laing and the Politics of Mental Illness', *Radical Philosophy* 197, nos. 5/6 (2016): 36–48; Vicky Lebeau, 'Psychopolitics: Frantz Fanon's Black Skin, White Masks', in *Psycho-Politics and Cultural Desires*, ed. Jan Campbell and Janet Harbord (London and Bristol, PA: UCL Press, 1998), 113–23; China Mills, *Decolonizing Global Mental Health: The*

Psychiatrization of the Majority World (London and New York: Routledge, 2014).

75. Byung-Chul Han, *Psychopolitik: Neoliberalismus und die neuen Machttechniken* (Frankfurt am Main: S. Fischer, 2014).
76. Ibid., 35.
77. Thomas Lemke, *Biopolitics: An Advanced Introduction*, trans. Eric Frederick Trump (New York and London: New York University Press, 2011).
78. Han, *Psychopolitik*, 35. Han's juxtaposition of bio- and psycho-politics alludes to French philosopher Bernard Stiegler's distinction between *biopouvoir* and *psychopouvoir*, see Bernard Stiegler, *Prendre soin: De la jeunesse et des générations* (Paris: Flammarion, 2008).
79. Ute Frevert, 'Neue Politikgeschichte: Konzepte und Herausforderungen', in *Neue Politikgeschichte: Perspektiven einer historischen Politikforschung*, ed. Ute Frevert and Heinz-Gerhard Haupt (Frankfurt am Main and New York: Campus, 2005), 26; Ulrich Meier, Martin Papenheim, and Willibald Steinmetz, eds., *Semantiken des Politischen: Vom Mittelalter bis ins 20. Jahrhundert* (Göttingen: Wallstein, 2012).

CHAPTER 2

Diagnosing the Revolution

When many of the leading psychoanalysts in Central Europe gathered in Budapest in September 1918 to discuss the consequences of the World War for the Freudian school, Sándor Ferenczi (1873–1933) opened the meeting with a topical anecdote.[1] A fellow Hungarian who had witnessed the Bolshevik revolution in Russia had told him about a town where the new rulers had encountered an unexpected problem. According to their materialist conception of history, they now were in control of political power and should have been able to swiftly introduce a new social order. But things were not going as smoothly as their doctrinaire computations had them believe. 'Irresponsible elements, enemies of every new order', gradually regained the upper hand and the new authorities were beginning to lose control. What had gone wrong? The local Bolsheviks went into a huddle to find out what their mistake had been and finally recognised that in all their economic and political considerations, they had overlooked something. 'This little thing was – emotional life, the people's line of thought, in a word: the mind'. As soon as they had found out what the problem was, they send their emissaries to the German-speaking countries to gather books about psychology to acquire the knowledge that they apparently lacked. Ferenczi concluded: 'Thousands of human lives have fallen victim to this forgetfulness of the revolutionists, perhaps in vain, but the failure of their efforts has helped them to make a discovery: the discovery of the soul'.[2]

D. Freis, *Psycho-Politics between the World Wars*,
Mental Health in Historical Perspective,
https://doi.org/10.1007/978-3-030-32702-6_2

The revolution that broke out in Germany two months after the Budapest conference had a similar effect. However, it was not so much the revolutionaries, but their adversaries who discovered the politics of the soul. Even as the upheaval was still going on, numerous psychiatrists and laypeople published their psycho-political diagnoses of what had happened. The behaviour of the revolutionaries and the predicament of the nation, they claimed, could only be understood in terms of psychology and psychopathology.

This conflation of psychiatric and political thought must of course be understood in a broader historical perspective. Generally speaking, the history of psychiatry, its diagnoses, and its therapies has always also been a history of social and political norms, beliefs, and imaginations. This has, in fact, been the gist of most of the historiography of psychiatry since historians and reform-minded psychiatrists introduced new methodologies and critical perspectives in the 1960s; the view that psychiatry is, in some way or another, political has since become a premise of most scholarship in the field. As a plethora of studies have shown, throughout its existence as a medical speciality, psychiatry was one of the institutions tasked with policing the contested boundaries of normalcy. From the subtle and not-so-subtle micro-politics of institutional spaces and diagnostic regimes to the deadly use of psychiatric expertise in the name of 'racial hygiene', psychiatry was involved with the wider politics of norms, order, power relations, inclusion, and exclusion. The most blatant politicisation of psychiatry happened when psychiatrists turned their clinical gaze directly on topics that they and their contemporaries unquestioningly considered to be political, that is, when politics and society themselves became the object of psychiatric diagnosis. Writings in which the diagnostic tools of psychiatry were used not to understand the pathologies of individuals, but to explain the state of society and the allegedly psychopathological causes and effects of political events instead, became a genre in medical scholarship and journalism as early as the beginning of the nineteenth century. Medical historian Volker Roelcke has argued that these writings should be understood as a medium of a 'bourgeois interpretation of the world and the self' and as a reaction to the crisis of bourgeois self-perception in the long nineteenth century.[3] However, as I show in this chapter, psycho-political diagnoses must also be understood as a performance of scientific expertise in a specific socio-political context. In the immediate post-war period of the First World War, the diagnosis of social and political events as psychopathological symptoms became a way to bolster psychiatrists' long-standing claims for an extension of their medical expertise into new areas.

The aftermath of the First World War was neither the first nor the last time that a revolution became a target of psychiatry. In moments of political, social, and cultural turmoil, diagnoses of contemporary events gained currency. In many cases, psychiatric arguments were not only used to decry moral decline and political chaos as forms of madness but were directly aimed at specific political groups, leaders, and ideas. German psychiatrists' talk of 'revolutionary psychopaths' in the aftermath of the 1918/1919 revolution was certainly a particularly blatant example for the medical stigmatisation of political adversaries. But as two very different examples in which political upheaval was diagnosed from a psychiatric perspective may show, allegations of madness were often directed against the legitimacy of radical political changes.

In 1850, shortly after the failed liberal revolutions in the German confederation, a doctoral thesis in medicine caused a stir at the University of Berlin.[4] The young physician Carl Theodor Groddeck (1826–1885) announced the discovery of a new kind of mental illness that had afflicted the nation—*morbus democraticus*, the 'democratic illness'.[5] Despite numerous references to authorities such as Wilhelm Griesinger (1817–1868) and Karl Wilhelm Ideler (1795–1860), Groddeck's dissertation hardly qualified as medical research. It lacked a well-defined vocabulary for the description of individual mental disorders, and Groddeck had little to say about the medical specifics of allegedly collective forms of madness such as the purported democratic illness. In fact, much of his argument appears rather muddled. Due to its obvious confusion of medical and political categories, Groddeck's *morbus democraticus* became a textbook example for the pitfalls of medical diagnoses of political life, and even the most fervent advocates of psychiatry's right to diagnose society and politics were eager to dissociate their own ideas from Groddeck's.[6]

When the global protests of 1968 reached Western Germany, psychiatric vocabulary became again widely used in political debates. While conservative newspapers and tabloids routinely denounced members of the student movement as dangerous madmen, the diagnosis that led to the most acrimonious debate came out of a very different direction. Like other protagonists of the Frankfurt school, the Federal Republic's chief philosopher Jürgen Habermas (*1929) had observed the student movement's actionism and radicalism with growing disconcertment and eventually published a sardonic opinion piece in which he castigated the 'pseudo-revolution and its children' (*Die Scheinrevolution und ihre Kinder*).[7] In the ensuing political father-son conflict, student activists were upset not just by Habermas's flagrant paternalism, but also by the fact that his political interjection tilted towards psychopathological diagnosis. Habermas's short text was spiked with concepts from clinical psychology. As he saw it, the student protests were driven by 'those foibles of the intellectuals that in quiet times are part of their *déformations professionelles*, but in more turbulent times, when they step out of the shadow realm of personal psychology and become political violence, really are a scandal'.[8] To student activists and their sympathisers, the centre-left philosopher's provocation was a painful betrayal and their replies were enough to fill a book. To former student activist and social psychiatrist Klaus Dörner (*1933), Habermas's rhetoric carried more than just a faint echo of earlier psychiatric defamations of left-wing revolutionaries—it was part of this very tradition. As Dörner argued, Habermas's diagnosis was just the latest iteration of a history of the 'psychiatric-clinical labelling of revolutionary movements' that was as old as bourgeois society, and thus modern psychiatry, itself.[9] Dörner assigned Habermas the part of the psychiatric mouthpiece of the reaction and drew a direct line between the Paris Communards of 1871, the Spartacist revolutionaries of 1918/1919, and the protesting students of 1968.

However, psychiatric diagnoses of politics were never as common or as fierce as in the years after 1918. The aftermath of the First World War saw a downright surge in psycho-political writings by German and Austrian psychiatrists. Shortly after the war had ended in a military defeat of the Central Powers and the revolutionary upheaval had swept away the Hohenzollern and Habsburg dynasties, leading psychiatrists drew on the concepts of their discipline to diagnose the current events as the work of antisocial 'psychopaths' or as the result of a national nervous breakdown and collective hysteria. While intellectual and political elites imagined the national body (*Volkskörper*) as a sick body, psychiatrists offered a psychological complement to this analogy of the political body.[10] In doing so, they could rely on long-standing traditions. Many of the concepts used after 1918 had already been part of psychiatric and popular discourse in the nineteenth century, such as Cesare Lombroso's category of the 'born criminal' or Gustave Le Bon's theories of crowd psychology. But while these concepts had been the expression of diffuse fears of an educated bourgeoisie towards the anonymous masses, degeneration, criminal 'inferiors', and anarchist troublemakers in the late nineteenth century, they now offered a seemingly scientific explanation for the very acute socio-political crisis of the post-war period.

As was often the case in discourses of crisis, pessimism and optimism went hand in hand.[11] The post-war crisis called for urgent action, but it also created opportunities to shape a new society that would finally overcome the problems of the old. In a political situation in which many conservative psychiatrists saw the nation in existential danger, older concepts were not only updated and politicised, but were also used to legitimise demands for far-reaching socio-medical interventions to salvage and regenerate the national collective. Diagnosing the political crisis as a medical urgency, and with a profound belief in the ability of the modern sciences to reform society, psychiatrists cast themselves in the role of socio-political experts, psycho-political leaders, and healers of the collective.

To some extent, this vision of psychiatry's role was a product of the experience of the First World War. The treatment of the so-called war neurotics had seemed like a therapeutic breakthrough, promising to finally end psychiatry's notorious inability to heal its patients and to usher in a new era of 'heroic therapies'.[12] The war also marked a new height in the prestige and political relevance of the discipline.[13] With the military stalemate along the Western front, the mental resilience of the fighting troops and the nation was considered as potentially decisive strategic assets. It was field marshal Paul von Hindenburg who had famously stated in 1916 that 'victory will go to him who has the best nerves'.[14] After the defeat and the armistice, and against the backdrop of growing patient discontent and public protests against the brutality of 'active treatment' and struggles over the allocation of veteran pensions, psychiatrists' claim for expertise was an attempt to use the post-war crisis to defend and extend the wartime gains of their profession after the demobilisation.[15]

This 'psychiatric need for expansion'—as an anonymous author in the 'anti-psychiatric' journal *Die Irrenrechts-Reform* called it in 1919—was part of a broader development in the inter-war period.[16] Psychiatrists' alarmist diagnosis of a collective 'nervous breakdown' and their warnings of an imminent collapse of German culture were part of a ubiquitous discourse about the 'crisis' of the Weimar Republic and a rampant 'dramatisation of the political imaginary'.[17] Political alarmism was used to mobilise and legitimise visions of national regeneration and the restructuring of society and politics through rational and scientific methods. Psychiatrists were only one among many groups of techno-scientific experts who tried to seize the newly created opportunities. The socio-medical interventions that they proposed in the immediate post-war period, ranging from education to eugenics, should be seen as part of a more general trend towards 'social engineering'.[18] Hence, psychiatrists' aspirations for a socio-political expert status led the discipline into a contested field, where experts from other disciplines had already successfully staked out their claims in an ongoing 'scientification of the social'.[19] As I show in more detail in the following chapter, the Viennese psychiatrist Erwin Stransky was convinced that psychiatrists' new expert status had to be gained not only against the anti-psychiatric bias of 'public opinion', but that they would also have to conquer positions where jurists had already entrenched themselves.

The example of Stransky's 'applied psychiatry' also illustrates how the claim for psychiatry's socio-political expert status could blur the lines between disciplines and create new fields of scientific inquiry. The Association for Applied Psychopathology and Psychology, founded in Vienna shortly after the war, became a site of interdisciplinary encounter *avant la lettre*. A first and only international conference in June 1930 brought together psychiatrists, psychologists, psychoanalysts, but also sociologists, jurists, and even literary scholars, to discuss different aspects of modern life and society from a perspective of psychopathology.[20]

This chapter, however, examines the socio-political writings of German and Austrian psychiatrists in the immediate aftermath of the First World War and the political upheaval of 1918/1919. A first section focuses on the diagnosis of individual participants of the German revolution as psychopaths, examining how an already morally charged concept that had emerged in forensic psychiatry and criminology before the war became explicitly politicised in the wake of the revolution. A second section looks at the transfer of medical concepts from individuals to the national collective and shows how psychiatrists construed a direct analogy between clinical and political phenomena to redefine themselves as physicians of the nation. A third and final section summarises the subsequent history of psychiatric expertise in the inter-war period and asks how, and psychiatry as a discipline could capitalise on the psycho-political diagnoses of the revolution.

The Revolutionary Psychopaths

'It has long been known', psychiatrist Eugen Kahn wrote in the Munich medical weekly in August 1919, 'that in times of turmoil, those prone to mentally disorders come forward, and after the experiences we psychiatrists have made during the war, it did not come as a surprise to us that in the latest upheaval such people have stood in the front'.[21] Kahn was not the only psychiatrist who had come to this conclusion. In the short period following the end of the war and the revolution, numerous articles appearing in different professional journals made an almost identical argument, claiming that 'inferior' or psychopathic individuals had been the driving force behind the recent upheaval.

As a member of Emil Kraepelin's German Research Institute for Psychiatry (*Deutsche Forschungsanstalt für Psychiatrie*, DFA, on which more in Chapter 4) in Munich, Kahn was particularly well positioned to examine the psychopathology of the revolution. Munich had been one of the centres of the German revolution and, for a short time in the spring of 1919, had been the capital of a Bavarian Soviet Republic. After loyal government troops and right-wing *Freikorps* militia had violently crushed the revolution in May 1919, many of the survivors were imprisoned and could thus become objects of forensic examination by the psychiatrists of the DFA, such as Emil Kraepelin and Ernst Rüdin.[22] However, the most assiduous diagnostician was Eugen Kahn, whose article was based on a sample of sixty-six individuals who had participated in the revolution.

On 3 August 1919, Kahn presented his findings at the yearly conference of Bavarian psychiatrists. Emphasising the historical relevance of his research, he situated the revolutionaries of Munich in a longer line that reached from Savonarola's Florence to the French Revolution and the Paris Commune into the present. At the same time, he also positioned himself as a medical expert outside and above of political struggles. To speak about recent events, Kahn argued, obviously held the danger of being caught up in the current political disputes. However, 'the idea that the psychiatrist always has to be ready to provide his judgment impartially and to the best of his knowledge, can and must help us to get over these concerns'.[23]

Among those cases that Kahn discussed in detail were prominent leaders of the Munich Soviet, thinly disguised behind the pseudonyms Otto Wasner (alias Kurt Eisner), Werner Leidig (Erich Mühsam), and Erwin Sinner (Ernst Toller).[24] Mühsam and Toller had probably been personally examined by Kahn when they were imprisoned shortly after the end of the Bavarian Soviet Republic. Eisner, however, had been assassinated by the far-right nationalist Anton Graf von Arco auf Valley on 21 February 1919, so that Kahn's *post mortem* diagnosis of Eisner as a 'fanatic psychopath' had to rely solely on newspaper reports and other publications. Ernst Toller, 26 years old, former president of the short-lived Munich Soviet, and an eminent Expressionist playwright, had already encountered Emil Kraepelin in the summer of 1918, some months before the revolution. Toller later remembered the episode in his 1933 autobiography, where he described the famous professor as someone with the 'pathos of a manic debater' who tried to convince him of the right-wing policies of the Pan-German League. Inverting the direction of the diagnosis, the lesson that Toller took away from this encounter was 'that there are two kinds of sick people, the harmless lying around in barred and clinic-less rooms are called insane, the more dangerous are those who prove that hunger educates the people and create associations for the subjugation of England, those may then lock up the harmless'.[25]

Although Kahn stressed that he did not consider the revolution a pathological event as such and that not every revolutionary was necessarily 'mentally inferior', he had no doubt that psychopaths had played a most important role during the upheaval. Of the sixty-six revolutionary leaders in his sample, 'scarcely one could be seen as mentally intact overall' and all of the fifteen cases on which he reported in detail had to be considered as model types of the 'revolutionary psychopath'.[26] There was, however, hardly a precise definition of the underlying concept of psychopathy, and the term 'psychopath' was mainly used to describe individuals with a whole range of perceived 'abnormalities' in the grey area between normality and full-blown mental illness. As Kahn defined the term for the non-psychiatrist readers of the Munich medical weekly:

> Psychiatry describes as psychopaths personalities who are mentally not fully intact, who, although generally of sufficient or in many cases even of good intelligence, have deficits in their way of feeling and wanting; deficits, which do not let these personalities appear as mentally ill, but which lead them to make wrong life decisions often enough and to fail with them.[27]

The diagnosis of psychopathy was evidently normative, since the decision whether someone was to be considered a psychopath had to be based on an assessment of their life choices in terms of right and successful or not. For conservatives like Eugen Kahn and many others, joining a socialist revolution obviously was a wrong choice in life. The notion of psychopathy replaced older and equally broad concepts of 'mental inferiority' and 'psychopathic inferiority' in the years after the First World War, but it remained insufficient as a conceptual tool for the scientific description of deviant behaviour,[28] even as numerous, and sometimes rather arbitrary sub-species of psychopaths were invented. Karl Birnbaum's textbook, for example, distinguished between almost thirty different kinds of psychopaths.[29]

The problem of how to define psychopathy had already occupied psychiatrists and criminal biologists long before the war. One of the earliest and most influential attempts to describe and categorise different 'psychopathic personalities' was made in the seventh edition of Emil Kraepelin's textbook, published in 1903. Kraepelin devoted an entire chapter to his distinction between four types of 'psychopathic personalities': born criminals, unstable personalities (*Haltlose*), pathological liars, and 'pseudo-querulous' individuals (*Pseudoquerulanten*).[30] Before the publication of Kurt Schneider's *Die psychopathischen Persönlichkeiten* ('the psychopathic personalities') in 1923, Kraepelin's classification remained of the crucial reference for all psychiatric thinking on mental abnormalities and deviant behaviour, rivalled only by Karl Birnbaum's 1914 *Die psychopathischen Verbrecher* ('the psychopathic criminals'). In contrast to previous approaches, such as those by Julius Koch or Gustav Aschaffenburg, Kraepelin and the theoreticians of psychopathy that followed him excluded lack of intelligence and feeblemindedness from their definitions and focused on abnormalities in emotional life and volition instead.[31] This new figure of the psychopath was not necessarily inferior, but inherently different and socially deviant.[32]

Kahn did not rigorously follow the system of classification provided by Kraepelin, but introduced a set of categories that was adapted to the revolutionaries of Munich, who in his view had been 'ethically defective psychopaths', 'hysterical personalities', 'fanatic psychopaths', or 'manic depressives'.[33] Throughout Kahn's detailed descriptions and despite all his attempts at conceptual differentiation, the psychopath remained an elusive category, so much that, once the light of psychopathy fell on an individual, virtually any aspect of his or her physiognomy, character, and biography could be read as a sign of abnormality. Different groups of perceived troublemakers could thus be identified with each other. Against the backdrop of wartime psychiatry and the growing criticism of its harsh methods of treatment by both patients and the public, Kahn drew a direct line between the experiences of military psychiatrists and the revolution when he claimed that the revolutionary psychopaths were part of the same group that previously had 'filled the military hospitals as war neurotics of all kinds' and had kept the military courts busy 'as elements that exceedingly threatened discipline'.[34]

Notably, Eugen Kahn singled out revolutionary leaders of Jewish origin when he presented a statistical overview of his cases. He did, however, not elaborate on what these numbers meant. Blaming Jews for their role in the revolution was a recurring theme in far-right propaganda, but there is a least some reason to be sceptical about such a reading of Kahn's numbers. While clearly not a supporter of the revolution, Kahn, who himself was Jewish, had at least one reason to avoid repeating the anti-Semitic stab-in-the-back myth. The rising anti-Semitism in Weimar Germany and the resulting informal restriction of academic career opportunities probably became one reason why Kahn accepted a position as professor of psychiatry and mental hygiene at the Yale School of Medicine in 1928.[35] More likely, Kahn's data reflected the influence of his superior at the German Research Institute for Psychiatry, Emil Kraepelin, who was fiercely anti-Semitic. Unlike Kahn, Kraepelin explicitly blamed Jews for allegedly playing an outsized role in the revolution, writing in 1919 that 'the strong participation of the Jewish race in these upheavals' was not only due to their 'frequent psychopathic disposition' but also due to 'their ability for undermining criticism, their verbal and theatrical capability as well as their tenaciousness and ambitiousness'.[36] Together with several of the most common stereotypes, the cliché of the 'nervous Jew' became a link between racial anti-Semitism and the figure of the psychopath as an internal political enemy of the German nation.

Another forensic examination of a revolutionary psychopath was published by Kurt Hildebrandt, a psychiatrist at the clinic of Dalldorf in the vicinity of Berlin. Like Kahn, Hildebrand had been an expert witness in the trials after the end of the revolution. When he presented the results of the forensic examination of the anonymous painter 'M.', who had participated in the Spartacist uprising in Berlin in January 1919, Hildebrandt highlighted the scientific value of this publication and his own impartiality: 'the psychopathic influence on the revolution and the following class struggles is so considerable that it cannot be ignored, regardless of the political orientation'. With a nod to future historians, he claimed that 'even for historiography the question of psychopathic influence in the revolution is not irrelevant'.[37]

Hildebrandt believed that two different types of psychopaths had played particularly important roles during the recent events, the first being the 'enemies of society and barraters', the second the 'impostors and braggarts', who, just for want of being great men (*Großmannssucht*), had forced themselves into leading positions. As he had not shown any interest in politics before the end of the war and his participation in the revolution had not brought him any material gains, Hildebrandt initially identified M. as a representative of the second type. But the more the exhaustive account advanced, the less clear and the less important the distinction between the different types of psychopaths became. 'M. shows the typical and very clear appearance of a mentally inferior person, a "psychopath". All of his pathological symptoms could be satisfactorily and completely explained by "psychopathy"', Hildebrandt wrote, but also noted that the painter showed the symptoms not only of one of the different types but of several of them. Without questioning the broader concept of psychopathy, Hildebrandt was quite aware of the constructedness of the categories and argued that 'these types are not separate units of illness, but for practical reasons and with a certain arbitrariness are singled out from the larger group of psychopaths'.[38]

Kahn and Hildebrandt were only two voices in a larger chorus of psychiatrists from all areas of Germany who believed that psychopaths of one kind or another had played an outsized, if not even a decisive role in recent history. Similar interpretations of the revolution appeared in many other contributions to medical journals. The physician Hans Brennecke from Hamburg for example published several articles in which he expounded on how psychopathy had shaped the revolution.[39] 'In the murky waves of upheaval', psychiatrist Helenefriderike Stelzner from Berlin wrote in 1919, psychopathic individuals who previously had been unable of finding their place in the 'social body' (*Sozialkörper*) were washed into positions of high responsibility. Like Kahn, she argued that this was not specific to the current situation but a fact well-known from earlier events like the French Revolution and the Paris Commune.[40] It was no coincidence that 'pathographies' of leaders of the French Revolution like Jean-Paul Marat were published shortly after the 1918/1919 revolution in Germany.[41] To Emil Kraepelin, it was evident that during the revolution, psychopaths had been the ones ruling Germany: 'We ourselves have shudderingly seen what fruits the rule of the mentioned groups has yielded'.[42] Likewise, another 'historical-psychological study' of the revolution, published by one Hans Freimark in 1920, devoted two entire chapters to the role of the revolutionary crowds and their pathological leaders.[43] Finally, the example of Max Glass's 1919 novel *Die entfesselte Menschheit* ('Mankind unleashed') illustrates how the psychiatric perspective quickly entered the right-wing conservative interpretation of the revolution.[44]

By using psychopathy as a diagnosis, psychiatrists drew on the conceptual framework of forensic psychiatry and criminal biology to explain individual deviant behaviour as symptom of an underlying pathology. For Eugen

Kahn, Kurt Hildebrandt, and Hans Brennecke, their examination of participants of the revolution was part of criminal proceedings and thus took part at the contested interface between penal law and psychiatry as two institutions occupied with 'abnormal' and deviant behaviour. The relevant legislation—§51 of the German criminal code—stipulated that an accused could not be punished for a deed committed while in a state of 'unconsciousness or pathological mental defect (*krankhafte Geistesstörung*), suspending his ability to make free choices (*freie Willensbestimmung*)'. This paragraph, which gave medical experts the possibility to affect a trial by declaring a defendant *non compos mentis*, was the source of psychiatry's power in the German juridical system. Yet, none of the psychiatrists writing about revolutionary psychopaths used this argument to exculpate the subjects of their examination. Kahn, for example, had no doubts that all his fifteen cases were psychopaths, but that none of them was to be granted the protection of §51. Hildebrandt came to the same conclusion in the case of the Spartacist painter M., arguing that the diagnosis of psychopathy alone did not affect the question of criminal liability, since 'a psychopath can be fully or limitedly responsible or not responsible at all'.[45] Conveniently enough, the diagnosis of psychopathy could be used to apply the stigma of mental illness to individuals without lifting any of their criminal, moral, and political culpability.

More than by legal considerations, the use of the elusive category of psychopathy was driven by political motives. Even when it was applied not to political adversaries such as Spartacist revolutionaries, but to common criminals, troublemakers, and misfits, the concept of psychopathy was inherently political. All attempts to introduce finely nuanced categories notwithstanding, and regardless of the transition from the notion of 'inferiors' to the more scientific and neutral sounding 'psychopaths' after the end of the war, the concept remained part of a morally charged 'dispositive of normality'.[46] Situated in a grey area between madness and normality, psychopathy allowed psychiatrists and criminal biologists to identify, construct, and pathologise perceived threats against bourgeois society and morality.[47]

In the tumult of the immediate post-war period, psychopathy became a way to reframe perceived political threats as objects of medical and psychiatric expertise. Seeing the nation and the moral and political order of bourgeois society in peril and fearing for their own careers, positions, and in some situations, even their lives, German psychiatrists eagerly employed the propagandistic potentials of their diagnostic tools. As historian Paul

Lerner wrote, 'associating the recent political events with the actions of hysterics and psychopaths was one way in which doctors used their medical expertise and status to discredit the Revolution and critique the nascent Weimar system'.[48] Generally speaking, diagnosing political adversaries as psychopaths offered a possibility to delegitimise their political claims by ascribing their actions not to any rational response to the current political situation, but rather to egoism, lust for power, the need to stand out, defects in volition and willpower, or even to outright insanity. By shifting the analytical focus from the political to the clinical sphere, psychiatrists claimed for themselves the status of experts in a heated public debate and in the shaping of post-war society.

Moreover, Lerner has rightly pointed out that the practice of military psychiatry during the war, the post-war pathologisation of perceived psychopaths, and psychiatrists' reaction to the public attacks against the practitioners of 'active treatment' very linked to each other. By equating the revolutionists with their former patients, psychiatrists identified them as enemies of the nation and as the ones who were responsible for the military defeat as well as for the violence and turmoil of the post-war period. In doing so, they not only denied their former patients their status as traumatised victims of the war but depicted them as the true perpetrators.[49] With the psychopaths threatening society, German psychiatrists saw their duty not in the healing of the mentally ill but in defending the nation against them. Doris Kaufmann has argued that this 'labelling and marking out of a group of so-called inferiors for their "failure in the war" has to be seen highly significant for the scientific legitimation and acceptance of some later practices of national socialist population policy'.[50]

Even before the war, the concept of 'psychopathic inferiority' had been part of a practice of 'making up people'.[51] Merging various forms of deviant behaviour and personality traits into a single diagnosis, psychiatrists and criminologists constructed the psychopath as a figure that could be blamed for a broad range of problems in modern society and urban life. The idea that the revolution was the work of an antisocial group of 'psychopathic personalities' was a continuation of a way of psychiatric thinking about deviant behaviour and its biological origins that could be traced back well into the nineteenth century. At the same time, however, diagnosing prominent socialists and communists as psychopaths also served a function in the present, as psychiatrists lent their voices to Weimar Germany's obsessive search for those responsible for the defeat of 1918 and the collapse of the Hohenzollern monarchy. The narrative of the revolutionary psychopaths was essentially a psychiatric variation on the stab-in-the-back myth, and it was used to blame the same people—socialists, pacifists, malingerers, and dissenters—for having caused the defeat and the revolution. When used to scapegoat a group of individuals for the present state of the nation and the discontents of modernity in general, the concept of psychopathy was clearly compatible with Weimar Germany's virulent anti-Semitism. Like Jews in the anti-Semitic imagination, psychopaths were an invisible interior enemy, undermining the fabric of society from within. Right-wing psychiatrists like Emil Kraepelin directly associated both groups, psychopaths and Jews, with each other and attributed the same characteristics to both.

As a kind of right-wing polemic in medical disguise, diagnosing the revolutionaries of 1918/1919 as psychopaths was a way to symbolically restore order in a political situation that challenged many of the certainties of the pre-war era. At the same time, however, these diagnoses also contained an argument about psychiatry's future role in society. In blurring the lines between medicine and politics, they delegitimised political actors by assigning them to the domain of psychiatry, but they also opened a gate for proactive socio-medical interventions. By depicting society as threatened by psychopathic subversives and troublemakers, psychiatrists eagerly positioned themselves in the first line of defence and claimed for themselves the status of socio-political experts. For psychiatrists Hans Brennecke, the observation that psychopaths had played an important role in the revolution raised the question of how to defend society: 'How can we effectively protect the general public against the dangerous, anti- and asocial psychopathic personalities and mentally inferior? The answer to this question lies equally in criminal law and in practical psychiatry'.[52] The measures that Brennecke proposed mainly consisted in the possibility to detain psychopaths not for juridical or medical reasons but for the protection of society. He also called for the creation of specialised institutions for dangerous and criminal psychopaths under the direction of psychiatrists, an idea that had already been flouted by some psychiatrists, lawyers, and criminologists in the decade before the war.[53] The establishment of specialised institutions for the custody and 'socialisation' of psychopaths was also advocated by Kahn.[54] Referring to the long-lasting psychiatric debates about the reform of criminal law, which had regained momentum after the end of the war, he highlighted the increased importance of psychiatric expertise: 'When in the course of the rearrangement of things our laws undergo the long-planned reforms, we will be there to participate and we will not forget what the revolution has told us about psychiatry'.[55] To Kahn, this also meant that psychiatry's long-lasting process of professionalisation was finally complete. Psychiatry, he reminded his fellow physicians in the Munich medical weekly, 'is no longer the poor cousin among the medical disciplines'.[56]

A National Nervous Breakdown

It was not only the actions of alleged antisocial psychopaths that worried many German psychiatrists in the months after November 1918. Surely, those had played their role in the upheaval, they argued, but had not the nation itself gone mad? In a 'medical emergency call' circulated in late 1918, Robert Sommer, chair of psychiatry at the University of Giessen, warned that the nervous system of the German nation had suffered a serious shock.[57] As malnutrition and the economic and political crisis drove the Germans deeper and deeper into a 'nervous mass illness', Sommer saw the imminent collapse of civilisation and expected mass suicides, general upheaval and devastation, and ultimately the descent into Bolshevism. This prognosis was obviously tinged by Sommer's own political and medical views, but his observations were not entirely wrong. In late 1918, Germany was in the midst of a profound crisis, as the collapse of political institutions, the return and reintegration of demobilised troops, the effects of years of malnutrition, and the raging influenza pandemic threatened the public order and the health of large parts of the population.[58]

In the course of the following months, other psychiatrists, among them leading representatives of the discipline such as Emil Kraepelin, Robert Gaupp, and, as late as 1923, Karl Bonhoeffer, joined in with Sommer's diagnosis and cast the current events as symptoms of a collective 'nervous breakdown', collective neurasthenia, mass psychosis, and mass hysteria.[59] This use of psychiatric categories had been prepared by a rhetorical mobilisation of both professional and general public debates during the war. In 1915, already Sigmund Freud had complained about his colleagues' eagerness to call the enemy nations 'inferior' or 'degenerated'.[60] Three more years of war and a revolution had done little to cool the minds. In 1919, notions like 'madness' and other more specific diagnoses were ubiquitously used throughout all political camps, in the press, and even in the national assembly. Irked by what they considered a form of psychiatric encroachment on public life, the 'anti-psychiatric' journal *Irrenrechts-Reform* tried to intervene and clarified: 'There is no such thing as political madness, no war psychosis and no revolutionary psychosis, no legal madness (*Rechtswahnsinn*), and also there is no mass madness'.[61] Many psychiatrists begged to differ, even if that meant stretching the epistemological validity of some medical concepts to their limits.

Psycho-political diagnoses offered a seemingly scientific interpretation of current events to an unsettled and disoriented public (of which their authors were themselves a part), especially when these views were legitimised not only by the abstract authority of psychiatry but also by the personal authority of individual experts. The use of psychiatric authority to explain the revolution had been relatively straightforward when individual revolutionaries were described as psychopaths—even if the diagnostic concepts were elusive, the judgement was politically biased, and the actual examination fell blatantly short of clinical standards, the diagnosis of individuals and their behaviour was inherently part of psychiatry's domain. However, many psychiatrists would not limit themselves to diagnosing individual behaviour but projected their medical categories from the individual patient to the nation as a whole.

The bridge between individual pathology and the nation was the idea of a collective 'national soul' (*Volksseele*). The *Volksseele*'s conceptual history can be traced back to early nineteenth-century political philosophy and late nineteenth-century 'folk psychology', but the term took on a new meaning when psychiatrists claimed that they could diagnose the metahistorical 'soul' of the nation like a disordered mind.[62] The result was an awkward tension between a metaphorical use and almost esoteric ideas of a supra-individual spirit. The Hungarian physician Jenő Kollarits was among the few who dared to explicitly argue that the existence of a diagnosable collective soul was an empirical fact, and even while they were at the margins of the scientific consensus, his views were still publishable in psychiatric and psychological journals.[63] Yet, most of the psychiatrists who used the concept cautiously avoided touching on its epistemological implications, much as their somatically oriented colleagues did when they casually spoke about the body politic as if the nation had a supra-individual body that could be afflicted by the same illnesses as their individual patients. Evidently, psychiatric invocations of the 'national soul' were driven by political motives. By projecting their medical categories from the individual patient to the collective, psychiatrists could discuss the social and political order in their own professional terms and thus extend their diagnostic and therapeutic authority onto society and the nation, claiming a formative role in the protection of the nation's collective health and the prevention of future 'hysterical' epidemics. Ultimately, the rhetoric of the 'national soul' legitimised an reinforced psychiatry's broader shift from the individual to the health of the collective, adding momentum to the bio-political project of eugenics, but also to the establishment and institutionalisation of new fields of research and practice, such as applied psychiatry and mental hygiene.

Collective mental states were an important part of the debate about revolutionary psychopaths. Beyond issuing individual diagnoses, psychiatric observers of the revolution also elaborated on the relationship between the leaders and the crowds they led, devaluing the political claims of the revolution, while at the same time expounding their visions of a future political and social order. By contrasting the psychopathic leaders of the revolution to the ideal of a 'true leader', they propagated an hierarchical state, a model that suited not only some conservatives' wish for a restoration of the monarchy or right-wing radicals' hopes for a dictatorial corporative state, but also reflected a general preoccupation of Weimar political culture with the figure of the 'leader'.[64] In other words, the debate about the alleged psychopathologies of revolutionary leaders was also a topical debate about political leadership that used the figure of the revolutionary psychopath as an antithesis of the 'true leader'. As mental illness became associated with political upheaval, the mental stability of a leader was equated with political stability.

Eugen Kahn developed the psycho-political implications of his findings in some detail. To answer the question how psychopaths came to play such important roles in recent politics, Kahn argued, one had to take into account 'the psychology of the two components which, in quiet and in tumultuous times alike, incarnate the lives of the peoples: the psychologies of the leaders and those that are led, that is, the crowd'.[65] Kahn's concept of collective psychology was directly based on Gustave Le Bon's influential theory of crowd psychology. A distinctive example of the antisocialist and elitist political ideas of late nineteenth-century French conservatives who saw their political and social order challenged by the emergence of an age of mass politics and the growing influence of the workers' movement, Le Bon's concept could easily be transferred and adapted from the French Third Republic to Germany after the First World War.

Following Le Bon, Kahn understood the crowd as an agglomerate of people where individual minds merged into a kind of primitive collective soul (*l'âme de foule*, or *Massenseele*).[66] Both saw the psychology of the crowd as a state of atavistic regression, where the intelligence of its members was greatly reduced, but violent urges and emotions were amplified. Characterised by its 'primitive affectivity', Kahn echoed Le Bon, 'the crowd has no conscious will; dark, unconscious instincts pull its strings'. Prone to all kinds of suggestive influence, the crowd was particularly susceptible to the leading figures that it recruited from its own ranks.[67] Apart from introducing the notion of the psychopath, Kahn added little to Le Bon, who in 1895 had already claimed that the leaders of the crowd usually are 'morbidly nervous, excitable, half-deranged persons who are bordering on madness'.[68] As 'true sons of the crowd', Kahn argued, the psychopaths knew and understood the coarse emotions of the crowd, which they could thus expertly manipulate and lead.[69]

Kahn found the exact opposite of the psychopathic leaders of the revolutionary crowd in the 'true leader', a larger-than-life figure with a mind characterised by 'outstanding creative and critical intelligence, by his unbending, unflinching and pure will and by the total control of all emotions, by the balance of his mind'.[70] If the recent chaos had been caused by mental disorder, mental stability was the key to political order. Unlike the psychopath, whose relation with the crowd was symbiotic, the 'true leader' would stand apart from and above the masses and only because of this opposition would they follow him, 'in awe and love, or in hate and fear'.[71] The difference between Le Bon and Kahn, however, was that for Kahn (as well as for his colleagues Brennecke and Kraepelin), the relation between leader and collective was no longer limited to crowds that were physically assembled in one place, but extended to the entire nation. The volatile, irritable, and suggestible 'crowd soul' and the metahistorical 'national soul' merged, and the search for an ideal leader became a nation endeavour. Kraepelin wrote: 'Why should [the German people] not again be able to bring forth a man who can satisfy our longings?'[72]

In the political imaginary of many conservative Germans in 1918/1919, including Kraepelin, this precedent of a 'true leader' was not the former German Emperor Wilhelm II, but the late chancellor Otto von Bismarck. Wilhelm II had lost much of his credibility and legitimacy when the German army was defeated and he unheroically absconded to the Netherlands in November 1918.[73] In a debate with striking parallels to that about the revolutionary psychopaths, the mind of Wilhelm II became the object of psychiatric diagnosis. Even before the war, Wilhelm's notorious impulsivity, his swaggering and passion for grandeur, and his diplomatic blunders had led to veiled speculations about his mental state. After August 1914, authors in enemy nations picked up on these earlier debates to paint the head of the German state as a dangerous madman. The topic returned to Germany as the war came to an end and the last Hohenzollern emperor left. In numerous newspaper articles, brochures, books, and articles in professional journals, psychiatrists and laymen alike discussed the mental state of the former emperor. Among others, renowned psychiatrists and neurologists like Auguste Forel and Adolf Friedländer diagnosed Wilhelm II as 'an unbalanced, impulsive, mentally abnormal person'.[74] Similar views were voiced by authors from all political camps, from Social Democrat pacifists to *völkisch* nationalists. Regardless of their political differences, all of them used the mind of the *Kaiser* as a foil to discuss the same topic: the question of German war guilt. The *Kriegsschuldfrage* was one of the key topics of Weimar Germany's political debates from 1918 onwards, and the diagnosis of Wilhelm II allowed to reframe this contested issue in the language of forensic psychiatry.[75] Declaring the former head of state mentally ill offered a way to exculpate Wilhelm and the Germans, but also to blame his entourage and the elites for manipulating him and the nation instead. As an ideal of political leadership, the former emperor became unsuited. The reputation of Otto von Bismarck, by contrast, had survived his forced resignation in 1890 intact and subsequently grew into a political myth that outlived him. Conservatives remembered the former chancellor as an ideal of tough-minded political leadership and strategic clear-sightedness. When the memory of Bismarck became a central element of antidemocratic ideology in the early Weimar Republic, Kraepelin and other conservative psychiatrists used their psycho-political diagnoses to support it.[76]

Even among psychiatrists who agreed that psychopaths had played an important role in the revolution, there was some pushback to the idea that this was a sufficient explanation for the recent events. Robert Gaupp, professor of psychiatry at the University of Tübingen, argued that from a medical perspective, it would be unjust to claim that 'the instigation of the masses by radical demagogues was the *only* source of the nameless distress which threatens to swallow Germany'. Instead, he pointed out, the truly important question was why the 'greatest part of our otherwise so thoughtful and thoroughgoing people has gotten into a state of mind in which it could fall prey to the influence of Russian agents and unscrupulous coffee house writers'.[77] To Gaupp, the answer to this question lays in the collective mental state of both the German army and the people at the home front in late 1918. As a military physician, he had observed the gradual decline of the morale of the troops due to the physical and mental strains of trench warfare, inequity, conflicts between officers and other ranks and, notably, due to 'the obvious injustices against Jewish volunteers'. Unlike other conservatives, Gaupp had no illusions about the military situation in 1918 and did not believe that the Central Powers had remained militarily undefeated, but argued that the declining morale of the troops had provided a fertile ground for the 'incendiary influences that, from 1917 onwards, increasingly came from home'.[78] As early as July and August 1918, he later claimed, he had seen the signs of the looming revolution. The hunger crisis at the home front, the deprivations, and the suffering of more than four years of war had brought about a mental state well known in clinical psychiatry: a 'neurasthenic' condition caused by fatigue and exhaustion, accompanied by 'nervous weakness, emotional instability and rootless surrender to the excitement of the moment'. Eventually 'the suffering of the last years, the despair of the lost and costly war, the anger about the years of deception have robbed the quivering nervous psyche of a half-starved people all interior restraints against the red flood sweeping over it'.[79] As a conservative nationalist, Gaupp refused to believe that the collapse of the Wilhelmine order had been brought about by the same idealised *Volk* that was at the centre of his political thought. He projected the diagnostic categories of clinical psychiatry from individual patients to the collective to exculpate the nation and blame both interior and exterior enemies instead.

After issuing a diagnosis, Gaupp recommended a treatment. Like Robert Sommer, who had argued that it was first and foremost the hunger that had driven the German people into 'nervous depression' and 'anarchistic political madness', Gaupp believed that without bread and economic and political security, recovery was impossible. It was the responsibility of the elites to sacrifice their money and their strength for the benefit of the whole nation in order to restore the nation's faith 'in its spiritual leaders, [...] the German men and women who by their formation and their education are entitled to win absolute authority and to impart the German culture to the whole of the people'. Without these sacrifices to restore the political legitimacy of the former and future elites, 'Germany's culture will perish, and all will sink into chaos'.[80]

Gaupp's visions of the future went beyond the restoration of the pre-war order. Addressing the medical students of the University of Tübingen on 23 October 1919, he took the medicalisation of politics one step further. When political and social problems were caused by individual and collective somatic and psychic illness, only the physicians would be able to save the nation. Driven by a profound sense of mission, he exclaimed: 'All call for the doctor, the strong-nerved leader and the saviour of a desperate people'.[81] Merging the vision of a strong-minded 'true leader', the professional ethos of medicine, and conservative hopes for forceful, charismatic political leadership, he conjured the almost messianic figure of a political physician who would heal the nation.

At the core of Gaupp's vision was the idea of an epistemologically privileged kind of psycho-political expertise. With the nation in a medical and psychological crisis threatening its very existence, physicians had a responsibility to come to rescue because they were the ones who really knew the people's soul. Propagating a far-reaching expert status for his profession, Gaupp called for the physician's 'right to be heard in all public questions'.[82] To save Germany, physicians had to become 'educators of the people' leading the nation on its way to regeneration in many ways, by combatting infant mortality, by propagating marriage and temperance with alcohol and tobacco, by opposing abortion, by educating the people in terms of hygiene, cleanliness, and the prevention of venereal disease, and by calling for land reforms. To realise all this, physicians—and psychiatrists in particular—would need to acquire charismatic leadership, providing new beliefs for a population that had had lost its religious orientation, thus becoming spiritual leaders and advisors of the nation.[83]

Thomas Mergel has accurately characterised the Weimar Republic's 'structures of political expectation' (*politische Erwartungsstrukturen*) as a 'constant, sometimes obsessive search for leaders', to the point of 'a messianic search for "Germany's saviour", who would lead the nation out of degradation and up to new glory'. This desire took was particularly pronounced on the far-right of the political spectrum, but it was anything but limited to the right.[84] But even against this backdrop, it is striking to see how Gaupp constructed the physician-leader as an authoritative public expert and as a real alternative to an unfit political leadership. Rejecting the wartime government and the new democracy, both of which he saw as a bureaucracy ignorant of the people's psychological needs, Gaupp was convinced that the 'destiny of our people' belonged in the hands of those who really understood the people. Against the fragmentation of the nation in competing interests and parties, he postulated an anti-political vision of a unified government of medical experts, legitimated by scientific knowledge as well as a deeper understanding of the human condition and a specific ethos of the profession:

> Above all the narrow and antiquated party systems, above all pathetic politics of interest, above all parliamentarian shallowness and vanity, based on a rich knowledge of human nature and a deep love of mankind stands the doctor's way of thinking, which in a daily struggle against poverty and distress and in

daily sight of the driving forces of human action learns how to rightly judge human concerns.[85]

To Gaupp's teacher Emil Kraepelin, the military defeat and the collapse of the monarchy had been a political catastrophe. 'The enormous events that have befallen the German people have deeply shocked its inner life', Kraepelin wrote shortly after the violent crackdown on the Munich Soviet in the right-wing monthly *Süddeutsche Monatshefte*.[86] Trying to make sense of recent events, he turned to the diagnostic categories of his discipline and authored the most exhaustive psycho-political analysis of post-war Germany.[87] Kraepelin shared much of Robert Gaupp's analysis of the situation, believing that the military and political collapse of November 1918 and the ensuing upheaval had been the result of a 'gradual attrition of the national soul (*Volksseele*)' in the course of the war.[88]

Referring to the Paris Commune of 1871 and the Russian Revolution of 1905, Kraepelin recognised a historical pattern behind the current events and applied the categories of clinical psychiatry to the collective: 'Every persistent and intense pressure on the collective psyche produces stresses which ultimately explode with enormous power and which in their blind rage can no longer be controlled by the forces of reason. In day-to-day psychiatric practice *hysterical disorders* are the counterpart to this behaviour'.[89] To Kraepelin, this was more than a metaphor. In every mass movement, he claimed, one could easily find traits which were closely related to hysterical symptoms.[90] Linking politics and individual mental disorder played a double role in Kraepelin's argument. By drawing the revolution into the clinic, he could not only subject it to a scientific analysis but bolster his 'psychiatric observations of contemporary events' with his scientific authority as Germany's most renowned psychiatrist.[91]

Apart from the effects of crowd psychology and the participation of psychopaths, Kraepelin found the reason for the collective hysteria in the demographics of the uprising. The revolution had mainly been supported by workers and other members of the lower classes, and in Kraepelin's biologistic world view, class was not a matter of political or economic relations but rooted in biological facts.[92] Consequently, he was convinced that the revolutionary masses had largely consisted of 'mentally underdeveloped compatriots'. Unfit of being rational political subjects, they lacked the 'ability for cool calculating consideration, self-control, foreseeing of future events, and the guidance of the will by rational insight'.[93]

Just like individual hysteria, collective hysteria would not only cause loss of control and rationality, it could also affect, alter, and suppress memories. This was Kraepelin's explanation for why the enthusiasm and the national unity of August 1914 had vanished from public memory and had been gradually supplanted by the opinion that 'the German people had unwillingly been driven into the war by a guilt-burdened government, bellicose military brass and greedy capitalists'.[94] Likewise, for Robert Gaupp the upheaval of 1918/1919 brought up feelings of 'nostalgic pain' when he remembered the national enthusiasm of 1914.[95] Imagined as an ideal moment of positive collective emotions, the mass mobilisation of August 1914 became the symbolic counterpoint to the hysterical revolutionary crowds of November 1918—like the 'true leader' was to the revolutionary psychopath.[96] For Hans Brennecke, the parallels between August 1914 and November 1918 were so obvious that they provided an argument *against* the psychiatric interpretation of the revolution:

> Otherwise one could, with the same right, also misinterpret the enormous, great, natural and true enthusiasm of the whole German people in these days of August 1914 as pathological, and thus do the whole of the people no greater injustice than by judging and dismissing its revolutionary movement as merely pathological.[97]

Kraepelin's polemics had political implications that went beyond the rejection of the revolution and the new political order. In the rule of the revolutionaries, he saw only the last consequence of the belief that all men were equal in their abilities and that only external factors such as oppression and exploitation prevented them from developing their potential.[98] Kraepelin believed in the exact opposite: the stratification of society reflected the hereditary biological characteristics of its members. On the one hand, he argued, nobility would not have become the ruling class if their ancestors had not possessed outstanding traits which they could pass on to their descendants. On the other hand, 'it is obvious that the ancestors of those who today belong to the lower social classes by and large did not have any traits that allowed them extraordinary achievements and thus they could not pass down such characteristics'. His social-Darwinist interpretation of social hierarchies based on a biologic meritocracy was not static but allowed for a certain degree of social mobility. 'We see old and glorious dynasties degenerate and [...] descend into the proletariat',

Kraepelin wrote, 'and at the same time new and vital families emerge without pedigree'.[99] As Eric Engstrom has observed, Kraepelin's social theory was 'conveniently double-edged' and 'reflected the conflicting interests of Kraepelin's own class, the *Bildungsbürgertum*. Confronted with a mass society which ultimately threatened to undermine its own social position, the *Bildungsbürgertum* erected barricades against the supposedly irrational threat from below, while simultaneously ensuring its own asset and hence the selective permeability of the social hierarchy'.[100]

'The rule of the people has to become the rule of the best' was the core of Kraepelin's political theory. Yet like many adherents of eugenics, Kraepelin had come to believe that the war had led to the opposite of eugenic selection, robbing the German nation of 'the men most gifted and most willing to sacrifice themselves (*opferbereit*)' while sparing 'the unable and the self-serving'.[101] Unwilling to content himself with 'the best' to emerge by chance or slow natural selection, he advocated active interventions and a far-reaching programme for the recovery of the nation. To avert degeneration, Kraepelin proposed a range of different measures, most of which had already been part of agenda of social hygienists before the war: early marriage, the promotion of fertility, the fight against alcoholism, syphilis, and the pathogenic influences of urban life. What was necessary now, he wrote, was 'by all means, to breed outstanding personalities who in the arduous days to come, may guide our fortunes'.[102] Kraepelin also stressed that the 'good parts of our people should not be ruined by the inferior ones' and that the 'inferiors' should not become a burden to the nation. Here, Kraepelin's socio-political ideas foreshadowed a 'negative' approach to eugenics which, following another wave of radicalisation after the world economy crisis, would ultimately lead to the coercive racial hygiene policies of the Nazi state.[103]

The situation after the war and the revolution, some psychiatrists came to believe, required an entirely new role of psychiatric and psychological knowledge in society. Asserting that 'the war [...] has been won by the Anglo-American psychologist', one doctor Hugo Marx from Berlin, who published his 'medical thoughts on the revolution' in early 1919, called for a turn away from the laboratory and towards 'applied psychology', 'cultural psychology and psycho-technology (*Psychotechnik*)'.[104] As the following chapters show in more detail, one of the most long-lasting and influential developments to directly come out of the wartime radicalisation of psychiatrists' psycho-political ambitions was 'applied psychiatry'. In the last months of the war, the Viennese psychiatrist Erwin Stransky emerged as the most vociferous propagandist of a new kind of socially and politically involved psychiatry. Going beyond the visions of Gaupp or Kraepelin, Stransky believed that psychiatrists were destined to become the ultimate psycho-political experts: 'There is no other human being, no other doctor, no one, whose work would allow him such deep insights into the deepest psychic matters of life, of individual men, of groups of men and even of the peoples [...] than the psychiatrist!' Yet, few psychiatrists were aware of their responsibility, while most remained stuck in the unworldly isolation of the asylum and the laboratory.[105] Stransky, a right-wing German nationalist,[106] merged the language and the concepts of national power politics with the professional policies of his discipline, calling for a 'healthy imperialism of the doctors' in the service of the protection of the nation and of racial hygiene, professional 'power politics', and transformed the political notion of a 'greater Germany' into a call for 'greater medical propaganda'.[107]

After the defeat and the collapse of the Central Powers, Stransky's radical rhetoric gained additional urgency. As he came to believe the experiences of the immediate post-war period had revealed how important the understanding of 'practical psychology' would have been to avoid this 'gruesome catastrophe'. Reconceived as an expansive programme for the bio-political and psycho-political re-education of common people and elites alike, Stransky began to advertise 'applied psychiatry' as psychiatrists' contribution to the 'mental reconstruction of the German people'.[108] On a practical level, Stransky's ideas were almost identical to the socio-medical interventions propagated by Gaupp, Kraepelin, and others, including the education of the people in *völkisch* virtues, positive eugenics, temperance, and the fight against syphilis. But more radically than his colleagues, Stransky not only advocated the expansion of the range of psychiatrists' expertise, but also claimed that psychiatry itself had to change to be able to seize this new kind of psycho-political authority.

Stransky's verbal radicalism provoked one of the few direct rebukes of post-war psycho-politics. In a 1921 article, the psychotherapist Arthur Kronfeld (1886–1941) positioned himself against contemporary attempts to extend the reach of psychiatric diagnosis and therapy into society and politics. 'Applied psychiatry', Kronfeld wrote, was one of the greatest threats to 'the factual and logical integrity of our discipline'.[109] His concerns were professional as much as political: Although Kronfeld went to great lengths to present himself as a scientist driven only by a concern for the objectivity of his discipline, his rejection of 'applied psychiatry' also had to do with his political views, which differed from the prevalent right-wing nationalism of German psychiatry. Kronfeld was a member of the Social Democratic Party and, in late 1918, had been a delegate in the Freiburg Soviet.[110]

Against the rampant politicisation of psychiatric expertise, Kronfeld propagated a disinterested scientific practice which had to remain 'above and apart of current opinions and political parties'. Psychiatric knowledge could not be entirely objective; Kronfeld was aware that every description of a mental process as 'abnormal, deformed or sick' relied on some kind of assumption about what was to be considered normal. The inherent normativity of its diagnostic tools was already challenging enough for the scientificity of psychiatry when applied to the mental processes of individuals. Kronfeld however attacked the key assumption of the diagnoses of the revolution by asserting that the specific norms of psychiatry were not the same as the norms of the socio-political realm. Psychiatry, including 'applied psychiatry', was bound by epistemological limits inherent to the discipline and its methods. To extend the diagnostic categories and norms of psychiatry into society and politics would not only mean to be unscientific and to repeat the mistake of Carl Theodor Groddeck, who in 1849 had announced the discovery of *morbus democraticus* as a new disease. As Kronfeld argued, Stransky's claim to psycho-political expertise was at risk of accomplishing the exact opposite of its goals and to confirm public preconceptions against psychiatry. Psycho-political claims for medical leadership were self-defeating and illegitimate: 'The national collective, whose fosterage we vindicate in this "applied" psychiatry, has not agreed'.[111]

Redrawing the Boundaries of Psychiatry

The persuasiveness of psychiatrists' warnings about a national nervous breakdown and rampaging psychopaths was linked to the specifics of the post-war situation. The defeat of the Central Powers after more than four years of brutal war, starvation and the Spanish influenza, the sudden collapse of the Hohenzollern and Habsburg monarchies, a series of revolutions, political violence, and fighting on the streets of major German cities felt to some like a 'disturbance of the psychic structure of the world' itself.[112] When the economy slowly recovered and the Weimar Republic and the Austrian First Republic consolidated themselves during the 1920s, clamouring psycho-political diagnoses fell out of fashion. Conservative psychiatrists reluctantly made their peace with the new order and the genre by and large disappeared from the pages of psychiatric and neurological journals. Nevertheless, the idea that concepts of psychopathology could be transformed into tools for the analysis of society remained very much alive. Erwin Stransky and the Association for Applied Psychopathology and Psychology in Vienna continued to extend the boundaries of the psy-ences. Other examples include Karl Birnbaum's sketch for a 'psychopathology of culture' (*Kulturpsychopathologie*) published in 1924 or the works of Arthur Kronfeld, who—his severe criticism of Stranksy's expansionist programme notwithstanding—ventured into the field of 'sociological psychopathology' and 'psychopathological sociology' in 1923.[113] Fischl Schneersohn, a Russian-born physician, psychologist, and Yiddish novelist in inter-war Berlin, laid out the outline of a new science of 'national and mass psychopathology' in 1925, based in part on a criticism of some of the psycho-political pamphlets of the immediate post-war period.[114] Psychoanalysis, too, began to explore the mental dynamics of groups, communities, and nations. Sigmund Freud's re-reading of Le Bon's theory of crowd psychology in *Group Psychology and the Analysis of the Ego*, published in 1921, should also be seen in the context of the psy-ences' increasing interest in socio-political matters in the early inter-war years.[115]

Equating communities, institutions, and states to the human body and its parts was a long-standing tradition in political thought, even before the rise of modern nationalism. And where there was a body, there was also illness. The idea of a malady of the collective body became one of the essential motives of the right-wing conservative discourse in the inter-war period. Conservatives and nationalists of every shade routinely evoked the image of national illness and national regeneration to bolster their political agendas.[116] After the First World War, psychiatric concepts played an increasingly prominent role in this discourse as psychiatric knowledge was adopted by a wider public. Although the use of elusive concepts such as the 'national soul' (*Volksseele*) can be traced back at least to the first third of the nineteenth century, the cataclysm of the First World War and its aftermath gave the psychiatrisation of society additional urgency and plausibility.[117] Psychiatrists actively promoted this popularisation of specialist knowledge: Hermann Oppenheim and Emil Kraepelin published their diagnoses of the revolution in high-circulation media like the *Berliner Tageblatt* and the *Süddeutsche Monatshefte*, respectively, disseminating their diagnoses to a broader educated public.[118] What direct impact their ideas had and if their authors could capitalise on them in terms of social and scientific prestige is, however, difficult to assess.

As a discipline, psychiatry successfully consolidated both its standing as a medical speciality and its interpretative authority for social and political affairs during the inter-war period. Apart from the creation of new university departments and the expansion of existing ones, the incorporation of the German Research Institute for Psychiatric Research (*Deutsche Forschungsanstalt für Psychiatrie*, DFA) in Munich, into the Kaiser Wilhelm Society in 1924 underlined the increasing scientific and socio-political relevance of psychiatry.[119] Founded in 1917, the DFA quickly became the most important institution in German psychiatry even before it was integrated into the major umbrella organisation for basic research in Germany. Its creation was, more than anything else, the result of the organisational efforts of Emil Kraepelin, who had already begun to campaign for a psychiatric research institute as early as 1912. Kraepelin's lobbying for a psychiatric research institute went hand in hand with his social and political views. When presenting plans for the future institute in November 1915, he stressed the necessity of basic research in psychiatry for the fight against the 'devastations that mental illness causes to our national body'.[120] Even more than about the mentally ill, he was concerned about the many 'slightly abnormal people, as the "nervous", eccentrics, psychopaths, or as the feeble-minded, inferiors, degenerates, and enemies of society'.[121] The 'weapons' against this threat to the very existence of the nation would not be forged in the messy everyday practice of insufficiently equipped psychiatric clinics and asylums, but required the resources of a specialised research institution. While the German army fought external enemies on the frontlines in the East and West, Kraepelin militarised the language of science and mobilised psychiatry for the fight against internal enemies.

Kraepelin's plan for a research institute came considerably closer to being realised in 1916, when a substantial donation by the Jewish-American philanthropist James Loeb provided a financial basis. In April 1918, research activities at the DFA commenced, only a few months prior to the end of the war and the revolution in Munich. As shown earlier in this chapter, two staff members of the institute, Kraepelin and his assistant Eugen Kahn, were among the most outspoken psychiatric diagnosticians of the immediate post-war period. In the following years the institute became a national and international centre of psychiatric and neurological research. Kraepelin's emphasis on the role of psychiatry for national regeneration was reflected in the DFA's organisational structure. From the beginning, the institute included a department for genealogy and demography led by Ernst Rüdin, one of the main representatives of psychiatric genetics and eugenics in Germany.[122] Under the direction of Rüdin, who himself became head of the DFA in 1931, research in heredity, eugenics, and genetics as well as in criminal biology and psychopathy became increasingly important for the profile of the whole institute.[123] After 1933, Rüdin was one of the most renowned psychiatric experts in the 'Third Reich', playing a pivotal role in the scientific legitimisation of Nazi' medical policies both domestically and abroad.

The inter-war period created new possibilities for expert activity, and psychiatrists were eager to seize these positions. The expansion and bureaucratisation of social welfare created a new market for scientific expertise from different disciplines both in Weimar Germany and in the Austrian Republic.[124] The question to which pensions mentally injured veterans should be entitled had already been one of the most contested topics in the debates about the epidemic of 'war neuroses' before 1918. In Germany, the passing of a pension law (*Reichsversorgungsgesetz*) in 1920 finally promised pensions for mental disorders caused by traumatic war experiences and work accidents. But as crucial passages of the law were open to interpretation, its implementation required the participation of psychiatric experts on every level, from testimonies in individual cases to high-level policy advice. With health officials in need of expertise and psychiatrists eager to extend their influence, the welfare system of the early Weimar Republic was a situation in which science and politics functioned as 'resources for each other'.[125] As Stephanie Neuner has shown, the pension question mobilised an active and stable network of health officials and psychiatric experts, in which a small and exclusive circle of conservative psychiatrists was able to exert considerable influence on national health and welfare policies in Germany.[126]

Another area in which psychiatrists were able to defend and extend their expert status was the judicial system. Beyond the continuing importance of forensic expert testimonies in the courtroom, the period after the First World War saw an increasing institutionalisation of psychiatric expert knowledge in the penal system. Psychiatric debates during and after the war strongly influenced the theory and practice of criminology in the inter-war period. The rising importance of criminal biology in Weimar Germany was closely connected to psychiatry's expansion beyond the clinic, as well as to psychiatrists' concern 'with the welfare and protection of society as a whole rather than the individual patient'.[127] The introduction of criminal-biological examinations in the Bavarian prisons from the early 1920s onwards was certainly one of the most striking examples of the entrenchment of psychiatric expertise in the penal system.[128]

Concepts like 'mental inferiority' and psychopathy were instrumental in the gradual 'medicalisation of penal law'. By situating 'mental inferiority' in the grey area between sanity and outright mental illness, psychiatrists could claim responsibility for all sorts of abnormalities beyond the confined medical space of the clinic and asylum. Even before the turn of the century, the idea that 'mentally inferior' individuals were to blame for a significant amount of crimes committed and represented a large part of prison inmates had been a rarely challenged consensus in psychiatric and criminological circles.[129] The introduction of the figure of the psychopath was the next step in the construction of a criminal, moral, and political menace to bourgeois society that only trained specialists could safely identify and assess. Notably, the narrative of psychopaths as protagonists of the revolution was readily adopted by political decision-makers in the post-war period. In September 1920, the Prussian minister of welfare, Adam Stegerwald, prompted the establishment of specialised counselling offices for psychopaths. Although these offices were not the same institutions for the custodial care for psychopaths that Eugen Kahn, Hans Brennecke, and others had proposed, Stegerwald used the same arguments to back his initiative: The recent upheaval, he wrote, was proof that 'juvenile psychopaths are to be found in the frontline of politically extreme movements'. Although these psychopaths were considered as a threat to the whole nation, Stegerwald believed that coercive medical treatment was not the right way. Counselling offices offering voluntary examination and guidance, which had to be strictly separated from asylums, would more effectively reach psychopathic individuals with their own consent.[130]

Counselling offices for psychopaths were but one facet of a more general trend towards the psychiatric prophylaxis. Notoriously unable of really healing their patients, psychiatrists discussed a wide range of different approaches for the prevention of mental illness and the preservation of both individual and collective mental health. As has been shown in the previous sections, different forms of socio-medical interventions had already been an integral part of psychiatrists' psycho-political diagnoses of the immediate post-war period when the threat of epidemic hysteria and the need for national regeneration became a legitimisation for the expansion of psychiatry's field of activity. Although the debate lost some of its alarmist edge and momentum, it continued during the inter-war years and contributed to the emergence of a movement for mental hygiene in the German-speaking countries. Parallel to related trends in many other countries, *psychische*

Hygiene became part of a highly diverse international movement for 'mental hygiene' in the second half of the 1920s.[131] An important step in the institutionalisation of this loosely defined concept was the creation of a German Society for Mental Hygiene (*Verband für psychische Hygiene*) in 1925 following the initiative of Robert Sommer, who also became its first president. The society's first conference in Hamburg in 1928 attracted many prominent psychiatrists but also state officials and representatives of the welfare authorities and the police.[132]

The development of mental hygiene in the German-speaking countries was closely related to the professionalisation of psychotherapy as well as to ideas of social reform. The General Medical Society for Psychotherapy (*Allgemeine Ärztliche Gesellschaft für Psychotherapie*) was founded in late 1927 in Hamburg with the participation of psychiatrists interested in psychotherapeutic approaches like Robert Sommer, Arthur Kronfeld, Karl Birnbaum, and Ernst Kretschmer.[133] The society's journal, the *Allgemeine ärztliche Zeitschrift für Psychotherapie und psychische Hygiene*, was first published in 1928 and explicitly connected psychotherapy to mental hygiene in its title. In the preamble to the first issue, the editors defined psychotherapy and mental hygiene as an interdisciplinary project and highlighted the social importance of their enterprise: the implementation of psychotherapy, they argued, was necessitated by the discontents of modern life and the epidemic (*Volksseuche*) of neuroses. Thus, psychotherapy and mental hygiene were not only meant to serve the suffering individual but were also presented as complementary parts of social-medical reforms for the benefit of the nation, the state, and the economy.[134]

However, mental hygienists' initial interest in psychotherapy was soon pushed aside by calls for more aggressive socio-medical interventions. As the history of the German Association for Mental Hygiene shows, the concept of mental hygiene itself was increasingly narrowed down to eugenics. This was not a change of direction: in the early days of the society, its inclusive concept of mental hygiene and the prophylaxis of mental illness had already explicitly contained eugenic ideas, which had already been prevalent among German psychiatrists before and during the war and had gained additional momentum against the backdrop of the post-war crisis. As Paul Weindling writes: 'Virtually any aspect of eugenic thought and practice – from "euthanasia" of the unfit and compulsory sterilization to positive welfare – was developed during the turmoil of the crucial years between 1918 and 1924'.[135] When mental hygiene emerged, it was not a synonym for eugenics, but an umbrella term covering a broader array of prophylactic approaches. Eugenics only came to dominate the psychiatric discourse both inside and outside of the Society for Mental Hygiene in the late 1920s, when the impact of the world economic crisis increased the pressure on the welfare system and brought an end to many reform projects in psychiatry.[136] In the early 1930s, the eugenic paradigm had entirely displaced alternative approaches in the Society for Mental Hygiene. At the First International Congress on Mental Hygiene, held in Washington, DC in May 1930, it was the delegation of the German society which most emphatically advocated eugenics as the royal road to mental hygiene with methods including the sterilisation of the mentally ill.[137] Two years later, the second national conference of the Society for Mental Hygiene in Bonn focused entirely on the 'eugenic duties of mental hygiene'. After the Nazis' rise to power, society's understanding of mental hygiene became indistinguishable from racial hygiene. The following chapters will follow more closely the actors who tried to reframe the boundaries of psychiatry in the years after the First World War and examine how their psycho-political projects engendered utopian visions of mental health as well as the worst abuses in the history of psychiatry.

Notes

1. Sándor Ferenczi, 'Die Psychoanalyse der Kriegsneurosen', in *Zur Psychoanalyse der Kriegsneurosen: Diskussion gehalten auf dem V. Internationalen Psychoanalytischen Kongress in Budapest, 28. und 29. September 1918* (Leipzig and Vienna: Internationaler psychoanalytischer Verlag, 1919), 9–30.
2. Ibid., 10.
3. Volker Roelcke, *Krankheit und Kulturkritik: Psychiatrische Gesellschaftsdeutungen im bürgerlichen Zeitalter (1790–1914)* (Frankfurt am Main: Campus, 1999), 204–5.
4. Carl Gustav Carus, *Ueber Geistes-Epidemien der Menschheit* (Leipzig and Meissen: F. W. Goedsche'sche Buchhandlung, 1852), 55–56.
5. Carl Theodor Groddeck, *Die demokratische Krankheit, eine neue Wahnsinnsform* (Naumburg: H. Sieling, 1850).
6. Karl Bonhoeffer, 'Inwieweit sind politische, soziale und kulturelle Zustände einer psychopathologischen Betrachtung zugänglich?', *Klinische Wochenschrift* 2 (1923): 598; Erwin Stransky, 'Keine Bedenklichkeit der angewandten Psychiatrie', *Zeitschrift für die gesamte Neurologie und Psychiatrie* 69 (1921): 330.

7. Jürgen Habermas, 'Die Scheinrevolution und ihre Kinder', in *Die Linke antwortet Jürgen Habermas*, ed. Oskar Negt (Frankfurt am Main: Europäische Verlagsanstalt, 1968), 5–15.
8. Ibid., 13.
9. Klaus Dörner, 'Über den Gebrauch klinischer Begriffe in der politischen Diskussion', in *Die Linke antwortet Jürgen Habermas*, ed. Oskar Negt (Frankfurt am Main: Europäische Verlagsanstalt, 1968), 60.
10. Moritz Föllmer, 'Der "kranke Volkskörper": Industrielle, hohe Beamte und der Diskurs der nationalen Regeneration in der Weimarer Republik', *Geschichte und Gesellschaft* 27 (2001): 41–67.
11. Rüdiger Graf, 'Optimismus und Pessimismus in der Krise: Der politisch-kulturelle Diskurs in der Weimarer Republik', in *Ordnungen in der Krise: Zur politischen Kulturgeschichte Deutschlands 1900–1933*, ed. Wolfgang Hardtwig (München: Oldenbourg, 2007), 115–40.
12. Hans-Walter Schmuhl and Volker Roelcke, '*Heroische Therapien*': *Die deutsche Psychiatrie im internationalen Vergleich 1918–1945* (Göttingen: Wallstein, 2013).
13. Volker Roelcke, 'Die Entwicklung der Psychiatrie zwischen 1880 und 1932: Theoriebildung, Institutionen, Interaktionen mit zeitgenössischer Wissenschafts- und Sozialpolitik', in *Wissenschaften und Wissenschaftspolitik: Bestandsaufnahmen zu Formationen, Brüchen und Kontinuitäten im Deutschland des 20. Jahrhunderts*, ed. Rüdiger vom Bruch and Brigitte Kaderas (Stuttgart: Franz Steiner, 2002), 119.
14. Alexander Watson, *Enduring the Great War: Combat, Morale and Collapse in the German and British Armies, 1914–1918* (Cambridge: Cambridge University Press, 2009), 1.
15. Paul Lerner, *Hysterical Men: War, Psychiatry, and the Politics of Trauma in Germany, 1890–1930* (Ithaca: Cornell University Press, 2003), 209–14.
16. Anonymous, 'Psychiatrisches Ausbreitungsbedürfnis', *Die Irrenrechts-Reform* 11 (1919): 197–99.
17. Moritz Föllmer, Rüdiger Graf, and Per Leo, 'Die Kultur der Krise in der Weimarer Republik', in *Die 'Krise' der Weimarer Republik: Zur Kritik eines Deutungsmusters*, ed. Moritz Föllmer and Rüdiger Graf (Frankfurt am Main and New York: Campus, 2005), 8.
18. Thomas Etzemüller, 'Social engineering als Verhaltenslehre des kühlen Kopfes: Eine einleitende Skizze', in *Die Ordnung der Moderne: Social Engineering im 20. Jahrhundert*, ed. Thomas Etzemüller (Bielefeld: transcript, 2009), 11–40.
19. Lutz Raphael, 'Die Verwissenschaftlichung des Sozialen als methodische und konzeptionelle Herausforderung für eine Sozialgeschichte des 20. Jahrhunderts', *Geschichte und Gesellschaft* 22, no. 2 (1996): 165–93.

20. Heinz Hartmann, Martin Pappenheim, and Erwin Stransky, *I. Internationale Tagung für angewandte Psychopathologie und Psychologie, Wien, 5.–7. Juni 1930: Referate und Vorträge* (Berlin: S. Karger, 1931).
21. Eugen Kahn, 'Psychopathie und Revolution', *Münchener medizinische Wochenschrift* 66, no. 34 (1919): 968.
22. Hanns Hippius et al., *Die Psychiatrische Klinik der Universität München 1904–2004* (Heidelberg: Springer, 2005), 90.
23. Eugen Kahn, 'Psychopathen als revolutionäre Führer', *Zeitschrift für die gesamte Neurologie und Psychiatrie* 52, no. 1 (1919): 90.
24. Peter Riedesser and Axel Verderber, *Maschinengewehre hinter der Front: Zur Geschichte der deutschen Militärpsychiatrie* (Frankfurt am Main: Fischer, 1996), 82–85.
25. Ernst Toller, *Eine Jugend in Deutschland* (Reinbek: Rowohlt, 1963), 78.
26. Kahn, 'Psychopathen als revolutionäre Führer', 91.
27. Kahn, 'Psychopathie und Revolution', 968.
28. Richard F. Wetzell, *Inventing the Criminal: A History of German Criminology, 1880–1945* (Chapel Hill and London: University of North Carolina Press, 2000), 145.
29. Ibid., 149.
30. Emil Kraepelin, *Psychiatrie: Ein Lehrbuch für Studierende und Ärzte*, 7th ed., vol. 2 (Leipzig: J. A. Barth, 1904), 815–41.
31. Wetzell, *Inventing the Criminal*, 146–53.
32. James Horley, 'The Emergence and Development of Psychopathy', *History of the Human Sciences* 27, no. 5 (2014): 91–110; Greg Eghigian, 'A Drifting Concept for an Unruly Menace: A History of Psychopathy in Germany', *Isis* 106, no. 2 (2015): 283–309.
33. Kahn, 'Psychopathen als revolutionäre Führer', 92.
34. Kahn, 'Psychopathie und Revolution', 968.
35. Volker Roelcke, 'Psychiatry in Munich and Yale, ca. 1920–1935: Mutual Perceptions and Relations, and the Case of Eugen Kahn (1887–1973)', in *International Relations in Psychiatry: Britain, Germany, and the United States to World War II*, ed. Volker Roelcke, Paul Weindling, and Louise Westwood (Rochester: University of Rochester Press, 2010), 166.
36. Emil Kraepelin, 'Psychiatrische Randbemerkungen zur Zeitgeschichte', *Süddeutsche Monatshefte* 16 (1919): 179; A. Sack, *Die geistigen Typen der Juden und die Revolutionsbewegung* (Heidelberg: Wolff, 1920).
37. Kurt Hildebrandt, 'Forensische Begutachtung eines Spartakisten', *Allgemeine Zeitschrift für die Psychiatrie und psychisch-gerichtliche Medizin* 76 (1919): 487.
38. Ibid., 507.
39. Hans Brennecke, 'Debilität, Kriminalität und Revolution', *Archiv für Psychiatrie und Nervenkrankheiten* 63, no. 1 (1921): 247–60; Hans Brennecke, 'Zur Frage der Psychopathologie der Revolution und der Revolutionäre', *Zeitschrift für Kinderforschung* 26, no. 5 (1921): 225–31; Hans

Brennecke, *Zur Frage der Psychologie und Psychopathologie der Revolution und der Revolutionäre* (Langensalza: Beyer, 1922).

40. Helenefriderike Stelzner, 'Psychopathologisches in der Revolution', *Zeitschrift für die gesamte Neurologie und Psychiatrie* 49 (1919): 393–94.
41. Hermann Schelenz, 'Jean Paul Marat', *Münchener medizinische Wochenschrift* 66, no. 27 (1919): 752–53.
42. Kraepelin, 'Randbemerkungen', 179.
43. Hans Freimark, *Die Revolution als psychische Massenerscheinung: Historisch-psychologische Studie* (Munich and Wiesbaden: J. F. Bergmann, 1920), 64–97.
44. Andy Hahnemann, '"Der Tod jagt durch die Straßen…": Zur Psychopathologisierung der Revolution in Max Glass' Die entfesselte Menschheit (1919)', in *Friede, Freiheit, Brot! Romane zur deutschen Novemberrevolution*, ed. Ullrich Kittstein and Regine Zeller (Amsterdam: Rodopi, 2009), 41–58.
45. Hildebrandt, 'Begutachtung', 507.
46. Wetzell, *Inventing the Criminal*, 145; Urs Germann, *Psychiatrie und Strafjustiz: Entstehung, Praxis und Ausdifferenzierung der forensischen Psychiatrie in der deutschsprachigen Schweiz 1850–1950* (Zurich: Chronos, 2004), 470.
47. Lerner, *Hysterical Men*, 210.
48. Ibid., 214.
49. Ibid.
50. Doris Kaufmann, 'Science as Cultural Practice: Psychiatry in the First World War and Weimar Germany', *Journal of Contemporary History* 34, no. 1 (1999): 142.
51. Ian Hacking, 'Making Up People', in *Forms of Desire: Sexual Orientation and the Social Constructionist Controversy*, ed. Edward Stein (New York: Routledge, 1992), 69–88.
52. Brennecke, 'Zur Frage der Psychopathologie der Revolution und der Revolutionäre', 228.
53. Ibid., 229–30; Silviana Galassi, *Kriminologie im Deutschen Kaiserreich: Geschichte einer gebrochenen Verwissenschaftlichung* (Stuttgart: Franz Steiner, 2004), 397–400; Christian Müller, *Verbrechensbekämpfung im Anstaltsstaat: Psychiatrie, Kriminologie und Strafrechtsreform in Deutschland 1871–1933* (Göttingen: Vandenhoeck & Ruprecht, 2004), 126–49.
54. Kahn, 'Psychopathie und Revolution', 969.
55. Kahn, 'Psychopathen als revolutionäre Führer', 105.
56. Kahn, 'Psychopathie und Revolution', 969; Dirk Blasius, *Einfache Seelenstörung: Geschichte der deutschen Psychiatrie 1800–1945* (Frankfurt am Main: Fischer, 1994), 117; Kahn, 'Psychopathie und Revolution,' 969.
57. Robert Sommer, *Aerztlicher Notruf zum Ende des Jahres 1918* (n.p.: self-published, 1918).

58. Richard Bessel, *Germany After the First World War* (Oxford: Clarendon Press, 1993).
59. Bonhoeffer, 'Politische, soziale und kulturelle Zustände'.
60. Sigmund Freud, 'Zeitgemäßes über Krieg und Tod', in *Das Unbehagen in der Kultur und andere kulturtheoretische Schriften*, 10th ed. (Frankfurt am Main: Fischer, 2007), 135.
61. Anonymous, 'Massenwahnsinn?', *Die Irrenrechts-Reform* 63 (1919): 181–84.
62. Egbert Klautke, *The Mind of the Nation: Völkerpsychologie in Germany, 1851–1955* (New York and Oxford: Berghahn, 2013); David Freis, 'Psyche, Trauma und Kollektiv: Der psychiatrische Diskurs über die erschütterten Nerven der Nation', in *Nerven und Krieg: Psychische Mobilisierungs- und Leidenserfahrungen in Deutschland 1900–1933*, ed. Gundula Gahlen and Oliver Janz (Frankfurt am Main and New York: Campus, n.d.) forthcoming.
63. Jenő Kollarits, 'Kann die Volksseele aus der Geschichte lernen?', *Deutsche Psychologie* 3 (1920): 177–83; Jenő Kollarits, 'Normalzustand und Ausnahmezustand in der Völkerpsyche', *Zeitschrift für die gesamte Neurologie und Psychiatrie* 66 (1921): 337–42; Jenő Kollarits, 'Die Störung im psychischen Weltgefüge', *Zeitschrift für die gesamte Neurologie und Psychiatrie* 65 (1921): 331–50.
64. Thomas Mergel, 'Führer, Volksgemeinschaft und Maschine: Politische Erwartungsstrukturen in der Weimarer Republik und dem Nationalsozialismus 1918–1936', in *Politische Kulturgeschichte der Zwischenkriegszeit 1918–1939*, ed. Wolfgang Hardtwig (Göttingen: Vandenhoeck & Ruprecht, 2005), 91–128.
65. Kahn, 'Psychopathen als revolutionäre Führer', 101.
66. Jaap van Ginneken, *Crowds, Psychology and Politics, 1871–1899* (Cambridge: Cambridge University Press, 1992), 130–87.
67. Kahn, 'Psychopathen als revolutionäre Führer', 103.
68. van Ginneken, *Crowds*, 177.
69. Kahn, 'Psychopathen als revolutionäre Führer', 104–5.
70. Ibid., 101–2.
71. Ibid., 103.
72. Eric J. Engstrom, 'Emil Kraepelin: Psychiatry and Public Affairs in Wilhelmine Germany', *History of Psychiatry* 2, no. 6 (1991): 131–32.
73. Martin Kohlrausch, *Der Monarch im Skandal: Die Logik der Massenmedien und die Transformation der Wilhelminischen Monarchie* (Berlin: Akademie, 2005), 414–43.
74. David Freis, 'Diagnosing the Kaiser: Psychiatry, Wilhelm II and the Question of German War Guilt', *Medical History* 62, no. 3 (2018): 273–94.
75. Ulrich Heinemann, *Die verdrängte Niederlage: Politische Öffentlichkeit und Kriegsschuldfrage in der Weimarer Republik* (Göttingen: Vandenhoeck & Ruprecht, 1983).

76. Robert Gerwarth, *The Bismarck Myth: Weimar Germany and the Legacy of the Iron Chancellor* (Oxford: Clarendon Press, 2005); Wolfgang Hardtwig, 'Der Bismarck-Mythos: Gestalt und Funktionen zwischen politischer Öffentlichkeit und Wissenschaft', in *Politische Kulturgeschichte der Zwischenkriegszeit 1918–1939*, ed. Wolfgang Hardtwig (Göttingen: Vandenhoeck & Ruprecht, 2005), 61–90.
77. Robert Gaupp, 'Der nervöse Zusammenbruch und die Revolution', *Blätter für Volksgesundheitspflege* 19, nos. 5/6 (1919): 43.
78. Ibid.
79. Ibid., 45.
80. Ibid., 46.
81. Robert Gaupp, *Die zukünftige Stellung des Arztes im Volke: Ansprache an die Studierenden der Medizin der Universität Tübingen (23. X. 1919)* (Tübingen: H. Laupp, 1919), 4; Robert Gaupp, 'Der Arzt als Erzieher seines Volkes', *Blätter für Volksgesundheitspflege* 19, nos. 9/10 (1919): 77–80.
82. Gaupp, *Stellung*, 20.
83. Ibid., 14–18.
84. Mergel, 'Führer, Volksgemeinschaft und Maschine', 105.
85. Gaupp, *Stellung*, 20.
86. Jens Flemming, 'Gegen die intellektualistische Zersetzung der alten moralischen Werte. Die Süddeutschen Monatshefte zwischen Krieg und Nationalsozialismus', in *Le milieu intellectuel conservateur en Allemagne, sa presse et ses réseaux*, ed. Michel Grunewald (Berne: Peter Lang, 2003), 165–201.
87. Engstrom, 'Psychiatry and Public Affairs', 128–32; Matthias M. Weber, Wolfgang Burgmair, and Eric J. Engstrom, 'Emil Kraepelin: Zwischen klinischen Krankheitsbildern und "psychischer Volkshygiene"', *Deutsches Ärzteblatt* 103, no. 41 (2006): 2685–90; Eric J. Engstrom, Wolfgang Burgmair, and Matthias M. Weber, 'Psychiatric Governance, Völkisch Corporatism, and the German Research Institute of Psychiatry in Munich (1912–26): Part 1', *History of Psychiatry* 27 (2016): 38–50.
88. Kraepelin, 'Randbemerkungen', 175.
89. Ibid.; translation by Engstrom, 'Psychiatry and Public Affairs', 129.
90. Kraepelin, 'Randbemerkungen', 176.
91. Engstrom, 'Psychiatry and Public Affairs', 129–30.
92. Ibid., 130.
93. Kraepelin, 'Randbemerkungen', 176.
94. Ibid., 177.
95. Gaupp, 'Der nervöse Zusammenbruch und die Revolution', 43.
96. Jeffrey Verhey, *The Spirit of 1914: Militarism, Myth and Mobilization in Germany* (New York: Cambridge University Press, 2000); Steffen Bruendel, *Volksgemeinschaft oder Volksstaat: Die Ideen von 1914 und die Neuordnung Deutschlands im Ersten Weltkrieg* (Berlin: Akademie, 2003).

97. Brennecke, 'Zur Frage der Psychopathologie der Revolution und der Revolutionäre', 227.
98. Kraepelin, 'Randbemerkungen', 180.
99. Ibid., 181.
100. Engstrom, 'Psychiatry and Public Affairs', 131.
101. Kraepelin, 'Randbemerkungen', 182; Stefan Kühl, *Die Internationale der Rassisten: Aufstieg und Niedergang der internationalen Bewegung für Eugenik und Rassenhygiene im 20. Jahrhundert* (Frankfurt am Main and New York: Campus, 1997), 41–58.
102. Kraepelin, 'Randbemerkungen', 182–83.
103. Ibid.
104. Hugo Marx, 'Aerztliche Gedanken Zur Revolution', *Berliner Klinische Wochenschrift* 12 (1919): 279.
105. Erwin Stransky, 'Angewandte Psychiatrie: Motive und Elemente zu einem Programmentwurf', *Allgemeine Zeitschrift für Psychiatrie und psychisch-gerichtliche Medizin* 74, nos. 1–3 (1918): 22–23.
106. Erwin Stransky, 'Großdeutschland und die Ärzteschaft', *Wiener Medizinische Wochenschrift* 69, no. 2 (1919): 117–25.
107. Stransky, 'Angewandte Psychiatrie', 35.
108. Erwin Stransky, 'Der seelische Wiederaufbau des deutschen Volkes und die Aufgaben der Psychiatrie: Erweiterter Vortrag, gehalten auf der Deutschen Psychiaterversammlung in Hamburg, am 27./28. Mai 1920', *Zeitschrift für die gesamte Neurologie und Psychiatrie* 60, no. 1 (1920): 277.
109. Arthur Kronfeld, 'Eine Bedenklichkeit der "angewandten" Psychiatrie', *Zeitschrift für die gesamte Neurologie und Psychiatrie* 65 (1921): 366.
110. Ingo-Wolf Kittel, 'Arthur Kronfeld zur Erinnerung - Schicksal und Werk eines jüdischen Psychiaters in drei deutschen Reichen', in *Arthur Kronfeld (1886–1941): Ein Pionier der Psychologie, Sexualwissenschaft und Psychotherapie*, ed. Ingo-Wolf Kittel (Konstanz: Bibliothek der Universität Konstanz, 1988), 8.
111. Kronfeld, 'Eine Bedenklichkeit der "angewandten" Psychiatrie', 367.
112. Kollarits, 'Störung'.
113. Karl Birnbaum, *Grundzüge der Kulturpsychopathologie* (Munich: J. Bergmann, 1924); Arthur Kronfeld, *Das seelisch Abnorme und die Gemeinschaft* (Stuttgart: Julius Püttmann, 1923).
114. Fischl Schneersohn, 'Zur Grundlegung einer Völker- und Massenpsychopathologie', *Ethos* 1 (1925): 81–120
115. Sigmund Freud, *Massenpsychologie und Ich-Analyse* (Leipzig, Vienna, and Zurich: Internationaler Psychoanalytischer Verlag, 1921).
116. Föllmer, 'Der kranke Volkskörper'.
117. Roelcke, *Krankheit*; Joachim Radkau, *Das Zeitalter der Nervosität: Deutschland zwischen Bismarck und Hitler* (Munich: Hanser, 1998).

118. Hermann Oppenheim, 'Seelenstörung und Volksbewegung', *Berliner Tageblatt*, 16 April 1919.
119. Roelcke, 'Entwicklung', 119.
120. Emil Kraepelin, 'Ein Forschungsinstitut für Psychiatrie', *Zeitschrift für die gesamte Neurologie und Psychiatrie* 32 (1916): 2.
121. Ibid.
122. Matthias M. Weber, 'Psychiatric Research and Science Policy in Germany: The History of the Deutsche Forschungsanstalt Für Psychiatrie (German Institute for Psychiatric Research) in Munich from 1917 to 1945', *History of Psychiatry* 11, no. 43 (2000): 235–58; Volker Roelcke, 'Psychiatrische Wissenschaft im Kontext nationalsozialistischer Politik und Euthanasie: Zur Rolle Ernst Rüdins und der Deutschen Forschungsanstalt für Psychiatrie/Kaiser-Wilhelm-Institut', in *Geschichte der Kaiser- Wilhelm-Gesellschaft im Nationalsozialismus: Bestandsaufnahme und Perspektiven der Forschung*, ed. Doris Kaufmann, vol. 1 (Göttingen: Wallstein, 2000), 112–50.
123. Weber, 'Psychiatric Research', 247.
124. Detlev J. K. Peukert, *Die Weimarer Republik: Krisenjahre der Klassischen Moderne* (Frankfurt am Main: Suhrkamp, 1987), 132–40.
125. Mitchell G. Ash, 'Wissenschaft und Politik als Ressourcen für einander', in *Wissenschaften und Wissenschaftspolitik: Bestandsaufnahmen zu Formationen, Brüchen und Kontinuitäten im Deutschland des 20. Jahrhunderts*, ed. Rüdiger vom Bruch and Brigitte Kaderas (Stuttgart: Franz Steiner, 2002), 32–51.
126. Stephanie Neuner, *Politik und Psychiatrie: Die staatliche Versorgung psychisch Kriegsbeschädigter in Deutschland 1920–1939* (Göttingen: Vandenhoeck & Ruprecht, 2011), 91–110; Lerner, *Hysterical Men*, 223–48.
127. Wetzell, *Inventing the Criminal*, 125.
128. Ibid., 128–37.
129. Richard F. Wetzell, 'Die Rolle medizinischer Experten in Strafjustiz und Strafrechtsreformbewegung: Eine Medikalisierung des Strafrechts?', in *Experten und Expertenwissen in der Strafjustiz von der Frühen Neuzeit bis zur Moderne*, ed. Alexander Kästner and Sylvia Kesper-Biermann (Leipzig: Meine, 2008), 66–67.
130. Franz-Werner Kersting and Hans-Walter Schmuhl, eds., 'Minister für Volkswohlfahrt an sämtliche Ober- und Regierungspräsidenten, 2. September 1920, Berlin', in *Quellen zur Geschichte der Anstaltspsychiatrie in Westfalen*, vol. 2 (Paderborn: Schöningh, 2004), 145–46; Paul Weindling, *Health, Race and German Politics Between National Unification and Nazism, 1870–1945* (Cambridge: Cambridge University Press, 1989), 381.

131. Mathew Thomson, 'Mental Hygiene as an International Movement', in *International Health Organisations and Movements, 1918–1939*, ed. Paul Weindling (Cambridge: Cambridge University Press, 1995), 283–304.
132. Volker Roelcke, 'Prävention in Hygiene und Psychiatrie zu Beginn des 20. Jahrhunderts: Krankheit, Gesellschaft, Vererbung und Eugenik bei Robert Sommer und Emil Gotschlich', in *Die Medizinische Fakultät der Universität Gießen: Institutionen, Akteure und Ereignisse von der Gründung 1607 bis ins 20. Jahrhundert*, ed. Ulrike Enke (Stuttgart: Franz Steiner, 2007), 395; Hans Ludwig Siemen, 'Reform und Radikalisierung: Veränderungen der Psychiatrie in der Weltwirtschaftskrise', in *Medizin und Gesundheitspolitik in der NS-Zeit*, ed. Norbert Frei (München: Oldenbourg, 1991), 193.
133. Uwe Zeller, *Psychotherapie in der Weimarer Zeit: Die Gründung der 'Allgemeinen Ärztlichen Gesellschaft für Psychotherapie' (AÄGP)* (Tübingen: Köhler, 2001); Christina Schröder, *Der Fachstreit um das Seelenheil: Psychotherapiegeschichte zwischen 1880 und 1932* (Frankfurt am Main: Peter Lang, 1995).
134. 'Zum Geleit', *Allgemeine ärztliche Zeitschrift für Psychotherapie und psychische Hygiene* 1, no. 1 (1928): 1–6.
135. Weindling, *Health, Race and German Politics*, 307.
136. Siemen, 'Reform und Radikalisierung', 196–99.
137. Thomson, 'Mental Hygiene', 288–89.

CHAPTER 3

Applied Psychiatry in Inter-War Vienna

Among the various inter-war-period attempts to shift the focus of psychiatry's activity from the asylum into society, one stood out for its radicalism, scope, and rhetoric: 'Applied psychiatry'. Introduced by the Viennese psychiatrist Erwin Stransky (1877–1962) in a programmatic article in 1918, applied psychiatry was supposed to extend the range of the discipline's expertise into every aspect of social, political, and cultural life. Psychiatry was to become the leading human and social science, explaining individual and collective life and intervening in it, advising and educating both the masses and their leaders. With his claim that the psychiatrist should become a 'supreme expert' (*Generaloberstsachverständiger*) for all aspects of life, Stransky was the most outspoken and radical propagandist of psychiatry's claim to socio-political expertise in the years after the First World War.[1] Over the following two decades, 'applied psychopathology'—as applied psychiatry was rebranded in late 1919—lost some of its political edge. Nevertheless, it grew into an association that became a place of interdisciplinary encounter in inter-war Vienna. But even as others became involved in applied psychopathology, it remained Erwin Stransky's personal project, and it is only through his biography that it can be situated in both political and medical history.

In the historiography of medicine, Erwin Stransky is sometimes remembered for his role in the emergence of the concept of schizophrenia and,

D. Freis, *Psycho-Politics between the World Wars*,
Mental Health in Historical Perspective,
https://doi.org/10.1007/978-3-030-32702-6_3

occasionally, as a pioneer of geriatric psychiatry.[2] To other historians, Stransky has been more interesting as a pan-German nationalist and prominent propagandist of eugenics in inter-war Austria. The existing research has, however, produced only an incomplete image of Stransky's work and life. The range of his medical interests was much broader, with exactly three hundred scientific publications touching on every major topic of contemporary psychiatry and neurology, from schizophrenia to bipolar disorders, and to the treatment of multiple sclerosis. During his long scientific career, which spanned from the Habsburg monarchy well into the Second Republic, he was among Austria's most prominent and prolific psychiatrists. The most important phase in his career was a period in which public health boomed in Vienna. In order to overcome the medical and political crisis of the post-war years and to realise an ambitious and utopian vision of social engineering, Vienna's socialist city government presided over an unprecedented expansion of social, medical, and counselling services which also provided new fields of activity for psychiatric experts. Stransky's political views were diametrically opposed to the political vision of 'Red Vienna', but he flourished in the environment that it had created and contributed to its network of public health institutions. When the socialist project was crushed by two subsequent fascist regimes whose ideologies were far more similar to his own, their racial anti-Semitism restricted Stransky's professional possibilities and eventually threatened his very survival. His vision of psychiatric expansionism explored in this and in the following chapter makes Stransky a particularly stark example of a broader trend of his time, but his biography and his politics set him apart from the categories of the visionary and the perpetrator as two common genres in the historiography of twentieth-century medicine.

Another reason why Erwin Stransky has not been more present in the historiography of medicine and psychiatry may be that he was well-known for his eccentric personality. The Swiss psychiatrist Max Müller (1894–1980), who encountered Stransky in the mid-1930s, sketched a vivid portrait:

> Hypomanic, overflowing to erratic, sometimes downright disjointed, he was a brilliant Viennese conversationalist (*Causeur*), as a Jew a professed National Socialist (!), and at the same time a gentleman of the old Austrian type. [...] On this evening, two by two in his ostentatious apartment, the old man – he was over sixty – showered me with a veritable flood of Jewish jokes, anecdotes, Viennese gossip and abstruse theories of blood and soil. This

monologue was exhilarant, but tiring in the long run, so that I later tried to avoid him whenever possible; for whenever he saw an acquaintance from afar, he would attack him with a stream of words and hold him by the arm or by the lapel, so that he couldn't slip away.[3]

Stransky later denied having ever been a Nazi, and, unlike many of his colleagues, he did not have to lie—he had been a far-right pan-German nationalist instead. Apart from this crucial detail, Müller's portrayal quite accurately reflects the impression that one gets when reading Stransky's published and unpublished writings with their baroque rhetoric, pathos, and hyperbole, his single-minded advocacy of applied psychopathology, and his unswerving loyalty to far-right politics even when he himself became the target of anti-Semitic discrimination. And yet, writing off Stransky as an odd and isolated figure would be a mistake. His eccentricities notwithstanding, he was well-known, well-educated, and well-connected, a university professor and a leading and renowned scientist in his field, who participated prominently in the founding of several associations, and was an honorary member of many others. Temporarily, he was the only Austrian honorary member of the American Psychiatric Association (APA).

Applied psychopathology eventually became part of the history of mental hygiene. Erwin Stransky's expansionist interpretation of the socio-political 'application' of psychiatry led him to the nascent movement for mental hygiene in the late 1920s. He authored the first German-language manual of mental hygiene in 1931, established himself as the leading expert for this emerging field in Austria and participated in the creation of the national branch of the movement. His notion of mental hygiene was extensive, encompassing not only the care for former patients and so-called psychopaths and the introduction of psychotherapy to psychiatric practice, but also the prophylaxis of mental illness in all segments of the population, including through eugenic measures.[4]

Stransky's vision of the psychiatrist as a socio-political authority directly affected his understanding of the causes and the treatment of mental disorders. In 1928, he proposed a psychotherapeutic method that was essentially based on a single premise: the physician had to be the leader of the patient. Unlike contemporary psychoanalysts, Stransky was convinced that delving into the individual subtleties of a patient's mind psychotherapy would not lead to therapeutic success. Instead, the therapist had to directly exert his medical authority to heal the patient—a set-up that Stransky described as the 'subordination-authority-relation' (SAR).[5] Although his method received positive feedback from at least some colleagues and patients, Stransky failed in inspiring a school of his own.

'SAR' psychotherapy was only one facet of another recurring theme of Stransky's biography, his long-lasting conflict with psychoanalysis. In inter-war Vienna, the influence of Freud and his school was impossible to ignore. For various reasons, psychoanalysis was particularly attractive to a younger generation of Jewish psychiatrist and physicians, many of leaning to the left. Stransky, who was of Jewish origin but had converted to Protestantism in 1901, took a different stance[6]: throughout his life, he remained a staunch and polemical adversary of psychoanalysis. To some degree at least, his opposition to psychoanalysis was political and motivated by Stransky's right-wing German nationalism—a conviction that not even the experience of Nazi rule after the annexation of Austria in 1938 was able to rattle.

And yet, applied psychopathology and psychoanalysis became closely entangled. This was not only the case because many of his Stransky's collaborators did not join into his ardent rejection of Freudian ideas. Despite all differences, psychoanalysis and applied psychopathology posed similar questions about psychology and society and even shared some common epistemological assumptions about the use of analytic categories derived from the study of individual psychopathology as tools for an interpretation of society and culture. On second sight, Stransky polemics against psychoanalysis often concealed a position that was—to use a term coined by Eugen Bleuler in 1910—far more ambivalent.[7]

In this chapter, I use the life of Erwin Stransky and the history of applied psychopathology to tell a larger story about psychiatry, psychotherapy, mental hygiene, and politics in Austria in the two decades between the world wars. To provide a framework for what follows and to situate Stransky in history, I begin with a general overview of his biography. Among many other published and archival sources, this biographic sketch relies on Stransky's unpublished manuscript for his memoirs, consisting of about 800 typewritten and heavily annotated pages.[8] Obviously, the author was anything but an impartial observer, and much of his account should be taken with more than just a grain of salt. And although they hardly qualify as a major work of literature, the memoirs are a relevant historical source in their own accord, providing a rich account of the Viennese medical school in the first two-thirds of the twentieth century, as well as of the First World War and the Nazi period in Vienna. Written in the years between 1938 and around 1947, the writing of the manuscript was closely linked to the profound impact that the *Anschluss* of Austria and the rule of the Nazis had on Stransky's professional life and personal identity. In the introductory remarks, he wrote about the 'mental crisis' that followed the experience of March 1938 and led him to begin working on his memoirs, as an act of self-assurance in unsettled times.[9] Regardless of his conversion to Protestantism in 1901, he was considered a Jew under the Nuremberg laws and stripped of his citizens' rights as well as his *venia legendi*.[10] Unlike many other Austrians of Jewish origin, he survived the Nazi period, and did so without emigrating, precariously protected only by the marriage to his 'Aryan' wife, the opera singer Josefine Stransky, née Holas (1899–1978). For Erwin Stransky, the annexation of Austria led to political and social discrimination, it brought an existential threat to his life and caused a profound crisis in his personal and political identity. For decades, he had supported a right-wing German nationalism, considered himself primarily as a German, and had fervently hoped for the unification of Germany and Austria in a Greater Germany. Like many Austrians, he had welcomed the *Anschluss* in March 1938, but his initial enthusiasm soon turned into profound disappointment.[11] The events that followed brought Stransky's Jewish origin to the fore and challenged his German nationalist *Weltanschauung*. In the end, however, this crisis of identity and faith was not enough to shatter his world view. When one compares his writings before and after the Nazi period, most of his views remained astonishingly stable throughout his life and through the cataclysms of the twentieth century. As I show in the following sections, these views formed early in Stransky's career, and both their content and their persistence in the face of profound historical changes must be understood in the context of his biography.

A Political Psychiatrist in Twentieth-Century Vienna

Erwin Stransky's parents both were Jews from Bohemia. His father, Moritz Stransky, had studied as an engineer at the technical universities of Prague and Berlin around 1848 and earned the family's living as the founder and owner of a small chemical factory in Brünn (Brno). In 1873, the family moved to Vienna, where, four years later, Erwin Stransky was born as the youngest of seven children. This family history was somewhat typical for a larger group of educated and assimilated middle-class Jews in the late days of the Habsburg Empire. The social advancement that had begun with the father continued in the next generation; two of the four brothers attended university and were economically successful. Erwin's considerably older brothers Siegmund and Felix were particularly prosperous, as they became vice president of an oil company and bank director, respectively.[12] After graduating from a gymnasium in the Viennese district Leopoldstadt (named today after its most famous student, *Sigmund-Freud-Gymnasium*), Erwin Stransky decided to become a physician. In autumn 1894, he enrolled as a student of medicine at the University of Vienna.[13]

Like his older brothers, Stransky converted to Protestantism as a young adult. While he attributed this decision to his areligious upbringing, it was not uncommon in early twentieth-century Austro-Hungary. Being religiously unaffiliated was not an option, and for many non-religious Jews Protestantism became the 'next best thing to atheism'.[14] This was certainly true in the case of Stransky, who was less concerned with religion as a source of transcendental truth, than with religion as a force of societal order.[15] However, as anti-Jewish prejudice had become racialised in the last third of the nineteenth century, it was no longer enough for former Jews to convert to escape their religious background. Over the following decades, the question of Jewish identity continued to haunt Stransky as it became the cause of discrimination and of an enduring struggle with his identity. Trying to distance himself from the perceived stigma of Jewishness, often in distinctly anti-Semitic terms, Stransky instead embraced pan-German nationalism.

He completed his medical studies just two days before his twenty-third birthday in June 1900.[16] After spending another two years as an intern in Vienna's general hospital, he joined the I. Psychiatric University Clinic as an assistant in 1902.[17] The director of the clinic, freshly appointed as successor of the venerable Richard von Krafft-Ebing (1840–1902), was Julius Wagner-Jauregg (1857–1940), the later Nobel laureate. Wagner-Jauregg and Stransky did not conduct much research together, but their scientific relationship would be of lasting importance to the latter. Throughout his life, Stransky remained an admirer and loyal follower of Wagner-Jauregg, with whom he shared many views about politics, racial hygiene, and psychoanalysis.[18] Moreover, Wagner-Jauregg's clinic proved to be a uniquely productive environment for psychiatric research. It was here that Wagner-Jaureggs's research in the treatment of progressive paralysis through the inoculation of malaria took place—a therapeutic breakthrough for which he was awarded the Nobel Prize in Medicine in 1927. However, another reason why the clinic became a veritable hothouse for psychiatric research in Vienna was the presence of numerous psychoanalysts. Wagner-Jauregg was an avowed adversary of the new psychological approaches to mental illness, but this did not stop many followers of Sigmund Freud and Alfred Adler to begin their careers as members of his staff, while making the clinic the site of vibrant interdisciplinary encounters.[19]

After his post-doctoral dissertation about *dementia praecox* in 1908, Stransky remained at Wagner-Jauregg's clinic as a *Privatdozent*.[20] He became a lead assistant (*dienstführender Assistent*), which meant that he was now in charge of the men's ward, while his same-aged colleague Otto Pötzl (1877–1962) was in charge of the women's ward.[21] At the same time, Stransky was making his name as a psychiatric expert beyond the university clinic. From 1906 on, he served as a regular expert witness for the regional criminal court, and from 1911 on as a neurological expert for the cooperative health insurances (*Verband der Genossenschaftskrankenkassen*).[22] He would continue to serve as a forensic expert throughout his life, taking part in several spectacular and high-profile cases.[23]

When the First World War broke out, Stransky, now thirty-seven years old and a reserve officer since his time as a one-year volunteer, was immediately drafted. He bought himself a Browning pistol, left his bachelor flat to his servant and his testament to his brother, and joined the East-Galician Corps in Lemberg (Lviv) on the day of mobilisation.[24] For the following year, he served as an army physician on the Eastern front, where he eventually became chief physician of the 55th infantry regiment.[25] Few parts of his memoirs are as detailed as the extensive account of his sometimes dramatic wartime adventures, for which he was decorated with the Knight's Cross of the Order of Franz Joseph.[26] Nevertheless, his front-line service ended as early as 1915, when his appointment as an associate professor, for which Wagner-Jauregg had already proposed him before the war, was signed by the emperor.[27]

Shortly after his return to Vienna, he received a new military assignment as psychiatric expert for the military courts of the Vienna division.[28] One of his first cases was a trial for high treason against the Czech political leader Karel Kramář, who in 1919 would become the first prime minister of the newly created Czechoslovakian state.[29] Apart from the occasional high-profile trial, the largest part of the daily routine of the military court consisted in cases of simulation, insubordination, and desertion.[30] Although he had already encountered some cases of 'war neurosis'—or *Kriegsknall*, as he called it—during his frontline service, a scientific interest in the characteristic psychiatric symptoms of the First World War began only at the military court.[31] From the start, Stransky was a proponent of the psychogenic aetiology of war neuroses, contending that the often severe symptoms of affected soldiers were 'deeply grounded in human wishes and desires' and not caused by physical trauma.[32] He also took part in the debates at the momentous wartime conference of German psychiatrists in Munich in 1916, where the controversy about the aetiology of war neuroses escalated. Notably, his participation as an Austrian psychiatrist was seen by some as problematic. Stransky recounted that some German colleagues argued that psychiatry, more so than neurology, was now involved with 'official matters' and thus objected to the presence of a foreign participant, even if he came from an allied country.[33]

With the end of the war came the end of the Habsburg Empire. For Stransky, like for many other inhabitants of the double monarchy, this was more than just a political caesura. As the map of Central Europe was redrawn, the political order in which Stransky had lived for his entire life fell apart, and so did the cultural and social fabric of 'Kakania'. In the course of just a few weeks in October 1918, Hungarians, Poles, Romanians, Czechs, Slovaks, Croatians, Serbs, Bosnians, and Slovenians declared their independence from the former Empire, which was now reduced to its small German-Austrian part with Vienna as an oversized capital and proverbial hydrocephalus. On 11 November 1918, Karl I resigned from the throne. On the following day, the national assembly proclaimed the Republic of German-Austria and revoked all privileges of the former emperor and the aristocracy. After more than four hundred years, the Habsburg Empire collapsed and ceased to exist in just a few days. In Vienna and Budapest in particular, the rapid political transformation went along with a social revolution. Workers' and soldiers' councils were formed, and mass demonstrations were held, which occasionally culminated in violent clashes with government troops.[34]

Although the transition from the Austro-Hungarian Empire to the Austrian First Republic was accompanied by some turmoil, the immediate postwar period was far less violent in Austria than in Germany. Even a steadfast conservative like Stransky noted that the socialist upheaval had, by and large, happened in 'an orderly manner'.[35] As a German nationalist, he did not have many tears to shed for the Habsburg monarchy. If anything, he now had reason to hope that its dissolution and the creation of German-Austria would bring Austria closer to unification with Germany.

Amid the upheaval, Stransky had his own little role to play, as recounted in his memoirs. When a revolutionary mob gathered in front of the parliament, he had intervened and confronted the crowd, still wearing his full officer's uniform. With a 'pithily speech', he claimed, he was able to convince the crowd of how senseless and undemocratic their actions truly were and soon got the people on his side. What had enabled him to do so was that he was a 'psychological authority'.[36] This small anecdote encapsulates some of the main themes of the psychiatric discourse about the events of 1918/1919, translating psychiatric authority into political authority and thus identifying the 'hysterical' crowd with the 'hysterical' patient. Moreover, the idea of a psychiatrist's 'natural authority' played a crucial role in Stransky's future work. It became a leitmotif not only in his first writings about applied psychiatry, but also in his approach to psychotherapy and mental hygiene. Many decades later, he would still return to this moment to illustrate the type of *auctoritas* that a physician had to use in 'SAR' psychotherapy.[37]

With the democratic transformation of Austria came the politicisation of many aspects of everyday life. Stransky, who despite his pronounced political views had kept a distance from politics before, now became involved in both the politics of the medical profession and in party politics. The economic devastation of the lost war and the accelerating inflation triggered the establishment of professional associations. Stransky joined the Physicians' Economic Organization (*Wirtschaftliche Organisation der Ärzte*)—the first step to a life-long involvement that would eventually lead him to the highest positions in medical professional associations both in Vienna and nationally.[38] Around the same time, he also began to attend political events and publish political opinion pieces in professional journals.[39] In late 1918, he became a member of the newly founded National Democratic Party (*Nationaldemokratische Partei*), whose programme he considered to be 'quite likeable'. Naively, Stransky assumed that the party was not anti-Semitic and chose to believe that a passage of the programme defining Jews as a 'separate people', as opposed to Germans, referred only to Zionist 'national Jews' and not to converts like himself. For a short period, he eagerly participated and spoke at party meetings. Yet, when invited as main speaker for a local event, he notified the organisers in advance that he was 'non-Aryan' and, as a result, was disinvited. Disillusioned, he left and never joined another political party again.[40] Despite this disappointing setback, the experience did not alienate Stransky from his German-nationalist views. Quite the contrary: in early 1919, shortly after the signing of the treaties of Versailles and St. Germain, he published *Der Deutschenhaß*, a book-length study of the pathological hatred that other European nations allegedly nourished against the Germans.[41] It was his most explicitly political publication, as well as a first attempt to actually apply the programme of applied psychiatry to a political and social topic (on which later more).

While Stransky continued to be a highly productive and versatile researcher and writer throughout the 1920s, his academic career during this period was less successful than he had initially hoped. Despite repeated applications, he did not reach the uppermost step of the academic ladder—the prestigious position of a full professor and director of a university clinic. Throughout his life, the fact that he did not get a chair during the inter-war period was a source of keen disappointment and frustration.[42] A particularly painful setback happened in 1928, when Stransky was not appointed as Otto Pötzl's successor at the German University of Prague. Stransky aspired for this position and was deeply frustrated by the rejection. Pötzl in turn left Prague to accept Wagner-Jauregg's former chair in Vienna, a position that made him the director of the psychiatric university clinic and thus Stransky's direct superior. Stransky suspected that the prevalent racial anti-Semitism of the faculty of the German University of Prague had prevented him from being appointed—an entirely plausible suspicion.[43] The situation in Austria was similar: after the collapse of the multi-ethnic Habsburg Empire, racial anti-Semitism was on the rise and fell on fertile ground in the universities. Throughout the inter-war period, anti-Semitism was a major obstacle for the careers of scientists of Jewish origin, regardless of assimilation and conversion.[44]

There is, however, also a more colourful and distinctly Viennese explanation for the stagnation of Stransky's career.[45] In 1927, few events captivated the Viennese public as much as the Grosavescu trial. Nelly Grosavescu stood accused of having murdered her husband, the famous Romanian opera singer Trajan Grosavescu. For several days in June 1927, the accounts of the sensational trial filled the front pages of major Vienna newspapers and tabloids.[46] In this trial, Erwin Stransky did not participate in his usual role as a forensic expert. Instead, he was called to testify as a common witness on 23 June, as was his wife, Josefine Stransky. They had married in 1919, when Josefine, twenty-three years his junior, was his secretary. After the marriage, she had begun a relatively successful career as an opera singer.[47] In the 1920s, the couples Grosavescu and Stransky became close friends, meeting both at social events and privately. Yet, Nelly Grosavescu grew convinced that her husband had an affair with Josefine Stransky and shot the 'prince of the Vienna opera' in a fit of jealousy.[48] After several days of court hearings, she was declared not criminally responsible due to mental issues.

Erwin Stransky was deeply concerned about the scandal's impact on his academic career and his reputation as a practising physician. After all, the defending lawyer of Nelly Grosavescu, Heinrich Steger (1854–1929), personally blamed Stransky for not having recognised the pathological traits in his client's personality in time, arguing that, as a psychiatrist, he should clearly have been able to do so.[49] To Stransky, always sensitive in matters of personal honour, having his medical authority publicly questioned in this way was a serious personal insult—even more so as he himself had emphatically claimed that 'there is no other human being, no other physician, no one, whose work would allow him such deep insights into the deepest psychic matters of life [...] as the psychiatrist!'[50] Only some decades earlier, a situation like this could easily have led to a duel. Stransky found another way to restore his honour. In June 1927, he appealed to both the medical chamber and the medical faculty, calling for the initiation of disciplinary procedures against himself. After both Stransky and Steger had defended their positions in front of the rectorate of the University of Vienna, it was unanimously ruled that no breach of professional conduct had occurred, thus clearing Stransky's name.[51]

The late philosopher Norbert Leser has claimed that the Grosavescu scandal seriously damaged the reputation of Erwin and Josefine Stransky and prevented him from becoming a full professor. This is likely exaggerated, as there is no archival evidence to back this assumption and there is ample reason to assume that other factors were at least as important. Nonetheless, the episode had caused quite a stir and rumours continued to linger long after the case was closed. When the Swiss psychiatrist Max Müller met Stransky in the mid-1930s, the Grosavescu murder was still talked about, privately, and with an interesting twist: 'One still whispered about the huge scandal, when his wife had shot her lover, a tenor at the Vienna opera, on stage. It is said that Stransky had stuck by her through thick and thin, in a most gallant way'.[52] Notably, Stransky avoided mentioning the entire episode in his memoirs.

Even though he did not receive the desired position as a full professor, Stransky's career continued during the inter-war period. Immediately after the war, he had first become engaged in professional organisations, now he advanced to leading positions in the association of medical specialists in Vienna (*Wiener Fachärzteverband*).[53] As psychiatric expert for the Vienna

Workers' Health Insurance (*Arbeiter-Krankenversicherungskasse Wien*), he was in charge of an outpatient clinic that served large parts of Vienna and parts of Lower Austria and was responsible for the cases referred to the Vienna central office of the insurance. In 1930 alone, the clinic had 2.234 patients.[54]

At the same time, Stransky became respected scholar in his field and received some important academic honours. Most prestigious was the honorary membership in the APA, which Stransky received as the first Austrian in 1933.[55] Two North American psychiatrists, I. V. May (Boston) and Clarence B. Farrar (Toronto), had noticed Stransky's earlier writings on *dementia praecox* and proposed him for an honorary membership in the APA. This award introduced Stransky to some American networks, and he would enter in a lasting and friendly correspondence with both Farrar and, until his death in 1947, May.[56] Farrar was the editor of the *American Journal of Psychiatry*, where Stransky published several articles.[57] He used this possibility to advertise applied psychopathology to an American professional audience in 1936.[58]

Meanwhile, the rise of the Nazis in Germany created an increasingly difficult environment for Stransky in Europe, long before the annexation of Austria in 1938. Unlike other colleagues of Jewish origin who emigrated from Austria to Palestine, the United States and to other destinations, Stransky underestimated the dangers and continued to believe that his conversion to Protestantism and his public German nationalism would put him in an entirely different category. Even as late as 1937, he still participated in academic life in Germany. He published an article about 'race and psychotherapy' in the *Zentralblatt für Psychotherapie*, then edited by the psychotherapist Matthias Heinrich Göring, director of the German Institute for Psychological Research and Psychotherapy and cousin of Hermann Göring.[59] Like Carl G. Jung, who had expressed similar views a few years earlier, Stransky maintained that the ethno-psychological differences between racially defined Jews and Aryans directly affected the relation between psychotherapists and their patients. This was a matter of utmost personal importance, as Stransky was treating both Jewish and non-Jewish patients. The problem was exacerbated by the ideological foundation of his own brand of 'SAR' psychotherapy: How could the crucial 'subordination-authority-relation' be maintained between a Jewish therapist and a non-Jewish patient when this would lead to a reversal of the hierarchy imposed by racial politics? The personal nature of the publication in this specific context forced Stransky to awkwardly position himself. He felt that he could not conceal his origin, stressing that he had always felt German in terms of 'language, culture, sentiments, sense of community, and *Weltanschauung*', but:

> [...] that I am, not in the religious-denominational sense used in former times, but following the anthropological definition that is predominantly used today, a Jew, and in fact a full-blood Jew (*Vollblutjude*) (as far as the family is concerned, originating from the Sudetenland; by birth and home of Viennese belonging and character).[60]

In 1937, Stransky travelled to Munich as member of the Austrian delegation at the conference of German psychiatrists. As an expert on schizophrenia, he had been asked by his Austrian colleagues to participate in a discussion. In his memoirs, Stransky wrote that he had not only gone up to speaker's desk without giving the Nazi salute, but had also reminded the audience of his doubts about attending the conference under the given circumstances, a statement for which he claimed to have received 'rapturous applause'.[61] And yet, this was no heroic repudiation of the Nazi regime. He left Munich with positive feelings and, back in Vienna, defended Nazi Germany against his wife's and other's 'unjust' criticism. There are no other sources to corroborate the details of this story, but it is another telling example of Stransky's long-standing willingness to underestimate and downplay Nazi anti-Semitism.[62]

Merely half a year after the Munich conference, the annexation of Austria was a profound shock. His initial reaction to the German ultimatum and the *Anschluss* had been mixed, after the dismissal of Austrian chancellor Kurt Schuschnigg he spends the night from 11 to 12 March on the streets with jubilant crowds, torn between nationalist exultation and vague fears over his own future.[63] The first disappointment already came on the next morning when Stransky found out that, as a Jew, he would not be able to participate in the referendum that was to take place on 10 April to legitimise the annexation post hoc. Outraged that he, unlike the 'gypsies, Mongolians, and negroes', would not be allowed to cast his vote, Stransky even petitioned to the newly appointed *Reichsstatthalter* Arthur Seyß-Inquart, stressing that he had actively and publicly campaigned for pan-Germanism and even sympathised with National Socialism. Josefine Stransky added in a subsequent letter that her husband had personally aided members of the then-illegal Nazi party had been persecuted under Schuschnigg.[64] Nonetheless, his request was rejected.[65] From then on, the deprivations followed in quick succession. First, he was forced to retire from his positions as a forensic expert witness and from serving as an expert for the health insurance. Soon after, he had to give up his professorship and other academic functions.[66] Stransky shared this fate with most of his colleagues: after 1938, at least 173 professors and lecturers at the Vienna medical faculty—more than fifty per cent of the academic staff—were forcibly removed from office.[67]

A conference of the International Society for Psychotherapy in Oxford, to which Stransky was invited as an honorary guest of the organising board, promised a last chance for emigration. After some inquiries, he was notified by the Nazi authorities that he would be allowed to leave the country, but not to return. Still misjudging the situation, Stransky decided to pass on the invitation, a decision he would later regret. Shortly after, his passport was revoked by the *Gestapo*.[68] The situation aggravated again on 30 September 1938, when an administrative order (the so-called *Ärzteverordnung*) revoked Jewish physicians' right to treat non-Jewish patients, thus abolishing the foundation of Stransky's economic existence.[69] Meanwhile, Josefine Stransky lost her permission to perform on stage because she was married to a Jew.[70] Erwin Stransky still hoped that they would be able to leave Europe.[71] However, the invitation for the annual conference of the APA in late 1939, where Stransky should have led a roundtable, arrived late, probably due to disturbances in the transatlantic postal system after the beginning of the war. Around the same time, he also petitioned for the legal status of a half-Jew (*Mischling*) and volunteered for a position as an army physician in the Wehrmacht. Both attempts to improve his situation failed.[72]

The following years were characterised by omnipresent discrimination and economic hardships, by the constant fear of deportation, and later also by the fear of air raids. During this time, Stransky was only protected by his marriage to an 'Aryan', and while this offered no protection against the countless forms of social, legal, and economical discrimination, it ultimately saved him from being deported and murdered.[73] Yet, even as deportations were concerned, the marriage offered no absolute security, and Stransky had every reason to feel threatened. In 1941, he closely evaded the forcible rehousing of the remaining Jews of Vienna to the traditionally Jewish second district (Leopoldstadt) but was forced to wear the yellow star badge from then on.[74] When he was informed about an impending deportation, he attempted suicide and survived only because the barbiturate turned out to be ineffective.[75]

In Vienna, the Second World War came to an end when Soviet troops, after days of fierce house-to-house fighting, conquered the city in April 1945. Stransky's medical activities restarted immediately after the arrival of the Red Army in his Josefstadt neighbourhood. As he remembers the scene in his memoirs, he woke early in the morning as someone violently rang the doorbell. It was the concierge of the building next door, asking him to tend to a sick child in his house:

> I answered that I would like to help, even though I was not a paediatrician, but that as a 'Jew,' as he well knew, I was not allowed to practice medicine. The man said: 'That's not in force anymore, *Herr Professor*, the Russians are already here.'[76]

His academic and professional status was quickly restored. In mid-April 1945, his medical licence was formally reinstated by a newly founded, provisory medical chamber. Little later, he was reappointed at the medical faculty of the University of Vienna, now finally as a full professor, but only to become an emeritus next year. Furthermore, he also began working as an expert witness for the criminal court again. In this function, he participated in the trial against Ernst Illing (1904–1946) and other physicians who had been involved in the 'euthanasia' murders of children at Vienna's Steinhof asylum.[77]

Neither the experience of Nazi rule nor his participation in the Steinhof trials could unsettle Stransky's firm belief in the necessity of eugenics. In an English-language lecture on mental hygiene for American exchange students in Vienna in 1951, he already called for the rehabilitation of eugenics:

> Ladies and Gentlemen, I hope you aren't annoyed about the abuse of science by the Hitler regime, you mustn't forget that we couldn't help it. The science of eugenics has been badly abused, but nevertheless we must clean it from every dirt and in spite of all think the best of it. It means in first place the protection of the best and healthiest and their descendants.[78]

The next step in Stransky's resumption of his interrupted career at the age of sixty-eight was his appointment as director of the Rosenhügel sanatorium on 14 May 1945.[79] The buildings of this institution in the western outskirts of Vienna had been used as a military hospital by the Wehrmacht during the war and were heavily damaged after an air raid and ground fighting in April. Stransky's first task was to organise the physical and institutional reconstruction. In the following years, Rosenhügel became one of the centres of Viennese neurology and psychiatry.[80]

Stransky retired at the age of seventy-four in 1951 but remained active in several organisations, nationally and internationally, and continued to publish on a variety of psychiatric topics. Until his death in January 1962, mental hygiene continued to play a major role in his work. Updating his 1931 manual, he published another much-noticed book on mental hygiene in 1955.[81] Around the same time, and in keeping with the zeitgeist, he began to lobby for mental hygiene as a means for the preservation of world peace. As he had already proposed back in 1918, psychiatric expertise held the key to better politics: arguing that the catastrophe of the Second World War could only be understood as a consequence of the destructive influence of 'psychopaths', he now called for the establishment of international psychiatric committees, which would have to screen economic and political leaders for mental abnormalities to prevent future wars.[82]

Erwin Stransky died on 26 January 1962 at the age of eighty-five. He was buried in a honorary grave on the vast Central Cemetery of Vienna; letters and telegrams of condolence were sent by leading medical men and politicians, including the mayor of Vienna, Franz Jonas (1899–1974), and federal president Adolf Schärf (1890–1965).[83] Extensive obituaries appeared in local medical journals as well as in the *American Journal of Psychiatry*. His marriage to Josefine Stransky, who survived her husband by 16 years, left no children.

Applied Psychiatry

Erwin Stransky was a political psychiatrist, in the general sense of being involved in the politics of his time as well as a researcher and physician specialising in psychiatry and its related fields. He was, however, also a political psychiatrist in a stricter sense, merging political and psychiatric ideas in a way that made him one of the most outspoken and radical psycho-political thinkers of the twentieth century. The key moment in this story was the publication of a programmatic article in 1918, shortly before the end of the First World War, in which Stransky proposed a new approach to psychiatric research and practice. His project, initially labelled 'applied psychiatry', and subsequently renamed 'applied psychopathology', became the intellectual lynchpin of much of his future work. Applied psychopathology was essentially an agenda for the aggressive expansion of the range of psychiatry's expertise into virtually any area of modern life and its transformation into a leading science with the ability to remake society and politics. Even as later reformulations gave the project a more moderate tone, the idea of an extension of psychiatry's expertise and the necessity of far-reaching psycho-political measures remained its essence.

Despite persistent lobbying, applied psychopathology did not grow into a significant trend in Austrian and German psychiatry and always remained closely connected to Stransky personally. And he was eager to assert his own role in its invention. The intellectual groundwork for his later ideas about applied psychopathology and mental hygiene, he claimed, had already been laid when he was still an assistant in Julius Wagner-Jauregg's clinic back in 1902. Applied psychopathology could only have emerged in the unique environment of an urban mental ward, were no unworldly isolation and no 'catatonia' could set in. Treating diverse groups of patients in the clinic while taking part in urban life, in the coffee houses and theatres of Vienna, at the same time, had led him to the insight that psychiatry offered the key to understanding society through complementary knowledge about pathological and normal mental states.[84] Nevertheless, Stransky succeeded in inspiring a group of dedicated followers and in creating an Association for Applied Psychopathology and Psychology that would remain active from its founding in 1920 until its dissolution after the annexation of Austria in 1938.

While some aspects of applied psychopathology have already been mentioned in the previous chapter, the following sections will tell a more complete story of its invention and beginnings. Starting from Stransky's 1918 manifesto for applied psychiatry, the story moves on to the increasing politicisation of the project in the tumultuous post-war period and the ensuing conflict between Stransky and the psychotherapist Arthur Kronfeld over the epistemological legitimacy of applied psychiatry.

When Stransky decided to call his new project 'applied' psychiatry, he entered an already crowded field of applied sciences. Applied mathematics and applied chemistry were well-established subdisciplines, and in the field of medicine, Julius Tandler (1869–1936), who would soon become the central figure of 'Red Vienna's' public health and welfare programmes, had already introduced the notion of 'applied anatomy' shortly before to the First World War.[85] Stransky was probably hoping that some of the increasing prestige of the applied sciences would also rub off on his pet project, but first and foremost, the name mirrored parallel developments in the psy-ences—and it was a jibe against his fellow psychiatrists.

The notion of 'applied' psychiatry implicitly meant that hitherto, psychiatry had not been applied. On the face of it, this was a nonsensical claim. The distinction between 'pure' and 'applied' does not apply to medicine, which has always been a social practice of treating and caring for the sick as much as a field of knowledge about the human body, its frailties and diseases. Psychiatrists had 'applied' their knowledge long before psychiatry even became a speciality of academic medicine in the last third of the nineteenth century, and much of this knowledge had itself been won through medical practice.

Against what type of psychiatry was Stransky's approach directed? On the one hand, the notion of 'applied' psychiatry could be read as an academic psychiatrist's slight against the asylums and the alienists, casually questioning whether the detention of patients in mental institutions had ever been an application of scientific knowledge. On the other hand, calling for a new kind of 'applied' psychiatry could also be understood as a self-criticism of psychiatry, both academic and institutional. Despite some groundbreaking advances in the nosology of mental illness in the decades before to the First World War, psychiatrists were still notoriously unable to ameliorate the condition of most of their patients, let alone to heal anyone. And while other fields of medicine had every reason to celebrate their scientific and therapeutic accomplishments, psychiatry remained stuck in a bygone era of 'therapeutic nihilism'.[86] In this view, applied psychiatry was part of psychiatry's broader 'therapeutic departure' after the First World War, precipitated by the apparent breakthrough in the mass treatment of 'war neuroses'.[87] The difference, however, was that for Stransky, the true 'application' of psychiatry and its knowledge would not consist in the healing of individual patients, but first and foremost in diagnosing and treating society at large. Nevertheless, Stransky soon realised that the idea that a medical speciality like psychiatry could itself be applied to a new set of problems was either tautological or a mistake of category and consequently rebranded his project as 'applied psychopathology'.

The most obvious inspiration for the notion of applied psychiatry came from the related field of psychology, where an 'applied' subdiscipline had emerged shortly after the turn of the century. Unlike psychiatry, academic psychology originated not at the medical faculties, but was originally a branch of philosophy. Hence, the idea that psychology had generated abstract knowledge about the human mind that only waited to be utilised in everyday settings was a lot more plausible than in the case of psychiatry, especially so as the dominant trend among German-speaking psychologists in the late nineteenth century was Wilhelm Wundt's (1832–1920) laboratory-based 'experimental psychology'. The narrative that psychology had been a 'pure' academic science before its knowledge began to be practically applied has since been challenged by historians, but when 'applied psychology' entered the stage, it could plausibly present itself as both a novelty and a significant shift in the discipline's priorities.[88] Two German psychologists were instrumental in the establishment of the new subdiscipline. In 1903, William Stern (1871–1938) published a programmatic article; a journal and an institute were founded in the following years.[89] At the same time, his colleague Hugo Münsterberg (1863–1916) propagated the implementation of psychological expertise in other fields such as law, medicine, and philosophy.[90] Stern and Münsterberg further subdivided applied psychology by distinguishing between cultural psychology (*Kulturpsychologie*), which analysed and explained cultural and social matters, and psycho-technology (*Psychotechnik*), which consisted of the practical application of psychological knowledge in society—a distinction unknown to Stransky's applied psychopathology, where psycho-political explanation and intervention—or, in medical terms, diagnosis, and therapy—were supposed to go hand in hand with each other.[91]

In 1913, Münsterberg further developed and refined the concept of *Psychotechnik*. Broadly, the term described the application of psychological knowledge for the 'forward-looking shaping of practical life', as opposed to the retrospective explanations provided by cultural psychology.[92] *Psychotechnik* was an umbrella term for different applications of psychology in virtually every area of social life; Münsterberg's examples included the work of teachers, lawyers, preachers, physicians, businessmen, fabricants, politicians, scientists, and artists.[93] Just a year later, this kind of psychological expertise was in high demand, as the mass mobilisation for the world war produced new organisational challenges for military institutions and industrial production had to be realigned towards the requirements of wartime economy. *Psychotechnik* was widely implemented in the examination of army conscripts and for the Taylorist rationalisation of economic and industrial processes.[94] Once it had found its place in organisations, *Psychotechnik* was there to stay. After the demobilisation and throughout the inter-war period, the notion of *Psychotechnik* was predominantly used to describe the use of psychological expertise for the rationalisation and efficiency enhancement of industrial workspaces down to seconds and specific movements.[95]

Applied psychology shared some of the expansionist traits of applied psychopathology, with *Psychotechnik* offering an outstanding example for the successful implementation of the expertise of the psy-ences in various areas of social and economic life. Stransky made no direct reference to Stern or Münsterberg, but there is little doubt that applied psychology lingered in the background when he devised and named his own project. When Stransky, Bernhard Dattner, Gaston Roffenstein, and others founded the Association for Applied Psychopathology and Psychology in 1920, 'applied psychology' became part of its name and purview.

Applied psychopathology's most direct competitor, however, was psychoanalysis, and the spatial proximity in Vienna ensured that this conflict was ever-present. Situated between psychology and medical psychopathology, Sigmund Freud and his followers had envisioned psychoanalysis as a practical science from the beginning on—the psychoanalytic setting combined the treatment of individual patients and the search for universal truths about the human mind. And psychoanalysis had always had an eye on the world beyond the couch. Even before the First World War, psychoanalysts pondered on the relation between individual neuroses and society and explored possibilities of using their psychological models to understand cultural, social, and political phenomena in past and present. The notion of 'applied psychoanalysis' appeared early on, although it was mostly used to refer to the application of psychoanalytical methods of interpretation to works of literature, an approach closely related to the contemporary genre of psychiatric 'pathography'.[96] Freud believed that applied psychoanalysis might play a strategic role in the development and acceptance of psychoanalysis and encouraged its development, although he occasionally bemoaned the rampant 'dilettantism' in this field of study.[97]

From 1907, Freud edited the series *Schriften zur angewandten Seelenkunde* ('writings on applied psychology'). In 1912, Hanns Sachs (1881–1947) and Otto Rank (1884–1939) founded *Imago* as a journal for non-medical audiences, dedicated to the 'application of psychoanalysis to the humanities'.[98] In the course of the following decades, many prominent psychoanalysts—among them Karl Abraham (1877–1925), Otto Rank, Ernest Jones (1878–1958), Carl G. Jung (1875–1961), and Freud himself—contributed to these two periodicals. While psychoanalytic interpretations of literature and cultural works remained the most common theme, studies of socio-political topics and mass psychology increased in frequency during the inter-war period. In the long run, Freud's hopes in applied psychoanalysis were not disappointed, and some of the studies first published in the *Schriften zur angewandten Seelenkunde* and *Imago* became the foundation of the lasting cultural influence of psychoanalysis in the twentieth century. And yet, even at its peak, psychoanalysis came not anywhere near of what Stransky expected applied psychiatry to become.

Medical Imperialism

As influential developments in the psy-ences in the decade before the war, applied psychology and applied psychoanalysis were both inspiration and competition when Stransky published his agenda for applied psychiatry in 1918. On a very general level, what all three approaches had in common was the premise that scientific knowledge about the human mind could be used in social, cultural, and political settings beyond the laboratory, the clinic, or the consulting room. Stransky's project, however, was far more radical, more extensive, and more political than its slightly older relatives.

The First World War had already been raging for four years and was not yet over when the main journal in German-speaking psychiatry published a manifesto for a new kind of psycho-politics. In his exuberant and metaphor-heavy style, Stransky claimed that psychiatry alone had the potential to solve almost any problem of society. And his idea of psychiatry as an 'applied' science was not limited to the use of scientific knowledge in culture and society. He had in mind a new public role for the psychiatrist that transcended the traditional idea of a scientific expert limited to one specific field of knowledge. Instead, psychiatrists were destined to become universal experts for virtually any aspect of modern life, educators, and spiritual advisors of the people. Claiming that psychiatry had a privileged access to the deepest facts of human life, Stransky wrote: 'There is no other human being, no other physician, no one, whose work would allow him such deep insights into the deepest psychic matters of life, of individual men, of groups of men and even of the peoples [...] than the psychiatrist!'[99] But while his optimism about the potentials of his discipline was boundless, he lamented that most of his colleagues were neither aware of the possibilities nor willing to live up to their responsibility. They limited themselves to work in clinics, laboratories, and asylums, which, to Stransky, were merely a prerequisite for psychiatry's true tasks, which lay beyond these confined spaces.

The juridical system was the first target in applied psychiatry's expansive campaign of disciplinary 'power politics', an objective likely defined by Stransky's animus against jurists and his own experiences as a forensic expert before and during the war.[100] He saw the juridical system, where psychiatrists had already firmly established themselves as experts in the course of the nineteenth century, as a stepping stone for the gradual extension of the range of psychiatric expertise into other areas of social life.[101] Stransky proposed a strategic ruse to gain influence in the juridical system: by ostensibly making concessions to the jurists on a formal level, psychiatrists could bring them to unknowingly adopt the premises of 'our superior reasoning'.[102] The therapeutic practice of psychiatry itself would provide the tools. By using 'benevolent suggestion', the psychiatrist should 'educate judges, prosecutors, and defenders so far as that he, gradually and gingerly, becomes the leading element of the process'.[103] Eventually, psychiatrists' new role in the courtroom would allow them to become leaders of civil society and 'educators of mankind' (*Menschheitserzieher*).[104] To illustrate his vision of a transformation of scientific experts into scientocratic rulers, Stransky resorted to a rather far-fetched early-medieval metaphor, the rise of the Carolingians from their functions as majordomos of the Merovingians to an imperial dynasty in their own right: '*Historia docet*! After Pippin followed Charlemagne and the sons of today's consulting experts will be tomorrow's leaders and judges of mankind'.[105]

Stransky's plan of colonising the juridical system was only one episode in the lasting border conflict between psychiatrists and jurists. From the eighteenth century to the present, representatives of both disciplines have continuously struggled about how to define, prevent, and sanction deviant behaviour, often claiming that only their respective discipline can provide the proper tools. Stransky was in good company when he polemically asserted that psychiatry was a natural science looking for objective truths, while the jurists could offer nothing more than 'the clueless safety of typing-room dogmatism and bureaucratic pseudo-empiricism'.[106]

Stransky's belief in the superiority of psychiatry was based not only on the epistemological quality of its findings but was also on a specific view of psychiatry's socio-political role. When praising the scientific truths that the discipline had to offer, what he truly meant was the commitment to the health of the national collective.[107] Most psychiatrists, Stransky complained, were hardly aware of their social responsibility and that 'every psychiatric expertise in the courtroom is an exercise of power for the protection of society and for racial hygiene, the only rational ground of everything that one calls "law"'.[108] Without providing many details of how eugenics were supposed to work in the courtroom, he had only contempt for the 'senseless inhumane philanthropy' that tried to show compassion towards the 'inferiors'.[109]

In the large scale of applied psychiatry's plan, the conquest of the juridical system would only be one skirmish in a larger war for psycho-politics that eventually was supposed to transform society as a whole. Stransky believed that the analytic concepts of psychopathology offered a key to the understanding of every human relation.[110] While psychiatry still suffered from images of straightjackets, padded rooms, and disenfranchisement, the psychiatrist had the potential to become the 'supreme expert (*Generaloberstsachverständiger*) for all forms and ways of life of the individual and the collective'.[111]

Without limits to the range of psychiatry's influence, Stransky's psychopolitics transcended the traditional domain of politics and entered the spiritual realm. For many, and not only for the mentally ill, he argued, the psychiatrist had to become a 'secular father confessor', and from there, expand his influence on 'the family, the friends, and the acquaintances'. In their midst, the 'medical pastor' would exert his guidance 'like an apostle'.[112] As the religious language indicates, the envisioned relationship between the psychiatrist and his patients would not only be based on the application of medical knowledge; instead, the psychiatrist would also have to become an expert of human nature (*Menschenkenner*). This was also about seizing a territory that the secularisation of society had left fallow before the competition could move in. For, if the psychiatrists would not respond to this need, others were ready to fill the gap—'quacks and semi-quacks and their "directions"', as Stransky wrote with a side blow against both psychoanalysts and non-medical practitioners.[113] In the early twentieth century, academic medicine was faced with increasing pressure from a broad variety of alternative approaches to health and illness—a situation that intensified after the end of the First World War, as the medical system was in a state of transformation and physicians diagnosed a profound 'crisis of medicine'.[114]

For Viennese psychiatry, psychoanalysis presented the most imminent challenge. Stransky responded by distancing himself from psychoanalysis while simultaneously appropriating elements of its method for his own approach to psychotherapy. In repudiating psychoanalysis, Stransky rejected its professional claims as well as its political anthropology. Whereas psychoanalytic therapy has often been described as an emancipatory practice aiming at the patient's self-empowerment, Stransky's vision of psychotherapy was distinctly patronising and outright authoritarian. The psychiatrist would have to meet his patient in a strictly hierarchical setting, 'like a warden with his ward', finally enabling him to become the 'professional custodian for everyone'.[115] When Stransky published his treatise on 'subordination-authority relation' psychotherapy in 1928, he still followed these same ideas first sketched in 1918.

From these relatively tangible uses of applied psychiatry in forensic and psychotherapeutic settings, Stransky moved on to the broader sociopolitical and scientific implications of his project. The political use of psychiatry was not in conflict with the treatment of individual patients, but a direct extension of it. 'Politics is *Menschenbehandlung*', Stransky wrote using an ambiguous notion that could mean dealing with people as well as treating them, 'and thus, strictly speaking, a sibling of psychotherapy'.[116] Consequently, psychiatry was not only about the mental health of individuals:

> No, for us psychiatrists in particular, it is imperative to put all branches of our experience in the service of broad and energetic cultural work (*Kulturarbeit*), the high-breeding of men, the mental hygiene and eugenics of our people, and thus of all mankind.[117]

These political and socio-medical tasks, Stransky claimed, were more important than any other part of psychiatric practice and certainly more important than 'the clinical, anatomical, and experimental filigree work' conducted in clinics and laboratories. Their realisation was, however, based on psychiatrists acquiring practical and theoretical knowledge about social, economic, and political matters and transforming this knowledge through their 'exceptionally deep understanding of the soul', so that it would become applicable to society. Through the political power derived from this kind of knowledge, the psychiatrist would then become 'the teacher and guide of future statesmen and diplomats'.[118]

When claiming that psychiatry should appropriate, revaluate, and refine the knowledge of the social sciences, Stransky had in mind ethnology, folk psychology (*Völkerpsychologie*), racial psychology, and, most of all, to history.[119] The pivotal episodes in the history of mankind were only waiting to be brought to life through the analytic touch of psychopathology 'like a cornfield awaits the rain'.[120] By examining history through the lens of their unique knowledge psychiatrists would be able to provide answers and expertise on many of the pressing questions of contemporary life, from women's rights to racial issues.[121] Apparently Stransky was particularly interested in the psychopathological study of Roman antiquity, claiming that the ramifications of late Roman degeneration and 'mass hysteria' were still shaping the modern world.[122]

Applied psychiatry as envisioned in 1918 was supposed to reach across disciplinary boundaries, but it was not supposed to be interdisciplinary in the sense of an eye-level encounter and exchange between different perspectives. Stransky's insistence that psychiatrists could and should appropriate all kinds of knowledge was based on an assumption of psychiatry's epistemological supremacy. Psychological and psychopathological experience could not be gained as simply as 'juridical, economic, sociologist, literary, or any kind of knowledge acquired in salons, on beer-benches, and in study rooms' but remained a privilege of trained and experienced psychiatrists.[123] And yet, as the further history of applied psychopathology shows, this was not where Stransky's project was headed. Ironically, Stransky's expansive contributed to moving the boundaries of psychopathology, but it also made them more permeable.

Hatred, War, and Mental Reconstruction

The first published example of applied psychiatry was the short treatise *Krieg und Geistesstörung* ('war and mental illness') written by Erwin Stransky in the final months of the First World War.[124] At this point in time, the topic was anything but unusual, as debates about the mental effects of the war and the epidemic of 'war neuroses' had dominated psychiatric discourse since the end of 1914. Stransky, however, promised a new perspective, using applied psychiatry to diagnose the events of the last four years through the lens of psychopathology. Applied psychiatry's expansive scope led Stransky to discuss a broad range of different topics, including the 'healthier nerves' of the Central Powers and the psychological roots of anti-German hatred, crowd psychology in 1914, the individual experiences of the war for both normal and 'psychopathic' individuals, and the mental and nervous disorders caused by the war. The thematic choices were evidently driven by psychiatric questions as much as by Stransky's far-right nationalism. The idea that European politics before and during the war were shaped by other nations' irrational and pathological hatred against the Germans became somewhat of an obsession during these years. Hatred against Germans, he believed, was the largest and most momentous psychological endemic in history.[125] The book-length study *Der Deutschenhaß* appeared in the following year.

The notion that other nations hated the Germans not because of the war, but that the war had been caused by this long-standing, historical hatred was not an entirely new idea. Partly in reaction to the depiction of Germany in British and French propaganda, the idea of *Deutschenhaß* was already a common theme among intellectuals in wartime Germany,[126] the most influential contribution to the debate being philosopher Max Scheler's (1874–1928) *Die Ursachen des Deutschenhasses* ('the origins of the hatred against Germans'), published in 1917.[127] Stransky picked up a popular nationalist trope and gave it a psychiatric twist. As a collective emotion, the hatred against Germans belonged to the field of mass psychology and could thus be understood in the same terms as individual psychology and psychopathology. Stransky found the French and Walloons' collective hatred of the Germans so deep-seated and intense that it could only be explained through processes akin to hysteria. To describe the underlying pathology, he borrowed a psychoanalytic concept when he alleged that the atrocity propaganda against Germany was mainly a 'projection' of the enemy's own deeds in past and present.[128] Stransky's use of psychiatric concepts to bolster a narrative of Germany's victimisation by irrational enemies was favourably received by Austrian and German conservatives.[129] A reviewer in the Vienna medical weekly praised that the book was written from the perspective of 'unprejudiced science' and would thus have a far greater impact on the public opinion than any politician's statement.[130]

From 1918 to 1920, Stransky was in a state of frantic activity. Apart from getting married, he became politically involved, authored a total of seventeen publications with topics ranging from applied psychiatry and politics to military and civilian forensic psychiatry, hysteria, epilepsy, and the creation of counselling offices for 'nervous' patients and tirelessly lobbied for the psycho-political expansion of psychiatry's domain. Due to these efforts, applied psychiatry began to gain traction, as Stransky gathered a small group of supporters and founded the Association for Applied Psychopathology and Psychology.

In Stransky's writings during this time, politics and medicine became virtually indistinguishable. This was certainly true for explicitly psychopolitical studies as the ones mentioned earlier, although he went to great length to present at least some of these political claims as the result of objective scientific reasoning. But politics also seeped into other writings, even when the genre called for clinical objectivity. When he published the second volume of his textbook of psychiatry in 1919, references to current politics were scattered throughout the book and the epilogue culminated in yet another appeal for applied psychiatry.[131] Stransky's style and vocabulary itself became a battlefield. Asserting the necessity of a 'healthy medical imperialism', professional 'power politics' of the physicians, and a 'greater-medical (*großärztliche*) propaganda', he merged the semantics of medicine and politics.

In May 1920, Stransky made another attempt to export applied psychopathology, as he was now calling it, to Germany. The world had changed since the publication of his 1918 manifesto in the final months of the war. The Central Powers had been defeated, the Austro-Hungarian Empire had vanished from the map, dissolving into numerous autonomous states, and the Hohenzollern and the Habsburg monarchies had been swept away. Germany and the new Austrian state were now democratic republics, their political landscapes still in upheaval and the memories of the post-war commotion still fresh. Economic and social recovery was only slowly beginning, as the consequences of several years of total warfare had to be overcome. As the previous chapter had already shown, this situation, in which a sense of existential crisis to the nation met new possibilities for experts of any kind, gave rise to new visions of psycho-politics. Stransky followed these debates closely, and when he presented applied psychopathology to an assembly of German psychiatrists in Hamburg, he presented it as a crucial part of Germany's national regeneration and the 'mental reconstruction of the German people'.[132] More clearly than in 1918, he stressed the concrete socio-political uses of psychiatry, promoting education, and mental prophylaxis on a national level.[133]

Many prominent psychiatrists believed that Germany's current predicament was, in part at least, the outcome of an insufficient use of what their discipline had to offer. Unsurprisingly, Stransky was no exception. If only the Germans and their leaders would have been more proficient in 'practical psychology' (*praktische Seelenkunde*), he argued, the 'gruesome catastrophe' would have been avoided or at least mitigated. Now, the duty of psychiatrists was to correct the mistakes of the past by educating and reforming 'our people of non-psychologists into a people of practical experts of the soul', starting at the top with the intellectual elites.[134] But before this ambitious programme could even begin, more immediate public health issues had to be addressed to 'save what can still be saved'. Stransky listed hunger, alcoholism, and venereal disease, the cost of essential medicines and concerns that reparation payments would limit the resources available for the health-care system.[135] First and foremost, however, psychiatry would have to restore the trust of both the elites and the masses. Stransky felt that psychiatrists were treated unjustly. Instead of being celebrated for their contribution to the war effort, they were being vilified and wrongly accused of mistreating patients as the 'active therapy' of 'war neuroses' was propagandistically used against them.[136] Stransky now considered the public sphere as the stage on which psychiatrists had to defend their claims for psycho-political leadership in a new age of mass politics:

> We psychiatrists have an enormous prophylactic duty; we must become the apostles of a better future for our people. But to reach this position, we must leave the ivory tower, we must get rid of the old and respectable methods of propaganda that do not reach the ears and hearts of the people. We must learn how to win souls (*praktische Seelengewinnung*), like the big political parties and the contenders of the Catholic Church.[137]

Winning the souls of the people would legitimise immediate socio-medical measures, but it would also prepare the ground for an educational 'enlightenment therapy' (*Aufklärungstherapie*) that was part of psychiatry's mission of mental reconstruction.[138] The time, however, was not yet ripe for this kind of collective therapy. As German psychiatrists blamed 'revolutionary psychopaths' and a collective 'nervous breakdown' for the recent upheaval, Stransky was convinced that the events of the recent past were reverberating as nervous disequilibrium and as a 'hystericisation' of the masses that were still susceptible to the irrational suggestions of psychopathic leaders. Notably, he stressed that these 'mentally abnormal' individuals could be found on the right as well as on the left. This departure from the anti-socialist consensus among psychiatric diagnosticians of German politics had likely been caused by the Kapp Putsch, an attempted coup against the fledgling Weimar Republic by various right-wing factions that had caused chaos and violence in many German cities little more than two months before the Hamburg conference. Stransky was an outspoken right-wing nationalist, but in the conflict between far-right insurgents and the state, his sympathies were with the side that promised to maintain order.

Alarmist rhetoric aside, Stransky was cautiously optimistic about the future. The present state of collective mental disequilibrium and nervousness would not endure. Sooner or later, he predicted, 'a gradual calming, the beginning of the regeneration of the people's collective soul' would set in. And then, psychiatry would begin its 'therapy by enlightenment'. The notion *Aufklärungstherapie* was borrowed from a talk by the sociologist and early adherent of applied psychopathology Gaston Roffenstein (on whom more in the next chapter), who had used it to describe educational measures to enlighten and emancipate the population. Stransky had something different in mind. Anticipating aspects of Edward Bernays's (1891–1995) concept of propaganda and Soviet psychology's visions of 'semantic conditioning', he proposed the psycho-linguistic use of Pavlovian conditioning on a societal scale. Recent examples of political propaganda had shown that the masses could be systematically influenced in such a way that even the sound of words like 'reaction' or 'bolshevism' would evoke feelings of displeasure.[139] Through skilful and systematic educational work, it would also be possible to

> [...] train the masses in the interior and exterior resistance against everything that is visibly psychopathic, and to educate them so that in the fanatic of every description they recognise the degenerate, who will not attract but repel their so trained emotional life.[140]

At the core of this psycho-linguistic vaccination against the suggestions of political 'psychopaths' was what Stransky called a 'transvaluation of the personality ideal', which had to set in early, in the nurseries and schools. To immunise the masses against the destructive political and cultural influence of the fanatics and the bohemians, psychiatrists would have to promote a holistic ideal of physical and mental health: 'They would have to teach the people that the mental degenerate should not be their mental model, as the physically degenerated is not their physical model'. This education would not only support the gradual mental recovery of the nation, it would also serve as a prophylaxis against any future relapse.[141]

Stransky's call for the 'mental reconstruction of the German people' was embedded in an idiosyncratic vision of German psycho-history in the longue durée. Psychiatry's reconstruction would rectify the mistakes of the past and set the psychological orientation of the nation back on the right track. For the last centuries, Stransky explained, the Germans had followed an individualistic ideal, they had neglected and marginalised their social 'exopsyche' and cultivated only an individualist 'endopsyche'.[142] Stransky blamed the Prussians. Instead of challenging individualism, their education system had only tried to superficially correct it, thus creating many of the traits that eventually contributed to other peoples' hatred against the Germans. The cultivation of the 'exopsyche' was, however, the precondition of any social bond and empathy and the basis for a 'true sense of national belonging'. For the German people to prevail in the social Darwinist 'struggle for survival', psychiatrists and educators would have to fight the prevalent destructive 'endopsychic' individualism and introduce 'life-affirming mental value judgments' to the mind of the nation.[143] Less than two years after the end of the First World War, Stransky saw the adherents of applied psychopathology at the frontlines of an existential struggle for Germany's survival. They were to become guides to other physicians, historians, social scientists, and political leaders, leading the way towards national regeneration. Stransky emphatically exclaimed: 'They will, in a double sense, lead Germany, and through Germany the world, upwards, from madness to truth'.[144]

A Threat to Psychiatry's Scientific Integrity

The initial response to applied psychopathology was mixed. Some, like the Viennese sociologist Gaston Roffenstein or the Swiss psychiatrist Walter Morgenthaler, were enthused the proposal and soon published their own works under the new label and actively participated in Stransky's efforts. Others did not make applied psychopathology a project of their own but used Stransky's call for the 'mental reconstruction of the German people' to support their own visions, nevertheless.

Oddly, this mostly happened in an area for which Stransky had shown little interest and even disdain, the asylum system. At the conference of German psychiatrists in Hamburg in May 1920, Gustav Kolb (1870–1938), a pioneer of 'open care' at the asylum of Erlangen, who would later become a protagonist of the mental hygiene movement, presented an extensive programme for the improvement of institutional care. Kolb believed that psychiatry's present problems could not be solved through reforms that remained within the asylum walls, but that measures with a wider range would be necessary. His sweeping agenda was characteristic for the psycho-political programmes of the immediate post-war period. It included the expansion of existing outpatient care, special education, and care for 'psychopaths' who had participated in the recent 'coup', measures against the economic loss caused by 'war neurotics' and brain-injured veterans, the struggle against superstition, homosexuality, and drug abuse, as well as negative eugenics for 'degenerates' and the education of the 'will'. Kolb immediately recognised Stransky as a potential ally, whose project of applied psychopathology reinforced his own ideas, while showing up additional areas of psycho-political activity.[145]

However, not everyone was as easily convinced. In 1922, the psychoanalyst Eduard Hitschmann (1871–1957) used a review of a recent book by Stransky to deliver a broadside against applied psychopathology.[146] Hitschmann, a long-time follower of Freud, was a protagonist of 'applied psychoanalysis' and among the first to use the methods of psychoanalysis for an interpretation of the lives of writers, poets, and statesmen.[147] Nevertheless, he had little sympathy for Stransky's ideas, which he considered to be a 'peculiar' reaction to wartime experiences. Apart from mocking such easy targets as Stransky's flamboyant rhetoric, his inflationary use of superlatives, and his 'superlunary proposals', Hitschmann also questioned whether the concept of 'applied' psychiatry actually had any scientific legitimacy. Unlike 'applied psychology' or 'applied psychoanalysis', he pointed out, psychiatry could not simply be 'applied' to culture, society, or politics: 'To do so, the notion [of psychiatry] is too narrowly defined in a medical and clinical sense; moreover, it does not describe any specific method'.[148] This was a criticism that Stransky had already anticipated by late 1919, when he renamed applied psychiatry into applied psychopathology, a term that he found to be 'more correct in terms of philology'.[149]

Whereas Hitschmann's criticism of Stransky amounted to little more than a short polemic, the German psychiatrist and psychotherapist Arthur Kronfeld (1886–1941) had more patience and took a nuanced look at applied psychiatry. In a response to the publication of Stransky's 1920 talk about the 'mental reconstruction of the German people' in the same journal, he complained that recent attempts to diagnose and treat the 'collective soul' were 'one of the most dangerous derailments to which we can expose the factual and logical integrity of our discipline'.[150] But despite this sharp criticism, he also fell for some of Stransky's swagger. To Kronfeld, applied psychopathology had in fact become the common enterprise of a larger group of 'important researchers', something that Stransky was still hoping to achieve. Without mentioning names, he implicitly identified Robert Gaupp, Helenefriderike Stelzner, Eugen Kahn, and others, who in fact had never used the notion of applied psychopathology to describe their own work, as followers of Stransky's programme.

It was not as if Kronfeld fully rejected the idea that the revolutionary upheaval might have brought latent psychopathologies to light or that manifest mental disorders might have become politically relevant. A revolution, like any incisive event in history, 'great wars, earthquakes, famines, the epidemics of the Middle Ages, or religious mass movements', could affect mass psychology.[151] Kronfeld agreed that psychiatry and psychology offered tools to analyse these effects. In fact, he would even publish a booklet on the question of 'mental abnormality and society' himself in 1923.[152] Neither did Kronfeld, who was a supporter of social hygiene and eugenics, reject many of the socio-medical measures proposed by his colleagues.

Instead, Kronfeld made his argument against applied psychopathology about the epistemological integrity of psychiatry. The problem with the psycho-political diagnoses of the immediate post-war period was that they overstepped the inherent epistemological boundaries of psychiatry as a science, confounding scientific research into the psychological and psychopathological causes and effects of historical events with subjective moral and political judgements about social movements and the ideas that they represented. As a branch of medicine, he argued, psychiatry necessarily was a normative science, but the norms that allowed to make qualified statements about the health or sickness of individual patients could not just be translated into social or political norms. By undermining the scientific credibility of psychiatry and reinforcing public reservations against the discipline, the epistemological transgressions of applied psychopathology would achieve the opposite of what Stransky intended.[153]

There were two reasons for Kronfeld's vehement opposition against applied psychopathology. The first one was political. As many examples clearly show, the psychiatric discourse about the mental state of the nation and the necessity of psycho-political interventions was dominated by right-wing conservative psychiatrists. Kronfeld, by contrast, had been a delegate of the Freiburg soviet in 1918, which made him one of the revolutionaries that his colleagues were eager to diagnose as 'psychopaths'. Since early 1919, he was part of Magnus Hirschfeld's (1868–1935) Institute for Sexology (*Institut für Sexualwissenschaft*) in Berlin; an institution that was the first of its kind and that, due to the fact that Hirschfeld was a Jew as well as an outspoken supporter of the emancipation of homosexuals, became a target of intense hatred by the far-right.[154] With this background, Kronfeld's misgivings about the nationalist and conservative thrust of most psycho-political diagnoses of the post-war period were hardly surprising. Even if he asserted that it was no specific political opinion that drove his opposition against applied psychopathology, but a 'deep and natural sense of responsibility' for the scientific integrity of psychiatry, the conflict between him and Stransky took place along a political divide. Their diverging political ideas entailed different concepts of the role of the medical profession in different present and future societies. Whereas Stransky was convinced that psychiatrists would take a lead role in the 'mental reconstruction of the German people' and the propagation of racial hygiene, Kronfeld had previously advocated the socialisation of medicine in a socialist society, 'of the whole medical profession, and of each and every physician's head in particular'.[155] Stransky's vision of political indoctrination through psychological methods was something that he firmly rejected as a form of 'patronising psychagogy'.[156]

Second, and perhaps more importantly, there was something else at stake for Kronfeld when he attacked applied psychopathology. With a 1920 book about the 'nature of psychiatric knowledge' (*Das Wesen der psychiatrischen Erkenntnis*), he had tried to establish himself as an authority on psychiatric epistemology by providing a logical philosophical foundation for the methods of both psychiatry and psychology.[157] The roots of this enterprise lay in Kronfeld's academic and intellectual formation before the war. After completing his medical studies in Heidelberg in 1909, he had also graduated in philosophy three years later. During this time, he had been part of the circle around the neo-Kantian socialist Leonard Nelson (1882–1927) in Göttingen, where he was strongly influenced by the works of Immanuel Kant (1724–1804) and Jakob Friedrich Fries (1773–1843).[158] Their theories became the foundation of Kronfeld's own reflections about psychiatric epistemology. The military service on the Western front and the tumultuous post-war situation prevented Kronfeld from completing his work in the systematic way that he had originally intended, so that the book that he published in 1920 was only a collection of essays. This, as well as psychiatrists' preoccupation with the more practical challenges raised by the post-war turmoil, may have been the reasons why the publication went largely unnoticed.[159] When Stransky began publishing his articles on applied psychopathology, they obviously were among the most blatant infractions against Kronfeld's understanding of psychiatry as a disinterested and epistemologically sound science. Yet, they also provided him with an occasion to present himself as an important voice in the philosophy of psychiatry and as a champion of scientificity in the psy-ences.

Erwin Stransky took Kronfeld's criticism personally, and even more than a decade after, he still spoke about Kronfeld as one of the 'wicked fairies' who had 'circled around [applied psychopathology's] cradle, threatening to finish it off'.[160] Following Kronfeld's article, he published a direct reply in the same journal. His defence of applied psychopathology, which he now defined as the 'attempt to analyse cultural, social, and political occurrences, not excluding present and recent events, from the perspective of psychopathology, and to draw conclusions from it', offered little new.[161] Stransky could not understand why occurrences that 'ultimately are based on psychological processes' could not be analysed by 'scientifically trained experts of the soul'. After all, he argued, it was a well-known fact that social and historical life was not of a different nature than the psychology of the individual, and psychiatry had always dealt with topics closely related to sociology and history, such as 'suggestion, mass psychology, mental contagion, addictions, psychological endemics, racial hygiene, degeneration, delusions in the life of nations, and so on'.[162] To Stransky, Kronfeld's demand that psychiatry should refrain from analysing current politics was 'somewhat squeamish'.[163]

In the decade that followed, Stransky repeatedly came back to the conflict with Kronfeld. In his view, there was more at stake than the boundaries of psychiatry's authority to interpret and intervene in society. Instead, he saw the conflict between Arthur Kronfeld and himself as a fundamental disagreement about nature and tasks of psychiatry. Like Kronfeld had done to applied psychopathology, Stransky accused Kronfeld of an unscientific understanding of psychiatry. As he claimed, Kronfeld was a representative of a recent trend to replace clinical empiricism by philosophical speculation, who arrogantly tried to delegitimise more practical approaches and narrow psychiatry down to a merely academic exercise.

Stransky's polemics against the influence of philosophy in psychiatry reached their peak in a 1929 talk to the Association for Applied Psychopathology and Psychology, subsequently published on the front page of the Vienna medical weekly.[164] He claimed that since the end of the First World War, speculative and philosophical thinking was gradually replacing the neurological foundations of clinical psychiatry. This trend had begun with the growing importance of psychoanalysis in psychiatry; then Karl Jaspers and others had introduced a philosophical and phenomenological approach that was more interested in patients' subjective experiences than in the neurological cause of their symptoms. Now, Stransky claimed, this development was spearheaded by Kurt Hildebrandt and Arthur Kronfeld, who called for nothing less than the subordination of clinical psychiatry under the primacy of philosophy.[165] To Stransky, this was far more than a conflict between different schools in psychiatry. He went as far as to frame the controversy itself in psychiatric terms when he argued that the diverging positions represented different types of character. Only 'syntonic' individuals were capable of being proficient psychiatrists and analysing symptoms in a systematic way, the phenomenological school, by contrast, consisted of 'personalities inclined to speculation and introspection'. He diagnosed his opponents as unfit of being proper psychiatrists and even resorted to outright pathologisation when he called them 'dystonic, schizoid psychopaths' threatening psychiatry's future as a science, an extremely polemic wording, even by his own standards.[166] When Arthur Kronfeld reviewed Stransky's talk for a psychotherapeutic journal, he left no doubt that Stransky's *ad hominem* attack was unworthy of any serious discussion. The review article was a compilation of the most outrageous quotes from the talk, without any further comment.[167]

In 1931, Stransky unilaterally returned to the controversy with Kronfeld, which he now depicted as a conflict between sciences and humanities. As he saw it, physicians were practical and empirical scientists, and their views should not be influenced by 'purely humanistic rules' such as Kronfeld's epistemological reflections: 'I refuse to be swayed by any methodology based on philosophy, and any objections arising from it'.[168] Accusing Kronfeld of wanting to reduce psychiatry to fruitless '*science pour la science*', Stransky presented himself as a practical physician in the pragmatic tradition of the Vienna medical school and his teacher Julius Wagner-Jauregg. As a practitioner of medicine, Stransky had already stressed in 1921, the psychiatrists had 'not only the right, but also the obligation to take a stand on contemporary mental occurrences, as soon as he becomes convinced that pathological or pathogenic moments […] play a harmful, or potentially harmful role'.[169] This was what applied psychopathology was essentially about: psycho-political interventions were not just a possible extension and application of psychiatry's expertise, but an integral part of its medical responsibility. Without being 'applied' to society, psychiatry would remain incomplete.[170]

Nevertheless, and despite its radial scope and rhetoric, Erwin Stransky's applied psychopathology would have remained a curious anecdote from a city rich in curious anecdotes, had he not been able to draw other people into his orbit. And he was in fact quite proficient in doing so. In 1920 already, applied psychopathology had become more than Stransky's one-man campaign in the name of psycho-political imperialism. It proliferated into a short-lived, but highly influential book series published in Switzerland, and a scientific association that became a hub for interdisciplinary encounters in inter-war Vienna. While this chapter has focused on Erwin

Stransky and his ideas, the next chapter widens the scope and tells the story of applied psychopathology's surprising development in the years before the world war. Its cast is large, varied, and sometimes famous, including the philosopher Karl Jaspers, the psychiatrist Hermann Rorschach, the artist Adolf Wölfli, the founder of ego-psychology Heinz Hartmann, the left-wing psychoanalyst Paul Federn, the medical historian Henry E. Sigerist, the Nobel Prize laureates Julius Wagner-Jauregg and Konrad Lorenz, two post-war presidents of the World Federation for Mental Health, André Repond and Hans Hoff, and others more.

Notes

1. Erwin Stransky, 'Angewandte Psychiatrie: Motive und Elemente zu einem Programmentwurf', *Allgemeine Zeitschrift für Psychiatrie und psychisch-gerichtliche Medizin* 74, nos. 1–3 (1918): 37; Thomas Beddies, '"Generaloberstsachverständiger für alle Lebensformen und Lebensgestaltungen": Zu gesellschaftlichen Vorstellungen von Ordnung und Normierung "angewandter Psychiatrie" nach dem Ersten Weltkrieg', in *Norm als Zwang, Pflicht und Traum: Normierende versus individualisierende Bestrebungen in der Medizin*, ed. Eva Brinkschulte and Mariacarla Gadebusch Bondio (Frankfurt am Main: Peter Lang, 2015), 103–34.
2. Lazaros C. Triarhou, 'Erwin Stransky (1877–1962)', *Journal of Neurology* 259, no. 9 (2012): 2012–13.
3. Max Müller, *Erinnerungen: Erlebte Psychiatriegeschichte 1920–1960* (Berlin, Heidelberg, and New York: Springer, 1982), 145.
4. Erwin Stransky, ed., *Leitfaden der psychischen Hygiene* (Vienna: Urban & Schwarzenberg, 1931).
5. Erwin Stransky, *Subordination, Autorität, Psychotherapie: Eine Studie vom Standpunkt des klinischen Empirikers* (Vienna: Julius Springer, 1928); David Freis, 'Vertrauen und Subordination: Das psychotherapeutische Ambulatorium der Universität Wien, 1918–1938', *Schriftenreihe der Deutschen Gesellschaft für Geschichte der Nervenheilkunde* 21 (2015): 557–85; David Freis, '"Subordination, Authority, Psychotherapy": Psychotherapy and Politics in Inter-War Vienna', *History of the Human Sciences* 30, no. 2 (2017): 34–53.
6. Daniela Angetter, 'Erwin Stransky: Mitbegründer der modernen Schizophrenielehre', 2012, https://www.oeaw.ac.at/fileadmin/Institute/INZ/Bio_Archiv/bio_2012_01.htm; Anna L. Staudacher, "*... meldet den Austritt aus dem mosaischen Glauben": 18.000 Austritte aus dem Judentum in Wien, 1868–1914: Namen - Quellen - Daten* (Frankfurt am Main: Peter Lang, 2009), 597.

7. Eugen Bleuler, 'Vortrag über Ambivalenz', *Zentralblatt für Psychoanalyse* 1 (1910): 266–68.
8. See also Milo Tyndel, 'In Memoriam: Erwin Stransky, M.D. 1878–1962', *The American Journal of Psychiatry* 119 (1962): 287–88; Hans Hoff, 'In Memoriam: Univ.-Professor Dr. Erwin Stransky', *Wiener Medizinische Wochenschrift* 112, no. 9 (1962): 181–82.
9. Erwin Stransky, 'Aus einem Gelehrtenleben um die Zeitenwende: Rückschau, Ausblick, Gedanken', n.d., 2, Josephinum Wien, Autographensammlung, no. 2065.
10. Ibid., 224–25.
11. Ibid., 1.
12. Ibid., 38–39.
13. Ibid., 132–206; Triarhou, 'Erwin Stransky (1877–1962)', 2012.
14. See the psychoanalyst Else Pappenheim's (1911–2009) account of the conversion of her father Martin Pappenheim (1881–1943) in 1908. He was a colleague of Stransky during the 1920s and early 1930s and was head of the Association for Applied Psychopathology and Psychology, Else Pappenheim, *Hölderlin, Feuchtersleben, Freud: Beiträge zur Geschichte der Psychoanalyse, der Psychiatrie und Neurologie*, trans. Wilfried Prantner, Else Pappenheim, and Stephen Frishauf (Graz and Vienna: Nausner & Nausner, 2004), 22–23.
15. Norbert Leser, *Skurille Begegnungen: Mosaike zur österreichischen Geistesgeschichte* (Vienna: Böhlau, 2011), 112.
16. Stransky, 'Gelehrtenleben', 205.
17. Triarhou, 'Erwin Stransky (1877–1962)', 2012.
18. Julius Wagner-Jauregg, 'Über Eugenik', *Wiener Klinische Wochenschrift* 44 (1931): 1–6.
19. Magda Whitrow, *Julius Wagner-Jauregg (1857–1940)* (London: Smith-Gordon, 1993); Stransky, 'Gelehrtenleben', 502; Julius Wagner-Jauregg, *Lebenserinnerungen* (Vienna: Springer, 1950).
20. Angetter, 'Erwin Stransky'; Erwin Stransky, *Über die Dementia Praecox: Streifzüge durch Klinik und Psychopathologie* (Wiesbaden: Bergmann, 1909).
21. Stransky, 'Gelehrtenleben', 307.
22. Ibid., 265; Angetter, 'Erwin Stransky'.
23. Stransky, 'Gelehrtenleben', 265–66.
24. Ibid., 354–61.
25. Ibid., 426.
26. Ibid., 443. The memoir largely follows his war diary, ÖNB HANNA, Cod. Ser. nos. 24125–24128.
27. Ibid., 352, 437.
28. Ibid., 442.
29. Ibid., 451.

30. Erwin Stransky, 'Kriegspsychiatrie und Kriegsgerichtsbarkeit', *Wiener Medizinische Wochenschrift* 69, no. 28 (1919): 1361–68; Erwin Stransky, 'Kriegspsychiatrie und Kriegsgerichtsbarkeit', *Wiener Medizinische Wochenschrift* 69, no. 29 (1919): 1425–30.
31. Stransky, 'Gelehrtenleben', 382.
32. Ibid., 453.
33. Ibid., 473–74.
34. Wolfgang Maderthaner, 'Die eigenartige Größe der Beschränkung: Österreichs Revolution im mitteleuropäischen Spannungsfeld', in… *… der Rest ist Österreich: Das Werden der Republik*, ed. Helmut Konrad and Wolfgang Maderthaner, vol. 1 (Vienna: Carl Gerold's Sohn, 2008), 187–206.
35. Stransky, 'Gelehrtenleben', 484.
36. Ibid.
37. Erwin Stransky, 'Menschenbehandlung und Menschenführung aus ärztlicher Schau', in *Menschenführung im Blickfeld der Pädagogik und Psychohygiene*, ed. Ludwig Hänsel, Karl Dienelt, and Erwin Stransky (Vienna and Munich: Österreichischer Bundesverlag für Unterricht, Wissenschaft und Kunst, 1960), 110.
38. Stransky, 'Gelehrtenleben', 493.
39. Ibid., 494; Erwin Stransky, 'Großdeutschland und die Ärzteschaft', *Wiener Medizinische Wochenschrift* 69, no. 2 (1919): 117–25.
40. Stransky, 'Gelehrtenleben', 496–98; Kurt Bauer, '"Heil Deutschösterreich!" Das deutschnationale Lager zu Beginn der Ersten Republik', in… *… der Rest ist Österreich: Das Werden der Republik*, ed. Helmut Konrad and Wolfgang Maderthaner, vol. 1 (Vienna: Carl Gerold's Sohn, 2008), 261–80.
41. Erwin Stransky, *Der Deutschenhaß* (Vienna and Leipzig: Franz Deuticke, 1919).
42. Stransky, 'Gelehrtenleben', 543; Erwin Stransky, 'Curriculum Vitae', n.d., 3, Autographensammlung, Josephinum Wien, no. 2064.
43. Stransky, 'Gelehrtenleben', 541–42.
44. Johannes Feichtinger, 'Kulturelle Marginalität und wissenschaftliche Kreativität: Jüdische Intellektuelle im Österreich der Zwischenkriegszeit', in *Das Gewebe der Kultur: Kulturwissenschaftliche Analysen zur Geschichte und Identität Österreichs in der Moderne*, ed. Johannes Feichtinger and Peter Stachel (Innsbruck, Vienna, and Munich: Studien Verlag, 2001), 317–21.
45. Leser, *Skurille Begegnungen*, 105–14.
46. See, for example, 'Frau Nelly Grosanescu vor den Geschworenen: Heute beginnt der Sensationsprozeß', *Die Neue Zeitung*, 22 June 1927.
47. Stransky, 'Gelehrtenleben', 486–90.
48. This title is used on a memorial plaque at the Grosavescus' former house in Lerchenfelder Straße.

49. Heinrich Steger, *Verteidigungsrede im Prozesse gegen Frau Nelly Grosavescu wegen Verbrechens des Gattenmordes, gehalten am 25. Juni 1927 vor dem Wiener Schwurgerichtshofe* (Vienna and Leipzig: Moritz Perles, 1927), 38–39.
50. Stransky, 'Angewandte Psychiatrie', 23.
51. Vienna University Archive, S 185.379.
52. Müller, *Erinnerungen*, 145.
53. Stransky, 'Gelehrtenleben', 547; Erwin Stransky, 'Der Fachärzteverband und die Kliniker', *Wiener Klinische Wochenschrift* 38, no. 46 (1925): 1241–43.
54. Erwin Stransky, 'Zur nervösen und psychischen Morbität der städtischen Hausgehilfinnen', *Wiener Klinische Wochenschrift* 44, no. 47 (1931): 1460.
55. Angetter, 'Erwin Stransky'.
56. Stransky, 'Gelehrtenleben', 511–12. See also ÖNB HANNA Cod. Ser. no. 24152.
57. Aldwyn Stokes, 'In Memoriam: Clarence B. Farrar (1874–1970)', *American Journal of Psychiatry* 127 (1970): 387–88.
58. Erwin Stransky, 'Remarks Concerning the Development of Applied Psychopathology', *American Journal of Psychiatry* 92 (1936): 1043–49.
59. Erwin Stransky, 'Rasse und Psychotherapie', *Zentralblatt für Psychotherapie* 10 (1937): 9–28; Stransky, 'Gelehrtenleben', 559; Regine Lockot, *Erinnern und Durcharbeiten: Zur Geschichte der Psychoanalyse und Psychotherapie im Nationalsozialismus* (Gießen: Psychosozial-Verlag, 2002), 179–82; Geoffrey Cocks, *Psychotherapy in the Third Reich: The Göring Institute*, 2nd ed. (New Brunswick and London: Transaction, 1997).
60. Stransky, 'Rasse und Psychotherapie', 10.
61. Stransky, 'Gelehrtenleben', 559–60.
62. Ibid., 560.
63. Ibid., 617.
64. Oliver Rathkolb et al., 'Forschungsprojektendbericht: Straßennamen Wiens seit 1860 als "Politische Erinnerungsorte"' (Vienna: Kulturabteilung der Stadt Wien (MA 7), 9 July 2013), 230.
65. Stransky, 'Gelehrtenleben', 619.
66. Ibid., 621–22; Angetter, 'Erwin Stransky'.
67. Kurt Mühlberger, *Vertriebene Intelligenz 1938: Der Verlust geistiger und menschlicher Potenz an der Universität Wien von 1938 bis 1945*, 2 (Vienna: Archiv der Universität Wien, 1993), 9. Michael Hubenstorf provides even higher numbers, according to which 77.5% (153 of 197) university teachers of the Vienna medical faculty were ousted, Michael Hubenstorf, 'Kontinuität und Bruch in der Medizingeschichte', in *Kontinuität und Bruch 1938 - 1945 - 1955: Beiträge zur österreichischen Kultur- und Wissenschaftsgeschichte*, ed. Friedrich Stadler (Münster: LIT, 2004), 312–13.

68. Stransky, 'Gelehrtenleben', 622–23. See also Vienna University Archives, Med. Fak. PA 509.
69. Ibid., 625.
70. Ibid., 640.
71. Ibid., 627.
72. See a letter by Erwin Stransky to Matthias Heinrich Göring (19 June 1940), quoted in full in Lockot, *Erinnern und Durcharbeiten*, 179–82.
73. On the legal regulations and definitions, and the debate on the possible deportation and annihilation of Jews living in 'mixed marriages' (*Mischehen*), see Raul Hilberg, *Die Vernichtung der europäischen Juden: Die Gesamtgeschichte des Holocaust*, trans. Christian Seeger et al. (Berlin: Olle & Wolter, 1982), 300–302. On their everyday life in Vienna, see Michaela Raggam-Blesch, '"Mischlinge" und "Geltungsjuden." Alltag und Verfolgungserfahrungen von Männern und Frauen halbjüdischer Herkunft in Wien 1938-1945', in *Alltag im Holocaust: Jüdisches Leben im Großdeutschen Reich 1941–1945*, ed. Andrea Löw, Doris L. Bergen, and Anna Hájková (Munich: Oldenbourg, 2013), 83–85. Kreuter's encyclopedia erroneously states that Stransky emigrated, Alma Kreuter, *Deutschsprachige Neurologen und Psychiater: Ein biographisch-bibliographisches Lexikon von den Vorläufern bis zur Mitte des 20. Jahrhunderts* (Munich: K. G. Saur, 1996), 1433.
74. Stransky, 'Gelehrtenleben', 652–53.
75. Ibid., 660.
76. Ibid., 680.
77. Ibid., 687–89. Ernst Illing was found guilty, and executed on 23 November 1946, Marianne Türk was sentenced to ten years, in 1949/1950 the prosecution dropped the charges against seven other defendants, Winfried R. Garscha, 'Euthanasie-Prozesse seit 1945 in Österreich und Deutschland', in *Medizin im Nationalsozialismus - Wege der Aufarbeitung*, ed. Sonia Horn and Peter Malina, Wiener Gespräche zur Sozialgeschichte der Medizin (Vienna: ÖÄK Verlag, 2001), 50–51.
78. Erwin Stransky, 'About Mental Hygiene', unpublished lecture manuscript, 1951, ÖNB HANNA Cod. Ser. 24072, 5.
79. For the history of the Rosenhügel sanatorium, which was founded in 1912 after a testamentary donation by Nathaniel Freiherr von Rothschild, see Gottfried Roth and Ruth Koblizek, 'Die Geschichte der Nervenheilanstalt Rosenhügel', in *50 Jahre Schlaganfallzentrum Rosenhügel - 90 Jahre Nathaniel Freiherr von Rothschild'sche Stiftung für Nervenkranke in Wien*, ed. Ruth Koblizek and Gernot Schnaberth (Vienna: Eigenverlag Verein MEMO, 2002), 27–36.
80. Stransky, 'Gelehrtenleben', 691; Angetter, 'Erwin Stransky'; Gernot Schnaberth, 'Das neurologische Krankenhaus Rosenhügel seit dem Ende des Zweiten Weltkriegs', in *50 Jahre Schlaganfallzentrum Rosenhügel - 90*

Jahre Nathaniel Freiherr von Rothschild'sche Stiftung für Nervenkranke in Wien, ed. Ruth Koblizek and Gernot Schnaberth (Vienna: Eigenverlag Verein MEMO, 2002), 58–69.

81. Ernst Brezina and Erwin Stransky, *Psychische Hygiene* (Vienna and Bonn: Wilhelm Maudrich, 1955).
82. Erwin Stransky, *Psychopathie und Staatsführung* (Vienna and Innsbruck: Urban & Schwarzenberg, 1952).
83. ÖNB HANNA, Cod. Ser. no. 24156.
84. Stransky, 'Gelehrtenleben', 248.
85. Tandler sought to reintegrate the findings of academic anatomy into clinical medicine, but also to connect it to theories of constitution and racial hygiene, 'Zur Einführung', *Zeitschrift für angewandte Anatomie und Konstitutionslehre* 1, no. 1 (1913): 1–3.
86. On therapeutic nihilism and the Vienna medical school, William M. Johnston, *The Austrian Mind: An Intellectual and Social History 1848–1938* (Berkeley: University of California Press, 1972), 223–29.
87. For a broader discussion of different forms of 'heroic therapies' in German psychiatry after the First World War, Hans-Walter Schmuhl and Volker Roelcke, eds., *'Heroische Therapien': Die deutsche Psychiatrie im internationalen Vergleich 1918–1945* (Göttingen: Wallstein, 2013).
88. Horst Gundlach, 'Reine Psychologie, Angewandte Psychologie und die Institutionalisierung der Psychologie', *Zeitschrift für Psychologie* 212 (2004): 195–98; Mitchell G. Ash and Thomas Sturm, 'Die Psychologie in praktischen Kontexten: Einleitende Bemerkungen', *Zeitschrift für Psychologie* 212 (2004): 177–82; Uwe Peter Kanning, 'Geschichte der Angewandten und Praktischen Psychologie', in *Jenseits des Elfenbeinturms: Psychologie als nützliche Wissenschaft*, ed. Uwe Peter Kanning, Lutz von Rosenstiel, and Heinz Schuler (Göttingen: Vandenhoeck & Ruprecht, 2010), 19–34.
89. William Stern, 'Angewandte Psychologie', *Beiträge zur Psychologie der Aussage* 1 (1903): 4–45; James T. Lamiell, *William Stern (1871–1938): A Brief Introduction to His Life and Works* (Lengerich and Berlin: Pabst Science Publishers, 2010).
90. Gundlach, 'Reine Psychologie', 196.
91. Hugo Münsterberg, *Grundzüge der Psychotechnik* (Leipzig: J.A. Barth, 1914), 6.
92. Ibid.
93. Ibid.
94. Siegfried Jaeger, 'Zur Herausbildung von Praxisfeldern der Psychologie bis 1933', in *Geschichte der deutschen Psychologie im 20. Jahrhundert: Ein Überblick*, ed. Mitchell G. Ash and Ulfried Geuter (Opladen: Westdeutscher Verlag, 1985), 96–103; Ulfried Geuter, 'Polemos panton pater - Militär und Psychologie im Deutschen Reich 1914–1945', in *Geschichte*

der deutschen Psychologie im 20. Jahrhundert: Ein Überblick, ed. Mitchell G. Ash and Ulfried Geuter (Opladen: Westdeutscher Verlag, 1985), 147–49.
95. Katja Patzel-Mattern, '"Dispositionen des Individuums" im Produktionsprozess: Die industrielle Psychotechnik der Weimarer Republik zwischen Selbstbehauptung, Unternehmererwartungen und Arbeiterinteressen', in *Das Selbst zwischen Anpassung und Befreiung: Psychowissen und Politik im 20. Jahrhundert*, ed. Maik Tändler and Uffa Jensen (Göttingen: Wallstein, 2012), 60–84.
96. Susanne Hilken, Matthias Bormuth, and Michael Schmidt-Degenhardt, 'Psychiatrische Anfänge der Pathographie', in *Kunst und Krankheit: Studien zur Pathographie*, ed. Matthias Bormuth, Klaus Podoll, and Carsten Spitzer (Göttingen: Wallstein, 2007), 11–26.
97. Elisabeth Roudinesco and Michel Plon, *Wörterbuch der Psychoanalyse: Namen, Länder, Werke, Begriffe*, trans. Christoph Eissing-Christophersen et al. (Vienna and New York: Springer, 2004), 34–35.
98. Peter Gay, *Freud: Eine Biographie für unsere Zeit*, trans. Joachim A. Frank, 2nd ed. (Frankfurt am Main: Fischer, 2006), 353.
99. Stransky, 'Gelehrtenleben', 23.
100. Ibid., 31, 266–67.
101. Esther Fischer-Homberger, *Medizin vor Gericht: Zur Sozialgeschichte der Gerichtsmedizin* (Darmstadt: Luchterhand, 1988); Michael Clark and Catherine Crawford, *Legal History in Medicine* (Cambridge: Cambridge University Press, 1994).
102. Stransky, 'Angewandte Psychiatrie', 31.
103. Ibid., 35.
104. Ibid.
105. Ibid., 31.
106. Ibid., 27.
107. Ibid., 30.
108. Ibid.
109. Ibid., 34.
110. Ibid., 36.
111. Ibid., 37.
112. Ibid., 37–82, 42.
113. Ibid., 39.
114. Michael Hau, 'The Humane Expert: The Crisis of Modern Medicine During the Weimar Republic', in *Experts in Science and Society*, ed. Elke Kurz-Milcke and Gerd Gigerenzer (New York: Springer, 2004), 105–22.
115. Stransky, 'Angewandte Psychiatrie', 40.
116. Ibid., 43.
117. Ibid. Stransky later claimed that he had been the first to introduce the term *Psychische Hygiene*, ÖNB HANNA Cod. Ser. no. 24054 a–c.
118. Ibid., 43–44.

119. On the history of 'folk psychology', see Egbert Klautke, *The Mind of the Nation: Völkerpsychologie in Germany, 1851–1955* (New York and Oxford: Berghahn, 2013).
120. Stransky, 'Angewandte Psychiatrie', 44, 47.
121. Ibid., 49–50.
122. Ibid., 45–46.
123. Ibid., 51–52.
124. Erwin Stransky, *Krieg und Geistesstörung: Feststellungen und Erwägungen zu diesem Thema vom Standpunkte der angewandten Psychiatrie* (Wiesbaden: J. F. Bergmann, 1918).
125. Ibid., 25.
126. Steffen Bruendel, *Volksgemeinschaft oder Volksstaat: Die Ideen von 1914 und die Neuordnung Deutschlands im Ersten Weltkrieg* (Berlin: Akademie, 2003), 189–90; Peter Hoeres, *Krieg der Philosophen: Die deutsche und britische Philosophie im Ersten Weltkrieg* (Paderborn: Schöningh, 2004), 255.
127. Max Scheler, *Die Ursachen des Deutschenhasses: Eine nationalpädagogische Erörterung* (Leipzig: K. Wolff, 1917). See also Thomas Mann, *Betrachtungen eines Unpolitischen* (Berlin: S. Fischer, 1918), XXXIV–XXXVI.
128. Stransky, *Der Deutschenhaß*, 95–99, 106–7.
129. Ibid., III–IV; Br, 'Der Deutschenhaß: Eine Studie von Erwin Stransky', *Deutsche Revue* 45 (1920): 93; Georg Weinländer, 'Stranskys Deutschenhaß', *Wiener Medizinische Wochenschrift* 70 (1920): 1017–18.
130. Weinländer, 'Stranskys Deutschenhaß'.
131. Erwin Stransky, *Lehrbuch der allgemeinen und speziellen Psychiatrie*, vol. 2 (Leipzig: F. C. W. Vogel, 1919), 367–71.
132. Erwin Stransky, 'Der seelische Wiederaufbau des deutschen Volkes und die Aufgaben der Psychiatrie: Erweiterter Vortrag, gehalten auf der Deutschen Psychiaterversammlung in Hamburg, am 27./28. Mai 1920', *Zeitschrift für die gesamte Neurologie und Psychiatrie* 60, no. 1 (1920): 271–80.
133. Similar ideas were also voiced by some German physicians and psychiatrists, for example, Gerhard Budde, 'Die seelische Gesundung unseres Volkes', *Blätter für Volksgesundheitspflege* 20, no. 1 (1920): 7–10; Julian Marcuse, 'Nervenkraft als Grundlage des Wiederaufbaus', *Blätter für Volksgesundheitspflege* 21, nos. 10–12 (1921): 117–18.
134. Stransky, 'Der seelische Wiederaufbau', 271.
135. Ibid., 272–74.
136. Ibid., 273–74.
137. Ibid., 274.
138. Ibid., 275.
139. Edward Bernays, *Propaganda: Die Kunst der Public Relations*, trans. Patrick Schnur (Freiburg: Orange Press, 2007); Willem J. M. Levelt, *A History of Psycholinguistics: The Pre-Chomskyan Era* (Oxford: Oxford University Press, 2013), 271–72.

140. Stransky, 'Der seelische Wiederaufbau', 275.
141. Ibid.
142. Elena L. Grigorenko, Patricia Ruzgis, and Robert J. Sternberg, *Psychology in Russia: Past, Present, Future* (Commack, NY: Nova Science Publishers, 1997), 23.
143. Stransky, 'Der seelische Wiederaufbau', 276–79.
144. Ibid., 280.
145. Gustav Kolb, 'Inwieweit sind Änderungen im Betriebe der Anstalten geboten?', *Psychiatrisch-Neurologische Wochenschrift*, nos. 21/22 (1920): 164; Adolf Groß, 'Zeitgemäße Betrachtungen zum wirtschaftlichen Betrieb der Irrenanstalten', *Allgemeine Zeitschrift für die Psychiatrie und psychisch-gerichtliche Medizin* 76, no. 1 (1923): 65. About Kolb, see Astrid Ley, 'Psychiatriekritik durch Psychiater: Sozialreformerische und professionspolitische Ziele des Erlanger Anstaltsdirektors Gustav Kolb (1870–1938)', in *'Moderne' Anstaltspsychiatrie im 19. und 20. Jahrhundert: Legitimation und Kritik*, ed. Heiner Fangerau and Karen Nolte (Stuttgart: Franz Steiner, 2006), 195–220.
146. Eduard Hitschmann, 'Prof. Dr. E. Stransky (Wien): Psychopathologie der Ausnahmezustände und Psychopathologie des Alltags', *Internationale Zeitschrift für Psychoanalyse* 8, no. 2 (1922): 222–23.
147. Roudinesco and Plon, *Wörterbuch der Psychoanalyse*, 411–12; Elke Mühlleitner, *Biographisches Lexikon der Psychoanalyse: Die Mitglieder der Psychoanalytischen Mittwoch-Gesellschaft und der Wiener Psychoanalytischen Vereinigung 1902–1938* (Tübingen: edition diskord, 1992), 149–51.
148. Hitschmann, 'Psychopathologie der Ausnahmezustände', 222.
149. Erwin Stransky, 'Angewandte Psychopathologie: Vortrag gehalten im Akademischen Verein für medizinische Psychologie in Wien am 10. Dezember 1931', *Psychiatrisch-Neurologische Wochenschrift* 16 (1932): 196.
150. Arthur Kronfeld, 'Eine Bedenklichkeit der "angewandten" Psychiatrie', *Zeitschrift für die gesamte Neurologie und Psychiatrie* 65 (1921): 366.
151. Ibid., 365.
152. Arthur Kronfeld, *Das seelisch Abnorme und die Gemeinschaft* (Stuttgart: Julius Püttmann, 1923).
153. Kronfeld, 'Eine Bedenklichkeit der "angewandten" Psychiatrie', 365–67.
154. Ingo-Wolf Kittel, 'Arthur Kronfeld zur Erinnerung - Schicksal und Werk eines jüdischen Psychiaters in drei deutschen Reichen', in *Arthur Kronfeld (1886–1941): Ein Pionier der Psychologie, Sexualwissenschaft und Psychotherapie*, ed. Ingo-Wolf Kittel (Konstanz: Bibliothek der Universität Konstanz, 1988), 9; Wolfgang Kretschmer, 'Arthur Kronfeld - ein Vergessener: Zu seinem 100. Geburtstag', *Der Nervenarzt* 58, no. 12 (1987): 737–42; Rainer Herrn, 'Vom Traum zum Trauma: Das Institut für Sexualwissenschaft, 1919–1933', in *Der Sexualreformer Magnus*

Hirschfeld: Ein Leben im Spannungsfeld von Wissenschaft, Politik und Gesellschaft, ed. Elke-Vera Kotowski and Julius Schoeps (Berlin: Be.Bra Wissenschaft, 2004), 173–200.

155. Arthur Kronfeld, 'Rätesystem, Klassenkampf und Ärzte: Eine Entgegnung', *Rätezeitung* 1, no. 10 (1919): 3; Magnus Hirschfeld, *Verstaatlichung des Gesundheitswesens* (Berlin: E. Berger, 1919).
156. Kronfeld, 'Eine Bedenklichkeit der "angewandten" Psychiatrie', 364.
157. Arthur Kronfeld, *Das Wesen der psychiatrischen Erkenntnis: Beiträge zur allgemeinen Psychiatrie I* (Berlin: Julius Springer, 1920).
158. Kittel, 'Arthur Kronfeld zur Erinnerung', 9–11.
159. Ibid., 11.
160. Stransky, 'Angewandte Psychopathologie', 196.
161. Erwin Stransky, 'Keine Bedenklichkeit der angewandten Psychiatrie', *Zeitschrift für die gesamte Neurologie und Psychiatrie* 69 (1921): 327.
162. Ibid., 328.
163. Ibid., 327.
164. Erwin Stransky, 'Psychiatrie und psychologische Methodik', *Wiener Medizinische Wochenschrift* 79, no. 21 (1929): 671–76; Erwin Stransky, 'Modeströmungen und Kurzschlüsse in der Psychiatrie', *Zeitschrift für die gesamte Neurologie und Psychiatrie* 101 (1926): 770–85.
165. Stransky, 'Psychiatrie und psychologische Methodik', 671.
166. Ibid., 671–72.
167. Arthur Kronfeld, 'Stransky, Erwin (Wien), Psychiatrie und psychologische Methodik', *Allgemeine ärztliche Zeitschrift für Psychotherapie und psychische Hygiene* 2, no. 12 (1929): 778–79.
168. Stransky, 'Angewandte Psychopathologie', 197.
169. Stransky, 'Keine Bedenklichkeit der angewandten Psychiatrie', 329.
170. Ibid., 331.

CHAPTER 4

Expansionism and Interdisciplinarity: Applied Psychopathology in the Inter-War Period

The history of applied psychopathology cannot be told without Erwin Stransky. He had coined the concept in two programmatic articles in 1918 and 1920, published the first studies in the new field, and remained its main representative and propagandist throughout the inter-war period and beyond. Nevertheless, he was not its only adherent. From 1919 onwards, a group of diverse scholars rallied around the flag that he had planted. The concept inspired a short-lived but influential monograph series as well as an association that remained active until its dissolution following the annexation of Austria in 1938. From the beginning on, the participation of other actors pushed applied psychopathology in new directions. What had started as Stransky's distinctly right-wing nationalist answer to the political and medical crisis of the immediate post-war period and a programme for the aggressive expansion of psychiatry's psycho-political expertise now became an increasingly open and interdisciplinary umbrella term for very different approaches to psychopathology, society, and culture.

This chapter examines the two strands of the institutionalisation of applied psychopathology in the inter-war period. The first part turns to Switzerland in the beginning of the 1920s, where the psychiatrist Walter Morgenthaler picked up Stransky's applied psychiatry as the inspiration for a monograph series. While the series as such is largely forgotten today, some major books of the period first appeared as part of the 'Studies in Applied Psychiatry' as, in particular, Hermann Rorschach's famous

D. Freis, *Psycho-Politics between the World Wars*,
Mental Health in Historical Perspective,
https://doi.org/10.1007/978-3-030-32702-6_4

inkblots and Morgenthaler's own study on the works of the artist and psychiatric inmate Adolf Wölfli. Morgenthaler and his board of editors—which included Stransky, but also psychiatrist-turned-philosopher Karl Jaspers—struggled to find a common definition of applied psychiatry as well as a political stance for the series in inter-war Europe. And even though the book series itself was only short-lived, Morgenthaler's involvement with applied psychiatry had a strong intellectual influence on his work for decades to come. At the same time, a part of the editing board of the 'Studies in Applied Psychiatry' became the nucleus of the mental hygiene movement in Switzerland.

In the second part, this chapter returns to Vienna, where the Association for Applied Psychopathology and Psychology was founded in early 1920 and soon became embroiled in the conflict between psychoanalysis and academic psychiatry. Many of Stransky's activities during the inter-war period were situated exactly where the lines between academic psychiatry and psychoanalysis became blurred and where open conflict, competition, and cooperation became possible. Since the early 1920s Stransky together with his younger colleague Heinrich Kogerer tried to break the Freudians and Adlerians' quasi-monopoly on psychotherapy by creating a therapeutic school of their own. While mostly forgotten today, they eventually established the first psychotherapeutic outpatient clinic at a university hospital in the German-speaking countries. Later in the 1920s the emergence of the mental hygiene movement in Europe pushed the idea of a prophylaxis of mental disorders to the fore and with it another issue over which psychiatrists and psychoanalysts could quarrel. Again, Stransky, who considered mental hygiene a part of applied psychopathology, was in the thick of it.

Nowhere were the histories of psychoanalysis and academic psychiatry as entangled as in the Association for Applied Psychopathology and Psychology. Although Stransky has often been painted as a fervent opponent of Freud, psychoanalysis played a considerable role in the history of the association. The co-founders Bernhard Dattner and Gaston Roffenstein were both former members of the Vienna Psychoanalytic Society. The first public event hosted by the Association for Applied Psychopathology and Psychology was supposed to prepare a rapprochement between representatives of the different psy-ences, and in the years to follow the association indeed became a sort of neutral meeting ground for the different schools. This cooperation was not without some friction, but it was the main reason for the association's success and rapid growth in the early 1920s. As Stransky's right-wing and anti-Freudian stance threatened to alienate the psychoanalysts, he decided to cede his position as chair to the left-wing psychoanalyst Martin Pappenheim in 1927. It was under the leadership of Pappenheim that the association, and with it applied psychopathology, reached its zenith. To celebrate the tenth anniversary of its founding, an international conference was held in 1930 in Vienna, with a thematic range unparalleled in the history of the psy-ences in the inter-war period. However, this experiment in interdisciplinarity remained a solitary event. With the rise of fascism in Germany and Austria, the political climate turned against applied psychopathology as an integrative project. Martin Pappenheim was forced to emigrate to Palestine in 1934 and Erwin Stransky retook his position as chair. Without the international contacts and the participation of the psychoanalysts, the association continued to exist but could not live up to the hopes that the 1930 conference had raised. Eventually, the annexation of Austria in 1938 brought the project of applied psychopathology to an end. And yet, what had begun as Erwin Stransky's jingoist reaction to the crisis after the First World War and as call for psychiatry's 'medical imperialism' against other disciplines, became an astonishingly open and interdisciplinary project during the inter-war period. The idea of applying the knowledge of the psy-ences to all aspects of cultural, social, and political life could appeal to representatives of the different disciplines, while still being just elusive enough to incorporate even contradictory approaches.

Inkblots and Society: Studies in Applied Psychiatry

Applied psychiatry was a radical psychiatric and political reaction to the experience of the war and the immediate post-war period in Vienna. And yet, it was also favourably received in Switzerland, which had not shared most of these experiences. For the Swiss psychiatrist Walter Morgenthaler (1882–1965), Erwin Stransky's manifesto became an inspiration to publish a monograph series with the newly founded publishing house of Ernst Bircher in Berne. Until 1922, five volumes of *Arbeiten zur angewandten Psychiatrie* ('Studies in Applied Psychiatry') appeared before the series was eventually cancelled when the publisher ran into financial problems.[1] But short-lived as it was, the series was influential. Some of the books of the series were among the most important psychiatric publications of the twentieth century and continue to be discussed, republished, and translated to this day.

The history of the book series began little more than a year after the publication of Stransky's manifesto. Inspired by the concept of applied psychiatry, Morgenthaler decided to publish psychiatric books that would explore topics beyond the usual boundaries of the discipline. His first step was to look for collaborators. In December 1919, he contacted Stransky to inform him about his plans. The aim of the series would be to 'provide the material & the experiences of the psychiatrist for other disciplines. The title & the direction come from a very interesting article in the All.Zeitschr.f.Psych. [*Allgemeine Zeitschrift für Psychiatrie und psychisch-gerichtliche Medizin*], whose author you doubtlessly know quite well'. Morgenthaler planned to sign on a number of co-editors and contributors who would represent different European countries and Stransky was his choice in Austria.[2] Stransky immediately cabled back: 'collaboration accepted' and showed himself very flattered in a subsequent letter.[3] Around the same time, Morgenthaler was already in touch with other potential co-editors. From Switzerland, Hans W. Maier (1882–1945) from Zurich, who was then an assistant at the Burghölzli clinic under director Eugen Bleuler, agreed to participate in the project.[4] From Germany, Morgenthaler picked Karl Jaspers (1883–1969) in Heidelberg. By then, Jaspers was not a practising psychiatrist anymore but had already accepted a chair in philosophy. Nevertheless, he agreed to coedit the series and submit a manuscript.[5]

Unbeknownst to Morgenthaler, having Jaspers and Stransky on the same board came with considerable potential for conflict. In his most important psychiatric work, *Allgemeine Psychopathologie* ('general psychopathology', 1913), Jaspers challenged Wilhelm Griesinger's (1817–1868) dogma that mental illness was brain disease and attacked the corresponding 'brain mythology'.[6] In what some still consider the basis of psychopathology as a science, Jaspers firmly argued against any biological and neurological reductionism and for an understanding, descriptive, and epistemologically reflected approach to the human psyche. To Stransky, this was philosophical speculation of a kind that threatened psychiatry's status as a part of scientific medicine. Later in the 1920s, he published several polemics against the new 'philosophical direction' in contemporary psychiatry in which he directly named and blamed Jaspers. The simmering tension between Stransky and Jaspers could have easily escalated, and on more than one occasion, Morgenthaler's diplomatic skills were the only reason that it did not.

Walter Morgenthaler was the uniting figure that kept the project together. Born in 1882, he had studied medicine in Berne, Vienna, and

Zurich. During a semester in Vienna in 1905/1906, he had followed Sigmund Freud's seminar on psychotherapy[7]; in Zurich, he was a student of Eugen Bleuler. After completing his studies, he worked in different Swiss clinics before becoming chief physician of the Waldau clinic in the vicinity of Berne in 1913, where he stayed until 1920. In 1917, Morgenthaler habilitated at the University of Berne. Between 1920 and 1925, he was director of the private Münchenbuchsee sanatorium, before opening his own private practice as psychotherapist in Berne.[8] Throughout his career, Morgenthaler published extensively on psychotherapy, mental hygiene, and the early modern history of psychiatry, while at the same time persistently campaigning for the professionalisation of psychiatric nurses.[9] In 1942, he became the founder of both the Swiss Society for Psychology and its Applications and the *Swiss Journal of Psychology*—an act that was later celebrated as 'a courageous act of intellectual national defence' against Nazi attempts to integrate Swiss psychologists into the German professional organisations.[10]

While Morgenthaler's life has received little scholarly attention, two aspects of his biography have. The first is his study *Ein Geisteskranker als Künstler* ('A Mental Patient as Artist'), which appeared in 1921 and in which he presented the artistic works of one of his patients at the Waldau clinic, Adolf Wölfli (1864–1930).[11] Wölfli was a violent schizophrenic who had been hospitalised after committing sexual assaults in several instances. After seeing that Wölfli painted the walls of his cell with his own excrements, Morgenthaler began to supply him with pens and paper. Over the following decades, Wölfli produced a great many drawings and paintings, and started to poetise and compose. Morgenthaler's 1921 book was an instant success and built Wölfli's reputation as the first 'outsider artist' of the twentieth century.[12] Together with Hans Prinzhorn's *Bildnerei der Geisteskranken* ('artistry of the mentally ill', 1922), which also included some reproductions of Wölfli's works, Morgenthaler's book became the starting point for a whole new reception of the artistic production of mental patients, both among psychiatrists and in artistic circles.[13]

Secondly, Morgenthaler also played a key role in the publication of Hermann Rorschach's (1884–1922) now-famous *Psychodiagnostik* in 1921.[14] In this study, Rorschach introduced what today is still commonly known and occasionally applied as the 'Rorschach test', a psychological method in which a person's associative interpretations of ten symmetrical inkblots are used to assess his or her personality. Morgenthaler had met Rorschach when the latter was an assistant at the Waldau clinic in 1914 and 1915. It was Morgenthaler who encouraged Rorschach to publish his work and proposed the catchy title *Psychodiagnostik*. After Rorschach's untimely death due to appendicitis in the spring of 1922, Morgenthaler took care of his friend's legacy; he supervised numerous reprints of the study, established a Rorschach commission, which later developed into an international Rorschach society, and eventually founded the Swiss Rorschach archive in Berne in 1956.[15] It is no coincidence that Wölfli's paintings and Rorschach's inkblots, both among the most iconic visual documents in the history of psychiatry, were published by the same person. Walter Morgenthaler, whose younger brother Ernst (1887–1962) was a successful painter, had a sense for art and occasionally evinced some artistic talent himself—for example by designing an educational frieze on mental hygiene, sixteen meters long, for the Swiss Hygiene and Sport Exhibition (Hyspa) in 1931.[16]

While the works of Wölfli and Rorschach have both received considerable attention, the existing research has ignored the context of their publication as parts of *Arbeiten zur angewandten Psychiatrie*. Morgenthaler's and Rorschach's studies were the first and the second volume of the series, respectively, to appear. The third was Erwin Stransky's *Psychopathologie der Ausnahmezustände und Psychopathologie des Alltags* ('psychopathology of the states of exception and psychopathology of everyday life'), with a title provocatively alluding to Sigmund Freud's 1901 *Zur Psychopathologie des Alltagslebens*.[17] It was followed by Gaston Roffenstein's *Zur Psychologie und Psychopathologie der Gegenwartsgeschichte* ('On the Psychology and Psychopathology of Contemporary History'), which was based on his opening talk for the Association for Applied Psychopathology and Psychology in Vienna.[18] The last volume of the series to be published by Bircher was Karl Jaspers's pathography *Strindberg und Van Gogh*, in which Jaspers also retrospectively examined the mental conditions of Emanuel Swedenborg and Friedrich Hölderlin.[19] At least one more publication, a book by Hans W. Maier on cinematographic studies of the facial expressions of the mentally ill, had been planned, but was never realised. Two decades later, in 1941, an isolated last instalment of the series appeared, an introduction to the Behn–Rorschach test by the Swiss psychoanalyst and educational theorist Hans Zulliger (1893–1965). Now published by Hans Huber's publishing house, which had also bought the rights of Rorschach's original study, the series was still edited by Walter Morgenthaler in cooperation with Hans W. Maier, André Repond, and Erwin Stransky; only Karl Jaspers had left the editing board and been replaced with the Swiss psychiatrist Oscar Forel (1891–1982).[20]

The diversity of the editors and topics begged the questions how 'applied psychiatry' could be defined. In the preface to the first volume of the series Morgenthaler laid out the aims of the 'Studies in Applied Psychiatry':

> 1. To make the vast *material* of the psychiatrist accessible not only for clinical-psychiatric purposes, but also for other fields of research and knowledge.
> 2. To use the *experiences* and *insights* that allow the psychiatrist to look deeper into mental occurrences than everyone else in such a way as that they become more useful for other sciences than they have been before.[21]

The second paragraph unmistakably echoed Erwin Stransky and his claims about the epistemological privileges of psychiatry. Initially, Morgenthaler had considered mentioning Stransky's manifesto in a footnote to the preface. However, Karl Jaspers refused to give Stransky credit for the invention of applied psychiatry—as he claimed, the term was merely an equivalent of 'applied psychology', and furthermore, it was commonly used in Heidelberg. Until now, Jaspers argued, he had not even heard of Stransky's article.[22] Although Stransky was disgruntled, Morgenthaler followed Jaspers's suggestion and removed the footnote from the draft.[23]

Two discrete strands of psychiatry's 'application' can be distinguished in the five volumes published in 1921 and 1922. One focus was on the visual, aesthetic, and artistic aspects of psychiatry. Morgenthaler and Jaspers wrote about the relation between individual mental pathologies and artistic production. Although Hermann Rorschach's *Psychodiagnostik* proposed a method for clinical use, it was closely related to these approaches. Like Morgenthaler and Jaspers, Rorschach was interested in the relation between art and psychopathology, but he reversed the roles. Instead of the patient producing art and the psychiatrists using it as a lens for diagnosis, the inkblot test had the psychiatrist producing art, the patient interpreting it, and the psychiatrist diagnosing the patient based on his or her interpretation. Hans W. Maier's proposed book on the diagnostic potentials of cinematographic techniques was further removed from art but it would have shared a visual approach. On the other side, Stransky and Roffenstein offered a distinctly psycho-political approach to 'applied psychiatry'. From different angles, they discussed the role of psychopathology in social and political life. Notably, Rorschach's alternative proposal, a psycho-historical study of various sects and heretics in Switzerland, would have fallen into the same category.[24]

However, while Morgenthaler did not contribute overtly psycho-political texts of his own, this does not mean that his own understanding of 'applied psychiatry' excluded society and politics. By the end of the 1920s, he became a member of the Swiss national committee for mental hygiene (*Comité national Suisse d'hygiène mentale*) and published extensively on the socio-medical importance of psychiatric prophylaxis.[25] Moreover, Morgenthaler's sympathy for more radical psycho-political ideas was not limited to his appropriation of Stransky's 'applied psychiatry'; he commented very positively on both Stransky's book *Der Deutschenhaß* and on his talk about the 'mental reconstruction of the German people'.[26] In fact, Morgenthaler and Stransky shared strikingly similar ideas about the role of psychiatric experts in society and politics, and Stransky's intellectual influence on Morgenthaler became visible in many of his later works.

In 1930, Morgenthaler used Stransky's 'subordination-authority-relation' to explain the social transformation in Europe after the First World War, advocating a more positive and sympathetic psychological attitude towards members of the proletariat, so that we 'might learn to organically and vitally incorporate ourselves in the whole of the people, each in the place where he belongs'.[27] In the same year, Morgenthaler presented two papers at the First International Conference for Applied Psychopathology and Psychology in Vienna, one on the 'artistic production of the mentally ill' and the second about 'psychotherapy and politics'. Stransky's influence was palpable here, although Morgenthaler shifted the focus from psychiatry to psychotherapy. Elaborating on the role of psychiatrists and psychotherapists in society and politics, Morgenthaler argued that they should use their position and their 'deeper knowledge and insights' to exert a positive psychological influence in many areas of life and beyond the 'asylum walls and the laboratories'. This also meant changing the hierarchies between different forms of expert knowledge. Starting with work environments, 'we should not simply parrot the engineers and businessmen, but we should bring technology and business into service for the psychological, and become leaders [...] for all questions that concern the personal, the mental, the human'.[28] Ultimately, the influence of psychotherapeutic knowledge, of 'healthy psychological opinions' and an understanding of the social relevance of psychotherapyand psychopathology would have to be transferred to other areas of social life, and to politics in particular:

'*Prinzhorn* rightly demands that the psychotherapist should be a *leader*. Conversely, it is of highest importance that our political leaders become, to a greater degree, *psychotherapists*'.[29]

Over the following decades, Morgenthaler repeatedly returned to these psycho-political tasks and each time his ideas went hand in hand with the zeitgeist. In 1935, as psychotherapy in the German-speaking countries—or, as it was now called, *deutsche Seelenheilkunde*—had largely fallen under the influence of Nazi ideology,[30] he published an article on the relation between neurology, psychiatry, and psychotherapy in the *Zentralblatt für Psychotherapie*, then edited by Matthias Heinrich Göring and Carl Gustav Jung. Morgenthaler argued that the psychotherapist, as a 'spiritual director based on biology', 'has a cultural mission, which arguably is rooted in biology, psychiatry, and psychotherapy, but which reaches far beyond these disciplines into what is universally human'. While psychotherapists could treat and guide disoriented individuals, in this new age of national reawakening, these methods had to be put into the service of the collective: 'What is sure, is that in a new culture [...] the foundations of psychotherapy, that up to now have been useful for the recovery of the individual, in some way have to come into their own for the whole of the people, as a restoration, and for its preservation and unfolding'.[31]

After the beginning of the Second World War, visions of social renewal coalesced with the defence of Swiss neutrality. In 1941, Morgenthaler discussed the collective mental disposition of the Swiss people and the conditions of the 'mental defence force' (*Geistige Wehrkraft*) needed for the preservation of its threatened neutral status. To Morgenthaler, this was not only a matter of mental health and mental force but also meant integrating the Swiss people into an organic community that could persist in this 'war of nerves' (*Nervenkrieg*).[32] With the end of the war, forging the Swiss people into a defensive community and mobilising their psychological defence powers suddenly became obsolete. In 1945, Morgenthaler turned to psycho-political explanations of recent events instead. Trying to explain what had happened in the previous years, he diagnosed the individual psychologies of Benito Mussolini and Adolf Hitler and their impact on the psychology of collectives, reframing politics as an extension of individual psychopathology.[33]

The Cold War offered yet another stage for psycho-political experts. Morgenthaler's last book was a psycho-historical study on Karl Marx published in 1962 by the Schweizerisches Ost-Institut, an anti-communist think tank in Berne. By examining the personality of Marx from a psychological and psychiatric perspective, Morgenthaler hoped to demystify the historical person and to lay bare the psychological roots of his doctrine and its lasting success.[34] Although he showed himself impressed by some of the qualities of Marx' personality, Morgenthaler still concluded that the founder of modern communism had exhibited traits of paranoia and other psychopathological disorders and could even be described as schizophrenic.[35] His last publication still followed the lines that Stransky had sketched in 1918. Morgenthaler stated that he was speaking from the standpoint of the psychiatric expert witness and defended his approach by arguing that, as all human affairs and products were always connected to the psyche, they could all be explained from a perspective informed by psychological knowledge.[36]

Beyond the appropriation of ideas, Morgenthaler was also institutionally connected to the Association for Applied Psychopathology and Psychology in Vienna. While his own attempts to establish a similar association in Berne never developed into anything larger than an informal circle, he became an honorary member of the flourishing association in Vienna on 14 April 1920, and after having presented two papers at the international conference in 1930, he also joined the 'permanence commission' that was tasked with preparing the association's future conferences.[37]

However, while Morgenthaler and Stransky agreed on the definition of applied psychiatry, national politics became one of the major points of contention among the editors of *Arbeiten zur angewandten Psychiatrie*. From the beginning, Morgenthaler had envisioned the series as a larger international project, not limited to the German-speaking countries. As he told Jaspers and Stransky in January 1920, he planned to enlist co-editors from France, from French-speaking part of Switzerland, the United States, and from England. Translations would appear in the other two languages—a widespread practice in Switzerland, where many publications were bi- or trilingual. For the United States, Morgenthaler had in mind Adolf Meyer (1866–1950). Meyer, of Swiss origin and a former student of Auguste Forel (1848–1931), was then a professor at Johns Hopkins University and a thought leader of mental hygiene in the United States.[38]

When Morgenthaler proposed to extend the international scope of the series, the war was less than one year and a half away, and this kind of international cooperation was still a topic fraught with emotion. Morgenthaler, who was well aware of the sensitivities of his colleagues, cautiously checked with his German and Austrian co-editors if they would agree to publish alongside Entente scientists. Political topics would be avoided wherever possible so that the series might become a neutral ground for scientific exchange.[39] Morgenthaler envisioned that this kind of scientific cooperation would gradually re-establish the severed connections between former enemies.[40]

However, Morgenthaler underestimated how fresh the wounds of the war still were, as neither Stransky nor Jaspers shared his Swiss sense of neutrality. Stransky grudgingly refrained from sending a manuscript about the psychopathology of anti-German resentment and agreed to select a more 'neutral' topic instead. While paying lip service to his belief in scientific cosmopolitanism, he left no doubt that while he could imagine cooperating with American, British, or Italian scholars, he drew the line at working together with the French—unless Morgenthaler could find someone who had not publicly denounced German culture or who had totally changed his 'mentality' since the war.[41] As Stransky reminded Morgenthaler, he had already severed his connections with the French scientific community in protest over the defamation of German culture early in the war when he had left the Société Médico-Psychologique whose corresponding member he had been since 1905.[42] For once Stransky and Jaspers agreed. Jaspers too appealed to the cosmopolitanism of the scientific community and claimed that discussions about 'political opinions, questions of [war] guilt, and submarine warfare' were out of place in the 'intellectual world'. But this 'humane feeling of solidarity' reached its limits where German science and culture had been attacked, as had often happened in France. Like Stransky, Jaspers emphatically stated that he would 'not tolerate any man who has expressed such defamations, unless he publicly recants'.[43] Faced with the emotional reactions of his co-editors, Morgenthaler had no choice but to abandon his original plan. As it was evidently still too early to include a scholar from France, he replied to Stransky and Jaspers, that he would instead choose the Swiss André Repond (1886–1973) to represent the French-speaking world.[44]

The activities of Repond, director of the psychiatric asylum Malévoz in the canton of Valais, show which direction the series might have taken if the publisher had not run into economic difficulties after only five volumes. Like Walter Morgenthaler and Hans W. Maier, who also were former students of Eugen Bleuler at Burghölzli, Repond was an adherent of social and prophylactic psychiatry and mental hygiene. Influenced by the American movement for mental hygiene as well as by the parallel French movement led by Édouard Toulouse (1865–1947), Repond later became a protagonist of the Swiss national committee for mental hygiene. At the First International Congress on Mental Hygiene in Washington, DC in 1930, Repond was a member of the Swiss delegation as well as one of the congress's numerous vice presidents.[45] A decade later, Repond, together with Heinrich Meng (1887–1972), published and introduced the first German translation of Clifford W. Beers's *A Mind That Found Itself* (1908)—the book that had jumpstarted the movement for mental hygiene in the United States.[46] Repond's commitment to psychiatric prophylaxis continued after the Second World War, when he became president of the World Federation for Mental Health in 1949,[47] making him one of the figures connecting psychiatry's inter-war period expansion in the name of applied psychiatry to the movement for mental hygiene and to post-war concepts of mental health.

Conflict, Competition, and Cooperation: Psychoanalysis and Applied Psychopathology in Red Vienna

When he died in 1962, Erwin Stransky was well known as a staunch adversary of psychoanalysis.[48] For half a century, he had rarely passed on an opportunity to verbally attack Freud and his followers, so much in fact, that his animus against psychoanalysis and its offspring became a constitutive part of his professional and even of his personal image. However, while polemics against psychoanalysis abound in his writings, he did not engage with it in any systematic way and rarely tackled any specific methodological or theoretical issues. Stransky's criticism of psychoanalysis was superficial and generalising and often did nothing more than reproduce common clichés. As his views—formed mostly in the early 1920s—changed little over time, they became increasingly anachronistic. In the 1950s and 1960s, he still criticised psychoanalysis in ways reminiscent of the anti-psychoanalyst rhetoric of the pre-war era.[49]

Behind the frequent polemics, however, Stransky's position towards psychoanalysis was less coherent. He repeatedly praised Sigmund Freud's 'genius' and acknowledged the importance of his contributions to psychology and psychopathology—and to his own project of applied psychopathology in particular.[50] His purported rejection of psychoanalysis was more than once undercut by the tacit appropriation of psychoanalytic concepts. As his colleague and rival Hans Hoff (1897–1969) wrote in an obituary for Stransky in the Vienna medical weekly, 'his position towards psychoanalysis was considerably more ambivalent than he perhaps had realised himself'.[51]

Stransky's difficulties in developing a consistent position towards psychoanalysis were the result of the troubled relationship between psychoanalysis and academic psychiatry in early twentieth-century Vienna, and thus of a conflict that took place among the sciences of the mind as well as inside a broader political context. While psychoanalysts and psychiatrists were often concerned with the same questions, the same problems, and sometimes with the same patients, the most striking aspect of their relationship was the rift between them. Psychoanalysis originated and developed on the margins and outside of the university and for a large part of the twentieth-century psychoanalysts were, and still are, a 'scientific subculture' separated from academic psychology and psychiatry.[52]

The quasi-official psychoanalytic narrative, propagated by Freud himself, according to which the nascent movement was met with nothing but uniform indifference and hostility in the first decades of the twentieth century, has since been refuted.[53] And yet, the other psy-ences did not welcome Freud and his followers with open arms. Most psychologists and psychiatrists found psychoanalysis to be incompatible with their disciplines, and while it is certainly not true that both disciplines simply ignored and scorned psychoanalysis, it was nonetheless given a 'fairly negative and apathetic reception'.[54] The rejection of psychoanalysis in German and Austrian academia, as well as his personal experiences, led Freud to pursue a strategy that relied on the development of an autonomous organisation outside the academy. In the years prior to the First World War, psychoanalysts successfully created their own associations, communication channels, and their own, separate system of training and teaching.[55] But despite some promising steps towards official recognition by state authorities for their contribution to the treatment of war neuroses, they were unable to gain a foothold in German or Austrian universities after the war.[56] In Switzerland, the situation was a little different. Eugen Bleuler (1857–1939) was one of the most renowned Swiss psychiatrists of his time, and together with Carl G. Jung, who had been his assistant from 1900 to 1909, he was among the 'early adopters' of psychoanalysis when he began integrating Freudian concepts in his works as early as 1904.[57]

In Vienna, where Erwin Stransky's encounters with psychoanalysis took place, the situation was particularly complex. Vienna was the political, social, cultural, and scientific centre of Austro-Hungary and, after the First

World War, of the Republic of Austria, but until 1938 it was also the world capital of psychoanalysis. Freud 'discovered' and developed psychoanalysis in *fin de siècle* Vienna and the majority of his early followers lived here. Personal contacts between psychoanalysts and other members of the medical community were hardly avoidable. This was obviously the case at the psychiatric university clinic where many psychoanalysts studied or were staff members.[58] However, the presence of the Freudians and Adlerians at the university clinic did little to bridge the gap between academic psychiatry and psychoanalysis.

The political transformations of 1918 profoundly changed the relation between psychiatrists and psychoanalysts in Vienna as well as the context in which they encountered each other. Political polarisation entered the internal politics of the sciences of the mind. While many psychiatrists fell in line with the mobilising right, psychoanalysis moved to the left. This development was not limited to the Austrian capital, but many of the ensuing debates in the psychoanalytic community originated in the specific social and political context of inter-war Vienna.

The military defeat of the Central Powers and the subsequent collapse of the Habsburg Empire had transformed the former centre of a multi-ethnic empire into the capital of a small republic in Central Europe; no longer a monarchy, but a democracy with universal suffrage and a pioneering social welfare agenda. Under its new socialist authorities, 'Red Vienna' became the site of a unique project of urban reconstruction and social reform. Today, large blocks of council flats and other public buildings, among them icons of modernist architecture, are the most visible traces of this era.[59] But Red Vienna was much more than new buildings and public housing; it was driven by a far-reaching reform agenda that encompassed economic, social, and cultural aspects, and by an expansive public health and welfare policy. The array of medical and social programmes designed by the anatomist Julius Tandler (1869–1936) created new opportunities for mental health experts.[60]

Psychoanalysis embraced the change and seized the new opportunities. This was neither opportunism nor a change of mind. Even before the war, psychoanalysts had tended towards moderate left-wing views. Some estimates assume that an overwhelming majority of the members of the Vienna Psychoanalytic Society were voters of the Social Democratic Party. Psychoanalysts and Social Democrats were connected by a certain degree of mutual sympathy and trust, as well as by a network of personal relationships.[61] However, the position towards politics and the workers' movement had rarely been discussed inside the psychoanalytic community before the war. A 1909 talk about 'the psychology of Marxism' by Alfred Adler (1870–1937) was one of the very few exceptions and probably the first attempt at a synthesis of Marxist and Freudian thinking.[62] More explicit reflections about the political potentials of psychoanalysis were reserved to outsiders and renegades like the psychoanalyst, anarchist, and libertine Otto Gross (1877–1920), who declared that 'the psychology of the unconscious is the philosophy of the revolution' in 1913 in what has been called the 'first psycho-utopian essay of the twentieth century'.[63] Even after the war, Gross's political and sexual radicalism would still have been outside any possible consensus among the psychoanalytic community—as the case of Wilhelm Reich (1897–1957), who was excluded from the Vienna Psychoanalytic Society for similar reasons after a decade of conflict in 1934, illustrates.[64]

The experience of mass violence and mass politics during and after the war created a demand for explanation. Like many psychiatrists, psychoanalysts were drawn to questions of mass psychology and the relations of psychology and politics. The best-known example for psychoanalysis' post-war occupation with society was Sigmund Freud's *Massenpsychologie und Ich-Analyse*, a critical re-reading of Gustave Le Bon's (1841–1931) crowd psychology published in 1921. While Freud's socio-political thought remained in the abstract and he was cautious to keep a certain distance from current affairs, other members of the psychoanalytic community were less shy of short-term political commentary. Paul Federn (1871–1950)—a socialist, senior member of the Vienna Psychoanalytic Society and a regular at the meetings of Erwin Stransky's Association for Applied Psychopathology and Psychology—coined the phrase of the 'fatherless society' in a 1919 essay about the psychology of the Austrian revolution. In this short essay, Federn used the conceptual framework provided by Freud's *Totem and Taboo* (1913) to explain the recent past, with the revolutionary horde of brothers overthrowing the patriarchal reign of the *Kaiser*-father.[65]

For members of the Freudian left emerging in the 1920s and 1930s, psychoanalysis was more than just a psychological theory and a therapeutic method, it was also a social science and, most importantly, a form of political practice. Throughout the inter-war period, many left-leaning psychoanalysts like Paul Federn, Wilhelm Reich, Siegfried Bernfeld (1892–1953), or Otto Fenichel (1897–1946) argued that socialism and psychoanalysis were not just compatible but complementary and that only a synthesis of Marxist and Freudian thought could guide the way towards a better society. These positions, however, were not necessarily shared by the whole of the psychoanalytic community; most psychoanalysts continued to consider their discipline as apolitical and the official line issued by Sigmund Freud was that psychoanalysis was a science, not an ideology and had to keep a safe distance from politics.[66]

The distance they kept from politics was one reason psychoanalysts were less successful than others in occupying the positions for psychological and psychiatric experts offered by Red Vienna. In particular, Alfred Adler and his followers could build on long-standing links to the socialist authorities in Vienna.[67] When the Austrian Social Democrats began their extensive reform of the schools and the education system, representatives of Adlerian individual psychology became involved on many levels, as for example through their network of child guidance offices (*Erziehungsberatungsstellen*).[68] In their consulting practice, the Adlerians sought to translate social ideas into psychological treatments. Rudolf Dreikurs (1897–1972)—who also was one of the individual psychologists to join the movement for mental hygiene—experimented with collective treatment and group counselling in a child guidance in the late 1920s. For Dreikurs, collective treatment was a 'democratisation' of psychotherapy, part of the social and democratic promises of Red Vienna and fundamentally incompatible with the authoritarian corporative state that succeeded it.[69]

The close affiliation with social democracy turned against individual psychology in 1934 when the First Republic was overthrown by the Dollfuß regime. After government troops had quelled the republican resistance in the Austrian Civil War of February 1934, the Social Democratic Party was banned and illegalised. This did not only spell the end of Red Vienna but also of individual psychologists' welfare and counselling projects.[70] Psychoanalysis, by contrast, remained relatively untouched by the political changes for the moment.[71]

The most important Freudian contribution to the expanding public welfare services of Red Vienna was the establishment of the psychoanalytic 'Ambulatorium', which opened its doors on 22 May 1922. The Ambulatorium was an outpatient clinic modelled after the psychoanalytic policlinic that Max Eitingon (1881–1943) and Ernst Simmel (1882–1947) had set up in Berlin in 1920. Like the Berlin policlinic, the Vienna Ambulatorium connected psychoanalysis to a social mission and provided free mental health care to those who could not afford treatment.

But before 'Freud's free clinic' could begin its operations in 1922, many barriers had to be overcome. For two years, Eduard Hitschmann, the driving force behind the attempts to create a psychoanalytic outpatient clinic in Vienna, led an uphill struggle against a lethargic medical bureaucracy and hostile functionaries.[72] The most important obstacle was the adverse position of academic psychiatry. In a 1921 expertise, Julius Wagner-Jauregg had come out in opposition to the Ambulatorium, arguing that a psychotherapeutic outpatient clinic would have to use treatment methods accepted by academic psychiatry.[73] The medical opposition to psychoanalysis in Vienna was so strong that the Ambulatorium was closed at the behest of the Vienna medical office (*Sanitätsbehörde*) on 30 November 1922 and only permitted to reopen after Eduard Hitschmann appealed to the Federal Ministry of Social Administration.[74] Even then, it did not receive any funds from the state or the city.[75]

Despite their opposition to psychoanalysts' social initiative, mainstream psychiatrists were not just passive bystanders or blockers, but actively took part in the extension of Vienna's public welfare and mental health-care system. As early as 1919, even before Eduard Hitschmann began lobbying for the Ambulatorium, Erwin Stransky had called for the establishment of a psychotherapeutic outpatient clinic. Arguing that the existing neurological outpatient clinics were already working to capacity to treat physical diseases like syphilis and sciatica, he proposed the creation of a specialised treatment and counselling office for 'nervous' patients and psychopaths. As it would operate without costly equipment, the creation of such a clinic would not be expensive, requiring only three to four rooms, furniture, a chief physician, one or two assistants, and a receptionist. Stransky did not miss the opportunity to offer himself for the position of a leading physician, who would be willing to work in an honorary role. With little investment, many of the 'lost' would receive help and would be saved from mental breakdowns, suicides, and—a side blow at psychoanalysis—from falling into the hands of 'quacks'.[76]

The psychotherapeutic outpatient clinic was eventually founded in October 1922 and was attached to the university clinic. It was led not by Stransky but by the psychiatrist and neurologist Heinrich Kogerer (1887–1958).[77] From 1922 to 1930, about 1.700 neurotics and 150 mostly schizophrenic mental patients received counselling or treatment. These numbers were below those of the Ambulatorium, which registered a total of 2.245 applicants between 1922/1923 and 1930/1931, but still significant.[78] And like the Ambulatorium, the psychotherapeutic outpatient clinic was connected to more encompassing socio-political ideas. Kogerer did not want to limit the activities of the outpatient clinic to counselling and treatment alone but tried to improve their economic situation where needed. From 1927 onwards, an agreement with the Industrial District Commission (*Wiener industrielle Bezirkskommission*) allowed the outpatient clinic to refer unemployed patients to the commission, where they would receive some limited support in their search for work.[79] As Stransky believed, this connection of psychotherapeutic and social thinking already pointed the way towards mental hygiene.[80]

And in fact, the psychotherapeutic outpatient clinic soon joined the Austrian branch of the mental hygiene movement. Like Stransky, Heinrich Kogerer was an active participant in the nascent movement and was convinced that psychotherapy would play a key role in mental hygiene. In a 1931 manual of mental hygiene, edited by Stransky, Kogerer laid out his ideas about the relation between individual psychotherapy and the societal prophylaxis of mental illness. As he acknowledged himself, his own approach had a lot in common with Stransky's 'SAR' psychotherapy. Both were the product of strikingly similar, conservative understanding of society that was directly translated into a treatment method. Like Stransky, Kogerer believed that the therapist had to retain control of the therapeutic process at all times, actively guiding it into the right direction. The therapy goal was to increase the patient's happiness, for: 'When someone is happier, it is easier for him to renounce his instincts and to submit to the demands of the community'.

The aim of Kogerer's method, which he described as an 'analytical-synthetic psychotherapy with suggestive symptomatic treatment',[81] was the integration of the individual into a demanding, organic society. At the centre of Kogerer's psycho-political ideas stood the notion of 'trust'; on the one hand, the therapist had to restore the patient's trust in society, and thus his or her willingness to submit to social demands. On the other hand, society could only subsist through the trust and loyalty of all its members. As a conservative critic of modernity, Kogerer closed the circle of his argument by claiming that the increase in mental disorders that threatened society's cohesion was itself a symptom of the disintegration of society and the bonds of trust between the individual and the whole. Once, religion had been able to maintain social cohesion. Now, mental hygiene would have to step forth and fill the gap.[82]

Against these high-flying ambitions, the actual attempts to spread the gospel of mental hygiene in Vienna fell flat. In April 1928, Otto Kauders (1893–1949), an assistant at the Vienna university clinic and another protagonist of the Austrian movement for mental hygiene, established a biweekly mental hygiene consultation at the university clinic.[83] However, attendance was disappointing. Until 1930, no more than 63 consultations took place. Moreover, the majority of attendants already suffered from mental disorders and were in need of treatment, so that the counselling office was unable to perform its prophylactic task.[84] The counselling hours were discontinued as early as January 1930, and the psychotherapeutic outpatient clinic again took over mental hygiene counselling.[85] As Kogerer saw it, this failure had two reasons. First, the propaganda for the counselling office had been ineffective in reaching a broader public. Second, Kogerer blamed public prejudices against psychiatry for having led many in need of counselling to use alternative offers instead—such as the counselling offices of the individual psychologists and the psychoanalytic Ambulatorium.[86]

While the creation of the outpatient clinic led to competition over the same patient groups, other attempts to popularise mental hygiene allowed for some cooperation between the different psychotherapeutic schools. From October to December 1930, the subcommittee for mental hygiene of the Austrian Society for Public Health (*Österreichische Gesellschaft für Volksgesundheit*) organised a series of radio lectures, using a medium that had only been introduced a few years earlier. The lectures were held by some of the most prominent figures in mental and social hygiene in inter-war Austria, including Josef Berze, Erwin Stransky, Heinrich Kogerer, Heinrich Reichel, Karl Gross, but also by the former individual psychologist Rudolf Allers and the psychoanalyst Martin Pappenheim.[87]

In the spring of 1932, Stransky organised another series of lectures on mental hygiene for middle school students, once again under the auspices of the subcommittee for mental hygiene. Addressing gender-segregated groups of students, the lectures dealt with the preservation of individual mental health, with questions of reproduction and eugenics, the relation of mental and bodily hygiene, and with drug abuse. To avoid conflict with Pappenheim, Stransky found himself forced to include a psychoanalytic perspective, and eventually, scholars from the three major psychotherapeutic schools in Vienna became involved in the lectures: Erwin Stransky, Heinrich Kogerer, and Otto Kauders as representatives of academic psychiatry,

Martin Pappenheim and Paul Federn as two avowed psychoanalysts, and the individual psychologists Rudolf Dreikurs and Lydia Sicher (1890–1962) as surrogate lecturers.[88]

This time however, the big-tent approach to mental hygiene led to considerable conflict between different actors in the field of public health. An initial offer to have the lectures held under the patronage of the Vienna Society for Eugenics was rejected, as the eugenicists, led by Julius Wagner-Jauregg, Ernst Brezina, and Heinrich Reichel, were unwilling to tolerate the participation of the psychoanalysts. The inclusion of psychoanalysis led to fierce criticism by pedagogues and hygienists who were afraid that the Freudian focus on sexuality might corrupt an audience of adolescents. Reichel, who had taken part in the 1930 radio lectures, lead the charge against Stransky, who found himself forced to grudgingly defend the psychoanalysts and their lectures against a kind of criticism that was very much his own.[89]

However, instances of cooperation such as these did not help psychoanalysts to gain a foothold in the university clinic. The scientific orientation of the psychiatrists at the university clinic had much to do with it. From the end of the nineteenth century on, psychiatry in Vienna rested on two pillars—the first was Emil Kraepelin's descriptive approach, the central conceptual paradigm for most of German-speaking psychiatry, the second was the long-standing local tradition of the Vienna medical school. The result was a biologistic and clinic-based approach to psychiatry, understood by its representatives as part of positivist science. Individuals mattered, too. Between 1902 and 1928, and thus during the period in which much of the institutional development of psychoanalysis in Vienna took place, the chair for psychiatry and neurology was held by Julius Wagner-Jauregg, a notorious adversary of anything that he considered as idle psychological speculation in general and of Freud's ideas in particular.

The best-known episode in the conflict between Wagner-Jauregg and Freud happened in 1919, as the former was accused of having mistreated 'hysterical' soldiers during the war by using the 'Kaufmann method' involving the painful electric currents.[90] While these accusations had been brought forward by a social democratic soldiers' newspaper in the context of a post-war reckoning with the brutal treatment of 'war neurotics', the inquiry soon turned into an arena for the long-standing conflict between academic psychiatry and psychoanalysis. Sigmund Freud had been appointed as the leading expert witness of the Commission of Inquiry on Derelictions of Military Duty (*Kommission zur Untersuchung militärischer*

Pflichtverletzungen), where this high-profile case was debated, and soon the individual case at hand was eclipsed by fierce polemics about the ethics of war psychiatry on one side, and the therapeutic efficiency of psychoanalysis on the other. Although Freud personally exonerated Wagner-Jauregg, he still used his testimony to make a case for psychoanalysis by arguing that the clinical experiences with 'war neuroses' offered conclusive proof for his theory. At the same time, he sharply criticised psychiatry's therapeutic methods, famously denouncing military physicians as 'machine guns behind the front line' whose task had been to push fleeing soldiers back to the trenches.[91] Representatives of academic psychiatry answered in like manner, calling into question both the effectiveness of psychoanalysis as a therapy and Freud's qualification as an expert witness on 'war neuroses'. Even Otto Pötzl (1877–1962)—then an assistant at the university clinic and a member of the Vienna Psychoanalytic Society—sided with Wagner-Jauregg and declared that psychoanalysis was of no use in military psychiatry, even if he was 'an absolute supporter of this method in theory'.[92]

After Wagner-Jauregg's retirement, the University of Vienna remained a stronghold of neuropsychiatry. Neurology and psychiatry were seen as two sides of the same coin, and until 1965, the principal lectures in both fields were held by the same chair. Only in the early 1970s was the old university clinic split into a neurological and a psychiatric clinic.[93] However, local traditions alone could not prevent psychoanalysis from taking root. Many members of the younger generation of psychiatrists and neurologists were interested in psychoanalysis, attended Freud's lectures, and tried to include psychoanalytic methods in their own work. During the inter-war period, several avowed psychoanalysts were part of the university clinic's non-professorial staff, among them some of Freud's closest and most prolific followers. This led to the paradoxical situation that academic psychiatry and psychoanalysis remained strictly separated as disciplines, even as individual physicians could walk on both sides of the divide.

A prominent example for these double affiliations was Paul Schilder (1886–1940), one of Erwin Stransky's most avid students before the war, and a member of the clinic's staff since 1918. Schilder was a dedicated psychoanalyst—Stransky considered him a psychoanalytic 'fanatic'[94]—seeking to combine neuropsychiatric, psychoanalytic, and depth-psychological perspectives. However, even though Schilder had his own, considerable group of followers at the clinic, his open advocacy for psychoanalysis was not well received. While Schilder became an extraordinary professor in 1925, Wagner-Jauregg refused to appoint him as his assistant and chief physician.

This was arguably the main reason why Schilder left the clinic in 1928 and continued his career in the United States after 1930, where he became one the key figures in the introduction of psychoanalysis to American psychiatry.[95]

As Schilder's case illustrates, the fact that psychoanalysis was unable to leave a mark at the Vienna medical school cannot be ascribed to the prevalence of neuropsychiatry alone. It was also a result of the hierarchical and highly centralised structure of Austrian universities in the early twentieth century and of the Vienna university clinic in particular. Decisions about teaching, training, and organisational issues rested in the hands of the chair holder, and his subordinates had few possibilities to change the clinic's scientific profile without his formal or informal consent.[96] Julius Wagner-Jauregg did not actively discourage or suppress psychoanalytic ideas among his staff and his students, but he would not acknowledge psychoanalysis as a worthy alternative or an addition to conventional neuropsychiatry, and continued to enforce a clear separation between the two approaches.

Psychoanalysis was tolerated—on condition that it remained a private pursuit and did not impinge on everyday medical practice. No psychoanalytical habilitation would have been accepted at the university clinic, and, for that matter, no individual psychological habilitation either, as Alfred Adler found out in 1915 when Wagner-Jauregg rejected his application for failing to meet scientific requirements and because it would not be desirable that his theories be taught at the medical faculty.[97] Under these circumstances, there was little chance for psychoanalysis to gain recognition as a specialised field in psychiatry.[98] Things changed a little when Otto Pötzl succeeded Wagner-Jauregg in 1928. Pötzl was a member of the Vienna Psychoanalytical Society from 1917 to 1933, and although he was mostly interested in neuropsychology, he was more sympathetic towards psychoanalysis than Wagner-Jauregg had ever been.[99] And yet, Pötzl did little to overcome the institutional separation of psychiatry and psychoanalysis.

However, the fact that most psychiatrists rejected Freud's ideas does not explain why they did so. There was more than reason, and not all of them were purely medical or scientific. Most importantly, psychoanalysis questioned two of the major premises of German psychiatry, in terms of both nosology and aetiology. Neither did it accept the idea that mental illness and mental health were discrete states that could be clearly distinguished, nor the claim that all mental illness necessarily was based on a physical substratum. But these were not the only reasons. Nationalism and anti-Semitism, and the competition between different types of psychotherapy played a role, as well as, as Hannah Decker has pointed out, the sometimes-provocative behaviour of the psychoanalysts themselves. The most fierce and emotional attacks against psychoanalysis usually had to do with the weight that Freudian theory placed on sexuality. A minority of psychiatrists were in fact scandalised by the psychoanalytic view of sexuality, while the majority (among them Stransky) thought that, while sexuality certainly mattered, Freud had clearly 'overshot the mark'.[100] Many, like the conservative psychotherapist Heinrich Kogerer, were ready to accept individual parts of the psychoanalytic theory, but did not consider it useful as a therapeutic method. As Kogerer argued, the insights of psychoanalysis had been of great value to psychotherapy but its methods of treatment were contraindicated in most cases.[101] The 'heedless stirring-up' of the deeper layers of the psyche, Kogerer claimed, might not only be dangerous to the patient, but also to the therapists themselves.[102]

Often, the psychiatric rejection of psychoanalysis was far from absolute. Psychiatrists adopted specific aspects of psychoanalysis (like the significance of dreams and the unconscious, or the psychological aetiology of neuroses) while rejecting others (like the pivotal role of sexuality and Freud's concept of libido). To Freud and his followers, for whom psychoanalysis was a coherent system in theory and practice in which all parts were necessarily interrelated, this piecemeal appropriation was evidently unacceptable.[103] Together with psychoanalysts' tendency to dismiss critical reactions to psychoanalysis as 'emotional resistance', and Freud's notorious unwillingness to engage in debates with his critics, this mindset may have contributed to alienating some physicians who otherwise would have approached psychoanalysis on better terms.[104]

The Association for Applied Psychopathology and Psychology

The Association for Applied Psychopathology and Psychiatry (*Verein für angewandte Psychopathologie und Psychologie*) was registered on 19 January 1920 in Vienna by Erwin Stransky and his colleague Bernhard Dattner. The association's aim was to foster research into 'the laws and experiences of scientific psychopathology and psychology, which pertain to mental processes in the life of individuals and of society, in history, and in cultural history'. What before had been an informal circle of 'physicians, jurists, and philosophers' who had gathered around Stransky and his idea of applied psychiatry now became an association that would remain an active part of intellectual life in Vienna until its dissolution in June 1939.[105] Many of its members and participants were recruited from the staff of Julius Wagner-Jauregg's clinic, but over the years, many non-psychiatrists became involved, too. It was this interdisciplinarity that set the association apart from a variety of medical and scientific organisations in inter-war Vienna and was the basis for its success. Less than three months after it was founded, the association had already about fifty members.[106] Over the following two decades, numerous lectures, seminars, and an international conference were organised by the association and many prominent psychiatrists, neurologists, psychoanalysts, psychologists, and scholars from other disciplines participated in its activities.

When one compares the association's founding statutes with Stransky's programmatic articles, three aspects are conspicuously absent. First, the association's statutes and its later proceedings cautiously avoided endorsing any political views. In stark contrast to Stransky's contemporaneous and later writings, the statutes contained neither any calls for the 'mental reconstruction of the German people' nor any commitment to pan-German nationalism. Second, the statutes spoke of no intention to conduct any of the socio-medical interventions for which Stransky had emphatically pressed in most of his writings of the immediate post-war period. Instead, the association was supposed to foster the extension and 'application' of psychopathological expertise on a scientific stage.[107] And third, while Stransky's vision of applied psychiatry had also entailed 'power politics' of the psychiatric profession, the association avoided this kind of rhetoric. In fact, membership was not limited to psychiatrists or physicians and, although those were in the majority, members of other disciplines joined in from the beginning. While Stransky was dreaming of 'medical imperialism' to remake society, the association's modest goal was to explore the social and political explanatory value of psychopathological concepts and to popularise them among scholars from other disciplines.[108]

The association's choice of honorary members told a similar story. Initially, this honour was bestowed on three scholars, attaching the association to the most prestigious names in Austrian and German neuropsychiatry: Julius Wagner-Jauregg, Heinrich Obersteiner, and Emil Kraepelin. On 14 April 1920, the members of the association added another five scholars to the list: Sigmund Freud, Robert Sommer, Gustav Aschaffenburg, Eugen Bleuler, and Walter Morgenthaler. Each of these names sent a different message positioning the association inside the psy-ences. Aschaffenburg was a leading authority in forensic psychiatry and psychiatric criminology, and

Sommer had established himself as a proponent of psychiatric prophylaxis; in the mid-1920s, he became the founder of the mental hygiene movement in Germany. While the story of Sommer and the German Association for Mental Hygiene will be told in the following chapters, it is notable that Stransky and Sommer were already connected before both of them became involved in the respective national committees of the international movement. Bleuler's name connected the association to Swiss psychiatry, as did Walter Morgenthaler's. The choice of Freud, who most likely never attended any meeting of the association, was not only meant to celebrate his achievements for applied psychopathology and psychology, which 'friend and foe equally must acknowledge', but also to present the association as a neutral and open ground amid the conflicts between the different psy-ences in inter-war Vienna.[109]

The association's political neutrality was a way not to scare away those who had other political or scientific views. Some years later, Erwin Stransky would even agree to step back as president of the association in favour of Martin Pappenheim for the same reason. But more importantly, despite Stransky's pivotal role in the creation of the association, he was not the only one involved. Others did not fully share his views and the contrast between his strongly political publications and the conspicuously neutral orientation of the association was the outcome of a tacit compromise. But if they did not agree with key aspects of Stransky's psycho-political agenda, for what reasons did others join an association that was unmistakably based on his ideas? To answer this question, it is worthwhile to take a closer look at the two most important collaborators in the founding phase of the Association for Applied Psychopathology and Psychology: Bernhard Dattner (1887–1952) and Gaston Roffenstein (1882–1927).[110]

In some respects, the biographies of Dattner and Roffenstein are strikingly similar. They were about the same age, both of Jewish origin, and had a primary background in a non-medical discipline, Dattner as jurist, Roffenstein as actuary. But more surprisingly, both had been promising young members of the Vienna Psychoanalytic Society prior to the First World War, and both had left the society around the same time in early 1914. At this time, three years had passed since Alfred Adler's secession from the Freudian circle and the reasons for Dattner and Roffenstein's break with psychoanalysis remain unclear. Most likely, it was disillusionment with psychoanalysis that led them to independently abandon the society. In 1919, both reappear as followers of Stransky and applied psychopathology. Again, one can only guess about what led them there. Despite Stransky's aggressive polemics and pan-German nationalism, he may have offered them a framework for interdisciplinary discussion and exchange that was more open than what the Freudians had to offer.

Ten years younger than Stransky, Dattner had only just finished his doctorate in medicine when he participated in the founding of the Association for Applied Psychopathology and Psychology in early 1920. Before becoming a physician, Dattner had already graduated in law. It was during his time as a law student that he became interested in psychoanalysis, first as an auditor in Sigmund Freud's lecture in 1910/1911, and from February 1911 as a member of the Vienna Psychoanalytic Society. Dattner was a productive and active member of the society; he presented a paper on 'psychoanalytic problems in Dostoyevsky's Raskolnikov', participated in the society's debate about onanism, and published two articles in the *Zentralblatt für Psychoanalyse*. Yet, he soon became estranged with psychoanalysis and left the society in May 1914.[111]

Around the same time, Dattner began his medical studies and encountered Stransky, who was appointed as an associate professor in early 1915.[112] Following his second doctorate in June 1919, he joined Julius Wagner-Jauregg's clinic as an assistant, specialising in neurology and participating in Wagner-Jauregg's groundbreaking research on the malaria therapy of neurosyphilis in the 1920s.[113] As Stransky remembered, Wagner-Jauregg held Dattner in high esteem and was ready to support his habilitation, unlike his successor Otto Pötzl, who personally disliked Dattner.[114] This may have been the reason that led him to open a private practice parallel to his position at the university clinic in the second half of the 1920s. During the same period, the relationship with Stransky turned sour and Dattner gradually retreated from the activities of the association.[115]

Dattner's medical career in Vienna came to a sudden end with the annexation of Austria in March 1938. As a Jew, he was disenfranchised and persecuted by the Nazis and, like many other 'thirty-eighters', emigrated from Vienna to New York.[116] His career in the United States was relatively successful. From 1943 to 1947, he was an associate professor of neurology at the New York University School of Medicine, after 1945 he worked at the Montefiore and Bellevue hospitals. And like many others involved in the psycho-political projects of the period after the First World War, he continued to be involved in public health, serving as an expert for the World Health Organization, the New York State Department of Health, and the US Public Health Service. Bernhard Dattner died in New York on 11 August 1952.[117]

Little is known about Gaston Roffenstein, who was born as Rosenstein but changed his surname after the First World War. Born in the Austro-Hungarian port city Trieste in 1882, his parents were Jews from Northern Germany. He quit the Jewish community in 1904 without joining another religion, and the name change likely was a belated attempt to distance himself from his origins by getting rid of the Jewish-sounding name Rosenstein.[118] He completed his studies as actuary at the Vienna Technical University in 1902 and was employed as a mathematician by the Gisela-Verein insurance company in the following years. During the same time, he also was secretary for a district *Volksheim* ('people's home') affiliated with the labour movement.[119] Although he published extensively and completed a doctorate in philosophy in 1920, Roffenstein's academic career was hardly successful. After his doctorate, he became a 'psycho-technic' vocational counsellor for the Vienna municipality in the 1920s. According to Stransky, Roffenstein had almost completed a postdoctoral thesis in philosophy and would have had good chances of being appointed as a professor soon. On 7 September 1927, however, Roffenstein was struck by a car while getting on a streetcar and died aged forty-five.[120]

Like Dattner, Roffenstein's came to applied psychopathology via psychoanalysis. In December 1910, he had joined the Vienna Psychoanalytic Society, where he participated in almost all meetings of the society in the following years. He published several articles and thirty reviews in the *Zentralblatt für Psychoanalyse* and the psychoanalytic yearbook.[121] Sigmund Freud apparently had a good opinion of Roffenstein, whom he described as a 'good mind, mathematician by profession, philosopher, etc.' in a letter to Carl Jung.[122]

During this time, Roffenstein made his mark as a theoretician of psychopathology for the first time. In 1912, Arthur Kronfeld, who would later become the most resolute adversary of applied psychiatry, published an extensive and widely read article scrutinising psychoanalysis from an epistemological perspective.[123] An alarmed Freud wrote to Jung that '[none] of the recent critiques has made more impression than Kronfeld's'. While Jung opined that 'Kronfeld is an arrogant gasbag who in my view doesn't even deserve refuting', Freud wanted a reply nevertheless.[124] As a member of the Vienna Psychoanalytic Society, it was Roffenstein who took on the task of defending psychoanalysis and to 'refute this shamelessly prejudiced paper in detail' (Freud)[125] with an elaborate riposte in the psychoanalytic yearbook.[126]

Freud and Jung were highly pleased with the 'excellent' result, although Freud had to admit that some 'things in it are of course no more intelligible to me than Kronfeld's attack, because I do not know the jargon'.[127] This was a promising beginning, and yet, Roffenstein's affiliation with psychoanalysis did not last. After 1913, his attendance at the meetings of the Vienna Psychoanalytic Society became rarer and ceased entirely in February 1914.[128] As Stransky claimed, 'Roffenstein was too independent and critical to be under the spell of any specific doctrine'.[129] In fact, Freud and the Vienna Psychoanalytic Society would probably not have welcomed the methodological eclecticism that came to characterise his later works.

Upon turning his back on psychoanalysis, Roffenstein continued his occupation with psychology and psychopathology. But unlike Dattner, he did not want to become a medical practitioner. Instead, he began a career in sociology, completing his philosophical doctorate at the University of Vienna with a dissertation about 'the sociological problem of equality' in 1920, although the authors of the faculty report cordially disliked that his approach was clearly influenced by psychoanalysis and Adlerian individual psychology.[130] This interest in the border areas between the psy-ences and sociology dominated Roffenstein's work and led him to join Stransky's circle as a founder and board member of the Association for Applied Psychopathology and Psychology. Stransky was full of praise; as he saw it, without being a clinical practitioner Roffenstein had penetrated the field of psychology and psychopathology like few others, in the association 'he was one of the leading thinkers, and in many regards even the leading one'.[131]

It was Roffenstein, not Stransky, who officially opened the association's scientific programme with a first lecture on 4 February 1920. This lecture on the 'psychology and psychopathology of contemporary history', which became the fourth volume of Walter Morgenthaler's Studies in Applied Psychiatry, showed that Roffenstein, despite his key role in the institutionalisation of applied psychiatry and his loyalty to the concept and the programme, was an thinker in his own right. Both politically and scientifically, Roffenstein went his own way. He never shared Stransky's staunch pan-German nationalism but held moderate left-wing views instead. He expressly opposed 'aggressive nationalism' and anti-Semitism and called for a 'reformed Marxism' that would overcome any materialist reductionism and would be able to approach sociological questions through 'multi-dimensional diagnosis'.[132]

Stransky was aware of the difference between his and Roffenstein's political opinion, and in the preface to the 1921 publication of the opening talk, he expressly cautioned against the 'less desirable political conclusions' that readers might come to.[133] Yet, he also stressed its importance to applied psychiatry and pressed for its publication. He had encouraged Roffenstein to publish the talk in the first place and had probably helped him in preparing the manuscript.[134] Despite what he considered Roffenstein's 'pessimism', he hoped that his ideas might also provide new ways for 'future prophylaxis and hygiene in social life'.[135]

However, Stransky probably underestimated the differences. Although he continued to use the concept of applied psychopathology until his untimely death in 1927, Roffenstein's understanding of the nature of psychiatry and psychology had little to do with Stransky's clinical pragmatism.[136] While Stransky vehemently rejected any philosophical tendency in psychiatry and attacked Arthur Kronfeld, Karl Jaspers, Karl Birnbaum, and others on various occasions, Roffenstein shared neither his views nor his enmities. He declared that he 'wholeheartedly' rejected that psychology should be understood as part of the natural sciences,[137] published two books in a series edited by Kronfeld and sided with him in a debate about the epistemological orientation of the psy-ences—despite Kronfeld's criticism of applied psychiatry and his own differences with Kronfeld about psychoanalysis before the war. Different from what Stransky's temper might give reason to expect, these political and scientific differences did not cause any personal conflict between the founders of the association. Behind Stransky's abrasive polemics against other psychiatric and psychological schools, scientific differences often mattered less than personal sympathies. And from the beginning, the association tried to reach out across the divides separating scholars in the psy-ences.

One of the first activities of the newly founded Association for Applied Psychopathology and Psychology was a meeting about psychoanalysis on 26 April 1920.[138] Stransky claimed that this 'serious, critical, and nonetheless dispassionate debate on the topic of psychoanalysis' was the first event of its kind to take place in the 'complex-laden atmosphere of Vienna'. He had high hopes in the meeting: 'Both sides – and the psychoanalysts in particular – have to come out of their [ivory] towers! [...] In the mutual complementarity of all schools lies the true progress'.[139] For this aim, the organisers had gathered a remarkable group of discussants, including the association's founders Stransky, Dattner, and Roffenstein, the prominent psychoanalysts Paul Federn, Paul Schilder, Eduard Hitschmann, Otto Pötzl, and Josef Karl Friedjung (1871–1946),[140] but also the fanatic anti-Semite Arthur Trebitsch (1880–1927).

The introductory lecture was given by Rudolf Allers (1883–1963), a key figure in inter-war period psychotherapy. At this time, Allers was a former psychoanalyst who had since joined the individual psychologists around Alfred Adler.[141] In 1927, he would also abandon this school following a political disagreement with Adler and his left-wing followers. After falling out with Adler, Allers, who was a Jewish-born convert to Catholicism, embraced religion. Recognising the Adlerian concept of community in medieval Christianity, he propagated an approach to psychotherapy based on the patient's submission under Catholic dogma.[142]

Allers referred neither to Adler nor to Catholicism but criticised psychoanalysis from an epistemological perspective, similar to what Arthur Kronfeld had done before the war. As he pointed out at the start, the clinical practice of psychoanalytic therapy was of no concern to his argument, as neither the failure nor the success of a therapeutic method could conclusively prove or disprove it. The only way to thoroughly examine a theory like psychoanalysis was to scrutinise its intrinsic argumentation for logical coherence. And from this perspective, he came to a withering judgement. Pointing out three fallacies of *petitio principii*, Allers concluded that the concepts of at the core of psychoanalytic theory—resistance, determination, and the meaningfulness of free association—were based on a kind of reasoning that presupposed the whole of the theory that it claimed to constitute. And if psychoanalysis was based on faulty reasoning, it had to be dismissed as a theory. However, Allers not only accused psychoanalysis of being based on logical fallacies, he also criticised its rationalising approach. Pessimistic about the possibilities of psychological analysis and treatment, he claimed that 'every living thing, including the soul, is essentially unanalysable'.[143]

Allers's epistemological attack against some of the cornerstones of Freudian theory triggered a heated discussion that revolved around two questions: Whether psychoanalysis provided a sound scientific method and what the relationship between psychoanalysis and academic psychiatry should be. The contenders of psychoanalysis, namely Paul Schilder, Paul Federn, Eduard Hitschmann, Otto Pötzl, and Martin Pappenheim, verbosely defended Freud's ideas against Allers's criticism and rejected both his approach and his conclusions. As the most vocal representative of the Freudian camp, Hitschmann, confidently declared, psychoanalysis was not on the defensive, but still had ground to gain. Ultimately, psychopathology as a science would not have to be complemented, but fully based on psychoanalytic principles: 'Psychopathology will either be understanding, that is: psychoanalytic, or it will – not be!' And he concluded: 'The triumph of psychoanalysis can no longer be stopped!'.[144]

On the opposite end of the debate stood Arthur Trebitsch, an outsider at the meeting. Unlike other participants, he was neither a physician nor a psychotherapist. Instead, Trebitsch, a prolific publicist, owed his reputation to the fact that he was probably the most fanatic anti-Semite that early twentieth-century Vienna could muster.[145] In his attack against psychoanalysis, which was by far the most aggressive at the meeting, he did not dwell on epistemology or therapeutic effectiveness, but claimed that the debate on psychoanalysis had, first and foremost, to be a debate about race. As Trebitsch alleged, Freudian psychoanalysis was an expression of deviant Jewish sexuality that had nothing to say about the mental life of non-Jews.[146]

Trebitsch's views were outside of the consensus at the meeting. Nevertheless, only Erwin Stransky came forward with a response, and it was anything but an unequivocal repudiation. He called Trebitsch's statement 'remarkable', but demurred that his ideas were certainly not universally valid, as the example of 'the large Swiss psychoanalytic school and its racial composition' showed. As the further history of psychotherapy in the twentieth century shows, Trebitsch anticipated views that would gain ground after the Nazis came to power in Germany in 1933. In the 1930s, the leading representative of the 'large Swiss psychoanalytic school' Carl Gustav Jung, as well as Erwin Stransky himself, among many others, would declare that racial differences between Jews and non-Jews also implied significant psychological differences that were an obstacle to psychoanalysis' claims to universality.[147]

Regarding the relationship between psychiatry and psychoanalysis, positions at the 1920 meeting diverged strongly. Hitschmann gave a particularly radical outlook on the future of psychoanalysis in psychopathology that was certainly not shared by all participants. Bernhard Dattner and Gaston Roffenstein, who were both former members of the Vienna Psychoanalytic Society, tried to formulate a mediating position, 'without the absolute rejection of most academic psychiatrists, without the fanatic belief of the psychoanalysts' (Roffenstein).[148] Erwin Stransky positioned himself in like manner. Although he agreed with much of Allers's epistemological criticism, he also acknowledged some important contributions of psychoanalysis to psychopathology, such as the idea of varying quantities of energy in emotional life, and—closer to actual psychoanalytic theory—the concept of sublimation. Psychoanalysis, he argued, had been an excessive but necessary and valuable reaction to the shortcomings of academic psychiatry. Psychoanalysis overrated the role of psychology and sexuality, but this was only possible because psychiatry had underrated them. Psychiatrists and psychoanalysts, Stransky believed, had much to learn from each other, and he was also ready to accept psychoanalysis 'on the full-worthy place in the realm of psychopathology and psychology, on which, as a valuable tool for the understanding of the human mind, it has every right'.[149] For a self-declared opponent of psychoanalysis, this was a rather diplomatic stance. However, Stransky's opinion about psychoanalysis would change soon, and political and personal factors were to play a significant role.

Only a few months after the 1920 meeting, the struggle between psychoanalysis and academic psychiatry continued on a more public stage. As has already been mentioned, public accusations of having mistreated 'hysterical' soldiers during the war led to an inquiry against Julius Wagner-Jauregg, with Sigmund Freud as a leading expert witness. Unsurprisingly, these hearings, which took place on 14 and 16 October 1920, came to revolve around the conflict between psychoanalysis and academic neuropsychiatry. Profoundly scandalised by the accusations against his superior, Stransky published a defence of Julius Wagner-Jauregg in the Vienna medical weekly and included a harsh critique of psychoanalysis.[150] This time, his criticism was not about scientific validity or therapeutic effectiveness, but about the role of medicine in society. As the question of military psychiatry was concerned, Stransky opined that psychoanalysis was not the proper method. Psychoanalytic therapy had to dwell on individual cases, while military physicians had to treat patients quickly, efficiently, and en masse.

The mass treatment of military psychiatry became the model for civilian psychotherapy as Stransky shifted the focus from the individual to the mental health of the collective. In this perspective, the public attacks against Wagner-Jauregg and psychoanalysts' repudiation of psychiatry's wartime methods were misguided and harmful to public health. Even more so, Stransky saw the accusations against Wagner-Jauregg as expressions of anti-medical prejudice firmly embedded in an effeminate, aestheticising and decadent worldview, which would culminate in the celebration of a right to antisocial neurosis and sickness. Juxtaposing egocentrism, hysteria, and the 'unhealthy aestheticism' of the Paris Salpêtrière to 'Nordic rigor', Stransky used the inquiry against Wagner-Jauregg to deliver a broadside of cultural criticism; promoting 'Nordic'—that is, Prussian and Protestant—rigour against the Frenchifying decadence of Catholic Vienna.

Building on his vision of the psychiatrist as a socio-political expert and his idea of the psychotherapist as a strict pedagogical leader, Stransky claimed that the public ideal of a gentle and caring physician was nothing but an expression of decadent 'pseudo-humanity'. Instead, the 'good man and physician' had to be unrelenting and forceful to heal and had to find self-evident the submission of the individual under the demands of society. Stransky's criticism of psychoanalysis was based on the idea of an authoritative physician devoted to the welfare of the body politic. Instead of merely engaging in the 'introspective dissolution' of the psyche, mental treatment would have to serve the 'organising therapeutic integration' of the neurotic individual into an organic community. The allegation that psychoanalysis had a corrosive effect on the cohesion of the national community became a recurring motive of Stransky's anti-psychoanalytic polemics even into the 1960s, with obvious anti-Semitic undertones.

Despite these ideological attacks against psychoanalysis, Stransky made one more attempt to reach out to the Freudians in the following year.[151] Replying to a negative review of one of his articles by Eduard Hitschmann, he again called for dialogue and cooperation between psychoanalysis and psychiatry in the Vienna medical weekly. This time, however, his offer was spiked with harsh criticism and betrayed a fairly ambivalent position. Ostensibly, Stransky repeated what he had already proposed in the previous year. Regardless of its scientific shortcomings, he acknowledged that psychoanalysis had every right to claim 'citizenship' in the community of the psy-ences. But more directly than before, he also blamed psychoanalysts for the persistent gap between the different schools. What stood in the way of psychoanalysis' academic acceptance was the comportment of its representatives:

> I want to say it frankly: The psychoanalytic school is, sadly, cultivating a very specific mentality, a mentality of sectarian and fanatic, limitless intolerance that in some cases develops into personal arrogance against anyone who does not confess himself in its favour; to them, psychoanalysis is not one of many, but *the* source of knowledge per se.[152]

In his private correspondence, Stransky's view of the Vienna psychoanalysts was even harsher and outright conspiratorial. Angered that the publisher had refused the proceedings of the 1920 meeting for the Studies in Applied Psychiatry, he complained to Walter Morgenthaler about what he considered the machinations of a sinister clique of malevolent psychoanalysts:

> In short, perhaps I am mistaken, but the impression cannot be shrugged off that a dark cloud is looming once again, because I am on the 'black list' of a certain, very powerful and diverse clique, whose tendency it is to 'finish me off' by hushing me up, by malicious reviews, and by other means, afraid that I eventually might get a chair, something that they try to thwart for different – not only personal – reasons. I hold this clique to be capable of spitting poison through channels which cannot be controlled.[153]

Unsurprisingly, Stransky's resentment against psychoanalysis soon led to conflict. From the beginning on, several psychoanalysts had participated in the seminars of the fledgling Association for Applied Psychopathology and Psychology, and the association had acknowledged them by naming Sigmund Freud and Eugen Bleuler honorary members. But soon, the psychoanalysts began turning their backs on the association and Stransky had to realise that they could not do without them, if they did not want to lose some of their brightest and most active members. The situation exacerbated when some psychoanalysts began to support a competing students' group.[154] Stransky understood that he himself, with his 'never un-objective, but sharp antagonism to the intellectual somersaults and the propaganda methods of the Freudian and Adlerian schools', was among the main reasons for the psychoanalytic exodus. However, he was also convinced that his rejection of the new psychotherapeutic approaches was not the only reason for the enmity that he faced. His psychoanalytic adversaries, he claimed, had found allies among those Jewish colleagues who disliked him for his conversion to Protestantism and accused him of being a 'Jewish anti-Semite' and a 'Nazi'—two reproaches that Stransky emphatically rejected.[155] And indeed, there is every reason to assume that his German-nationalist and anti-Jewish views did not sit well with many left-leaning, Jewish psychoanalysts and individual psychologists. Stransky found himself in an ironic situation. In late 1918, he was forced to leave a pan-German nationalist party for being Jewish; some years later, the problem, as he saw it, was that he was not considered Jewish enough.

To save the association, a radical step became necessary. In the summer of 1927, Stransky resigned as head of the association and left the position to Martin Pappenheim (1881–1943).[156] He remained a member of the association's board and an active participant, but the decisions were from now on made by Pappenheim. The change in management turned out to be successful. The psychoanalysts returned and the association flourished again. In 1930, the association could celebrate its tenth anniversary with a large international conference in Vienna—the 'I. International Conference for Applied Psychopathology and Psychology'.

Martin Pappenheim is almost forgotten today but was an eminent and well-connected figure in the medical and political worlds of inter-war Vienna. During his military service in the First World War, he was prison physician in the fortress Theresienstadt where he attended to the imprisoned Sarajevo assassin Gavrilo Princip (1894–1918).[157] From the second half of the 1920s, Pappenheim became one of three professors of the medical school affiliated with the Freudian school, the other two being Otto Pötzl and Paul Schilder.[158] This double affiliation made him a uniting figure for members of both camps in the Association for Applied Psychopathology and Psychology. For Stransky, this was not the only reason that qualified him as his successor. 'Influential circles', he wrote, had not only tried to obstruct the association because of the conflict between academic psychiatry and psychoanalysis, but also due to Stransky's political convictions and his rejection of his Jewish origins. Pappenheim as an 'emphatic Jew and a warm friend of psychoanalysis', Stransky believed, had a 'vastly better "press"' than he.[159]

Concerning Pappenheim's relation to psychoanalysis, Stransky was certainly right. Pappenheim had attended his first meeting of the Vienna Psychoanalytic Society in 1912, beginning a gradual rapprochement with psychoanalysis. In the 1920 debate, he had cautiously positioned himself in favour of psychoanalysis, but also declared that he was neither a member of the circle around Freud, nor agreed with psychoanalytic theory in its entirety.[160] Later in the 1920s, Pappenheim moved closer to the psychoanalytic establishment in Vienna as he became a frequent guest of the Freud and a full member of the Vienna Psychoanalytic Society in 1928.[161] After his emigration to Palestine, Pappenheim was one of the eminent psychoanalysts in the Yishuv, counting among his patients the first mayor of Tel Aviv, Meir Dizengoff (1861–1936) and the Hebrew poet Hayim Nahman Bialik (1873–1934).[162]

Yet, despite Pappenheim's emigration to Palestine in 1934, at a time when Jews in Austria did not yet face state persecution, he was not an 'emphatic Jew' as Stransky claimed. Stransky later described Pappenheim's emigration as the return of a religious Jew to the 'land of his fathers' in anticipation of 'the onslaught of Hitlerism'.[163] There are, however, good reasons to be sceptical about this account. Pappenheim's anticipation of the annexation of Austria in 1934 would have been an unlikely feat of historical clairvoyance. Moreover, Stransky's account is contradicted by the memoirs of Martin Pappenheim's daughter of the first marriage, the psychoanalyst Else Pappenheim (1911–2009), who remembered that her father grew up in a non-observant family and was anything but a religious Jew. After his arrival in Palestine, he frequently complained about the importance of religion in the Yishuv in his letters to his friend Karl Grosz.[164] Moreover, Pappenheim did not consider himself Jewish in political terms and was never part of the Zionist movement.[165] For his first marriage in 1908, Pappenheim converted to Protestantism—as being without denomination and civil marriage were no options in the Habsburg Empire, his daughter would later argue, Protestantism had just been the 'next best thing to atheism'.[166] Before his second marriage in 1918, and under changed political circumstances, he finally could rid himself of any religious denomination.[167]

The weight that Stransky's placed on Pappenheim's Jewishness conceals a different story. Instead of a religious Jew or a secular Zionist, Pappenheim was a socialist and an eminent representative of the Freudian left. From September 1920, he had spent a year on a study tour through post-revolutionary Soviet Russia and Ukraine, where he visited numerous clinics and hospitals, among them some newly founded psychoanalytic institutions, and made the acquaintance of the eminent Russian neurologist Vladimir Bekhterev.[168] After returning to Vienna in autumn 1921, Pappenheim spoke very positively about his experiences, and while he acknowledged manifold problems, he also highlighted the 'good will' of the Soviet authorities to improve public health as much as possible under the present circumstances.[169] In the following years, he was an active social democrat, well-connected with the party leadership and worked for the city government of Red Vienna.[170] His younger sister, the physician Marie Frischauf (1882–1966), was also politically active on the left. Together with Wilhelm Reich, she founded the Socialist Society for Sexual Counselling and Research in 1928, which operated six sexual counselling offices for workers in Vienna.[171]

His political involvement became the cause for Martin Pappenheim's emigration in 1934. From late 1933, Pappenheim was on a six-month lecture tour in Palestine, from which he intended to return to Austria in February 1934. Shortly before his scheduled return, however, the Austrian Civil War broke out. In Vienna, leading social democrats, many of them friends and acquaintances of Pappenheim were arrested by the triumphant Austro-Fascists. Among others, Otto Bauer (1881–1938), then the deputy chair of the Social Democrats and leading theoretician of Austro-Marxism, warned him not to return to Austria. Pappenheim heeded his advice and stayed in Palestine.[172]

In the beginning, Martin Pappenheim and his third wife, Rose, struggled to adapt to their new life in Tel Aviv, with its unfamiliar climate and a cultural life that was a far cry from Vienna.[173] He nevertheless hoped to make a career in Palestine, and although numerous physicians fleeing from Germany were crowding the job market, the prospects initially seemed good. A new psychiatric hospital was planned in the vicinity of Tel Aviv. As the first professor of neurology to immigrate to Palestine and with his excellent connections to the psychoanalysts and the movement for mental hygiene, Pappenheim was well-positioned to become director of the new institution. He prepared detailed plans for a clinic following the principles of 'open care', and Jewish and British authorities already promised him a position as head of a future medical faculty.[174]

These hopes were, however, quickly dashed. Shortly after his arrival, Pappenheim's renunciation of Judaism and the fact that his immigration was motivated by domestic politics in Austria rather than by Zionist convictions caught up with him. Members of the Vienna Jewish community had informed the authorities in Tel Aviv that Pappenheim had cut his ties to the local community and, moreover, even claimed that Pappenheim considered leaving Palestine for Soviet Russia. Consequently, the city authorities of Tel Aviv broke off negotiations with Pappenheim and declared in an open letter in the Zionist journal *Die Neue Welt* that they refused to work with people who 'are considered to be traitors to our people'.[175] Although he neither became director of the clinic nor received the promised professorship, Pappenheim remained in Palestine, where he died in the autumn of 1943.[176]

Why did Stransky chose to see Martin Pappenheim as a deeply religious Jew instead of the secular socialist he actually was? As a long-time colleague of Pappenheim at the medical faculty, he presumably knew better. Notably, he had acted in a similar way in 1927 when his obituary for Gaston Roffenstein omitted the fact that his closest collaborator in the early days of applied psychiatry had been involved with the Vienna social democrats.[177] Politics and Jewishness were both emotional topics for Stransky. And while he apparently had difficulties to acknowledge that the political views of his two closest collaborators in the Association for Applied Psychopathology and Psychology were at odds with his own, the narrative of Martin Pappenheim as a profoundly Jewish psychoanalyst must have fitted his worldview better—regardless of the fact that, while many early psychoanalysts were indeed Jews, none of them were deeply religious.[178]

The International Conference for Applied Psychopathology in 1930

Under the leadership of Martin Pappenheim the Association for Applied Psychopathology and Psychology experienced its heyday. Like mental hygiene, applied psychopathology reached its apogee with an international conference held in 1930. Just one month after the congress in Washington, DC in early May, the adherents of applied psychopathology gathered for a three-day conference in Vienna.[179] Despite the similar-sounding name, the I. International Conference for Applied Psychopathology could match neither the size nor the internationality of the mental hygiene congress. With a very few exceptions, 'international' here meant the German-speaking countries. Nevertheless, it became a singular event in the history of the psy-ences in the inter-war period; singular because the 'permanence committee' created after the model of the International Committee for Mental Hygiene failed to convene a second conference, but also because it was a uniquely interdisciplinary meeting that brought together an astonishingly diverse group of participants.

This diversity had already been a hallmark of the association even before Stransky proposed that its tenth anniversary should be celebrated with a large-scale conference.[180] In a decade, applied psychopathology had come a long way from Stransky's aggressive psycho-political expansionism in the aftermath of the First World War and was now the elusive approach of an association serving as a neutral meeting ground for adherents of different psy-ences. Throughout the 1920s, psychoanalysis played a far larger role than Stransky would have expected and liked. The same was also true for the organising committee preparing the 1930 conference. After Martin Pappenheim had keenly picked up Stransky's proposal, he enlisted the help of three colleagues—Karl Grosz, Gottfried Engerth, and Heinz Hartmann.[181]

Of these names, the last one is particularly noteworthy, as Heinz Hartmann (1894–1970) was about to become one of the key figures in the history of psychoanalysis.[182] The son of a history professor, who from 1918 to 1920 served as Austrian ambassador to Germany, Heinz Hartmann came from a well-to-do Viennese family with good political relations. After his medical studies, he joined the psychiatric clinic of Julius Wagner-Jauregg as an assistant—a position that he would keep until 1934. Through the influence of Paul Schilder, Hartmann became interested in psychoanalysis. In 1925, he became an associate member of the Vienna Psychoanalytic Society, in 1927, after undergoing training analysis with Sándor Radó (1890–1972) in Berlin, he was accepted as a regular member. By the time of the I. International Conference on Applied Psychopathology, he was the author of a psychoanalytic textbook and among the rising stars of the psychoanalytic community. In 1934 however, Hartmann was forced out of his position at the university clinic after the rise of the Austro-Fascists and had to flee the country in 1938. Via France and Switzerland, he arrived in the United States in 1941, where he became one of the most eminent psychoanalysts of the post-war period. Hartmann's Neo-Freudian 'ego-psychology' was the dominant paradigm in American psychoanalysis for decades to come—to the point that this time was later called the 'Hartmann era'.[183]

By including Hartmann in the organising committee, Pappenheim shifted the association further towards psychoanalysis. However, as the proceedings show, the interdisciplinary of the conference went beyond the question of psychoanalysis versus academic psychiatry.[184] The elusive idea that the knowledge generated by the psy-ences could and should be applied to society brought together eminent German-speaking scholars from diverse fields such as psychoanalysis (Paul Federn, Heinz Hartmann, Martin Pappenheim, and Eduard Hitschmann), independent psychotherapy (Rudolf Allers, Heinrich Kogerer, Johannes Heinrich Schulz, and Hans Prinzhorn), psychology (Karl Bühler and Julius Suter), theology (Karl Beth), medical history (Henry E. Sigerist), psychiatric genetics (Hans Luxenburger), and law (Siegfried Türkel). The announcement of the conference in the Vienna medical weekly also included the names of other prominent scholars who apparently did not attend, such as Robert Gaupp, Willy Hellpach, Kurt Goldstein, and Arthur Kronfeld.

But what did applied psychopathology mean in 1930? In his opening address, Martin Pappenheim struggled to piece together an overarching definition from different sources, one of which was psychoanalysis: 'Applied psychiatry and psychopathology in the present-day sense – the concept and the term were introduced and developed as a programme by Stransky – cannot be conceived without the work of Freud'.[185] Pappenheim listed the names of a number of scholars, many of them present at the conference, who in one way or another had applied the concepts of psychopathology to topics beyond the traditional boundaries of medicine. While Pappenheim was unclear about the definition of applied psychopathology, he was also ambiguous about its scope. On the one hand, he renounced the 'medical imperialism' of Stransky that sought to conquer territory from adjacent disciplines:

> As important as applied psychopathology is, we should not overstretch its ambit. We should beware of encroaching on foreign territory, because it would be a mistake to try to explain human life from our position alone. Rather, we have to be aware that other sciences, let us take the example of sociology, gain their insights through methods that are strange to psychopathology, and that psychopathology in these sciences can only gain insights inside its determined boundaries.[186]

On the other hand, Pappenheim believed that applied psychopathology had a mission. It would allow to bring together different scholars to create 'the complete knowledge of the human soul'. As one of the 'distinctive cultural movements of our time', applied psychopathology would create a circle of people interested in mental life and stimulate their research. However, despite his own involvement with the movement for mental hygiene, and in sharp contrast to Stransky, Pappenheim's idea of an 'application' of psychopathology was limited to an intellectual endeavour and did not extend to treating and remaking society.

Talking about 'psychopathology and contemporary civilisation', Stransky took the opposite position.[187] Using many of the common tropes of conservative cultural criticism, he argued that the emergence of applied psychiatry at the end of the First World War had not only been an answer to growing public interest in psychological and psychopathological questions, but also coincided with a very real increase of psychopathological influences on modern society. Folding together older concepts of 'degeneration' and the post-war debate about the 'revolutionary psychopaths' into a diagnosis of 'modern urban and industrial civilisation', Stransky claimed that mentally abnormal individuals were gaining influence through a culture endorsing their views and mannerisms and through media like the press, radio, and advertisement that spread their pathologies into every corner of society. And this was only one aspect of a broader crisis of modern civilisation, which was also caused by the suspension of natural biological selection through welfare services as well as by pathogenic urban living and working conditions, substance abuse, materialism, the acceleration of social life, and the dissolution of family structures and traditions. Against the backdrop of this alarming scenario, the application of psychopathology to society was not merely a way to better understand some aspects of social life and the human condition, but the first step towards an effective therapy:

> Therefore, applied psychopathology can amply show the sources from which so much of the maladies of our time arise; however, as I see it, with such a purely analytic work, it only partially accomplishes its purpose. The supreme objective of every pathology, also when it is applied psychopathology, is therapy, of which again prophylaxis is often the most important part. As the psychiatrist as an applied psychopathologist sees better and more profoundly where there is good and where there is ill, in the sense of a truly active therapy he should not shy away from becoming a called leader in the best sense of the word, and to purposefully intervene in the system of the lines of desire (*Sehnsuchtsliniensystem*) of our time; even if sometimes it seems like the pathological in it, the pathological influences on it, have already become so overwhelming that they cannot be countered any more.[188]

Which kind of psychopathological knowledge was to be applied, and where the boundaries of this application lay, was a question that remained unresolved during the conference. As the list of participants and lectures shows, there hardly was a consensus about what psychopathology meant. A Viennese psychoanalyst like Paul Federn had an understanding of mental illness and its causation that was very different from the views held by Hans Luxenburger as a geneticist in Ernst Rüdin's department at the German Research Institute for Psychiatry in Munich.[189] The same could, in some way or another, be said about most of the other participants. Bringing together scholars from many divergent backgrounds was a remarkable achievement, but it was also the underlying problem of the I. International Conference on Applied Psychopathology and Psychology.

Rudolf Allers, who had accompanied the activities of the association since 1920, tackled these questions directly. In the aftermath of the conference, he used a report of the meeting to contemplate what its topic actually meant—and to reframe the political metaphors that Stransky liked to use.[190] As Allers saw it, like a political territory dispute, every debate about an emerging 'applied' discipline revolved around three elements: first, one discipline had to have a 'need for expansion' that pushed it into the traditional territory of another discipline; second, the discipline that was to be 'conquered' would try to repel this intrusion; and third, in doing so it would try to expand the range of its own approaches and methods. What had set the conference in Vienna apart was that members of both sides—'conquerors' and 'conquered'—were present and had their say.[191] Allers was pleased that the conference had allowed to delineate the boundaries of the project of applied psychopathology—'downwards' towards biology and 'upwards' towards more intellectual and spiritual ways of thinking. To accept these boundaries was not an externally imposed constraint, but a rational necessity. Repeating Arthur Kronfeld's earlier critique of applied psychopathology, Allers wrote:

> To cross these [boundaries] would not only mean a violation of the new subject area and the eventual failure of such an enterprise, but also—as in a sense the solid ground of independent research is abandoned—a threat to the academy itself. All too ambitious expeditions into foreign lands have often also turned into a catastrophe for the homeland.[192]

Even as the exact definition remained up for discussion, the participants of the conference were convinced that applied psychopathology was a project worth continuing. During the final reception, a 'permanence committee' was tasked with publishing the proceedings and with periodically organising similar meetings in the future. The committee was as international and interdisciplinary as the conference had been. Hartmann, Pappenheim, and Stransky were elected as the committee's 'executive', while the committee included, among others, Paul Federn, Hans Luxenburger, Hans W. Maier, Walter Morgenthaler, and Henry E. Sigerist.[193] Like the Studies in Applied Psychiatry a decade earlier, what had begun as Stransky's personal quest for an aggressive expansion of psychiatry's ambit, once proved again surprisingly capable of integrating highly diverse perspectives and approaches. The 'permanence committee' was, however, more short-lived than its name promised. The conference proceedings were printed in the following year, but the first international congress would be the last.

Erwin Stransky blamed the failure of the 'permanence committee' on the rise of the Nazis in Germany.[194] This analysis was not mistaken. After 1933, the political climate in Germany strongly limited the possibilities for the international cooperation of German scholars, and for meetings with left-wing, Jewish psychoanalysts like Paul Federn and Martin Pappenheim in particular. This was certainly the case for Hans Luxenburger, who was closely connected to the racial hygiene policies of the 'Third Reich'. Another member of the committee, Alfred Hauptmann, a professor of psychiatry at Halle, was forced to emigrate because of his Jewish background.[195] The political changes in Germany were not the only reason why the committee fell apart. After the triumph of Austro-Fascism in early 1934, Martin Pappenheim did not return from Palestine and Heinz Hartmann had to resign from the university clinic—a double blow to the committee and the Association for Applied Psychopathology and Psychology, severing its connection with psychoanalysis.

After Pappenheim's emigration in 1934, Stransky returned to his former position as chair of the association. The task that he assumed was a challenging one. The 1930 conference had given ample reason to hope that applied psychopathology was becoming a vibrant international movement. By contrast, the reality in 1934 was sobering, and with the connection to German psychiatry and to psychoanalysis cut off, applied psychopathology again became a Viennese speciality. Nevertheless, the association continued to be a neutral meeting ground for representatives of the different psy-ences. In the spring of 1934, it became the vehicle for a cooperation between Karl Bühler's psychological institute and Otto Pötzl's psychiatric clinic as they established a 'seminar-like working group' as part of the Association for Applied Psychopathology and Psychology.[196] Over of the next years, the association continued its own programme of lectures, but as the published proceedings in the Vienna medical weekly show, the working group increasingly eclipsed its host organisation.[197] And while the association flourished, without the participation of the psychoanalysts it also lost much of its characteristic profile and its broad understanding of an application of the concepts of psychopathology to all aspects of cultural, social, and political life.

The annexation of Austria by Nazi Germany in 1938 led to another change in the association's leadership. Again, Erwin Stransky resigned from his position as chair. As he wrote in his autobiography, this was the second time that he had to defer to 'save the cause' of applied psychopathology.[198] Stransky was succeeded by Alfred Auersperg (1899–1968), a young psychiatrist and university lecturer from an aristocratic background. Immediately after the Nazis came to power in Vienna, 132 of the 197 professors and lectures of the medical school were forced out for racial reasons and the non-Jewish Auersperg was one of the remaining few.[199] Hans Hoff, who would emigrate from Austria to Iraq in the same year, became the association's last vice chair; after his return from the United States, where he was an associate professor at Columbia University since 1942, he became the central figure of Viennese and Austrian psychiatry well into the 1960s.[200]

This time, however, Stransky's resignation was not enough to save the association. As part of the forcible coordination (*Gleichschaltung*) of all aspects of Nazi society, the Association for Applied Psychopathology and Psychology was abolished and struck from the register in June 1939.[201] This was the end of applied psychopathology as an interdisciplinary project. After the Second World War, Stransky would not re-establish the association, but devote his energy to the reconstruction of the general psychiatric association and the Austrian branch of the mental hygiene movement.[202]

Notes

1. Walter Morgenthaler to Karl Jaspers, 21 March 1922, Walter Morgenthaler papers.
2. Walter Morgenthaler to Erwin Stransky, 10 December 1919, Walter Morgenthaler papers.
3. Erwin Stransky to Walter Morgenthaler, 29 December 1919 (cable), Walter Morgenthaler papers; Erwin Stransky to Walter Morgenthaler, 29 December 1919 (letter), Walter Morgenthaler papers.
4. In 1927, Maier succeeded Bleuler as director of Burghölzli,Vera Koelbing-Waldis, 'Maier, Hans Wolfgang', in *Historisches Lexikon der Schweiz* (Berne, 2008), https://hls-dhs-dss.ch/de/articles/014531/2008-02-27/; Hans W. Maier, 'Zum gegenwärtigen Stand der Frage der Kastration und Sterilisation aus psychiatrischer Indikation', *Zeitschrift für die gesamte Neurologie und Psychiatrie* 98 (1925): 200–19.
5. Karl Jaspers to Walter Morgenthaler, 15 December 1919, Walter Morgenthaler papers. Morgenthaler also tried to persuade Ernst Kretschmer and Karl Bonhoeffer to submit manuscripts for the series, Walter Morgenthaler to Erwin Stransky, 18 October 1921, Walter Morgenthaler papers.
6. Giovanni Stanghelleni and Thomas Fuchs, eds., *One Century of Karl Jaspers' General Psychopathology* (Oxford: Oxford University Press, 2013).
7. Diary 1905/1906, Walter Morgenthaler papers.
8. Heinz Balmer, 'Walter Morgenthaler 1882–1965', *Verhandlungen der Schweizerischen Naturforschenden Gesellschaft* 146 (1966): 227–28; Christian Müller, 'Morgenthaler, Walter', *Historisches Lexikon Der Schweiz*, 2008.
9. Balmer, 'Walter Morgenthaler', 230–34; Oscar Louis Forel, 'Walter Morgenthaler als Pionier der Pflegerausbildung', *Schweizerische Zeitschrift für Psychologie und ihre Anwendungen* 9, no. 1 (1952): 5–10; Eva Knechtle, 'Walter Morgenthaler (1882–1965) als Pionier der Ausbildung des Psychiatrie-Pflegepersonals in der Schweiz' (MD thesis, University of Berne, 1992).

10. Hanns Spreng, 'Zum Geleit', *Schweizerische Zeitschrift für Psychologie und ihre Anwendungen* 9, no. 1 (1952): 1–2.
11. Walter Morgenthaler, *Ein Geisteskranker als Künstler*, Arbeiten zur angewandten Psychiatrie 1 (Berne and Leipzig: Bircher, 1921).
12. Elka Spoerri, *Adolf Wölfli: Draftsman, Writer, Poet, Composer* (Ithaca: Cornell University Press, 1997); Katrin Luchsinger, *Die Vergessenskurve: Werke aus psychiatrischen Kliniken in der Schweiz um 1900: eine kulturanalytische Studie* (Zurich: Chronos, 2016); Hartmut Kraft, *Grenzgänger zwischen Kunst und Psychiatrie*, 3rd ed. (Cologne: Deutscher Ärzte-Verlag, 2005), 195–204; Angela Fink, *Kunst in der Psychiatrie: Verklärt - Verfolgt - Vermarktet* (Vienna and Berlin: LIT, 2012).
13. Hans Prinzhorn, *Bildnerei der Geisteskranken: Ein Beitrag zur Psychologie und Psychologie der Gestaltung* (Berlin: Julius Springer, 1922). The correspondence between Morgenthaler and Jaspers (who, like Prinzhorn, was at the University of Heidelberg) shows the competition between Prinzhorn and Morgenthaler during the time when both books were to be published shortly, Walter Morgenthaler papers.
14. Hermann Rorschach, *Psychodiagnostik: Methodik und Ergebnisse eines wahrnehmungsdiagnostischen Experiments (Deutenlassen von Zufallsformen)*, Arbeiten zur angewandten Psychiatrie 2 (Berne and Leipzig: Bircher, 1921); Walter Morgenthaler, 'Der Kampf um das Erscheinen der Psychodiagnostik: Hermann Rorschach zum 70. Geburtstag (8. November 1954)', *Rorschachiana* 2, no. 3 (1954): 255–62; Naamah Akavia, *Subjectivity in Motion: Life, Art, and Movement in the Work of Hermann Rorschach* (New York and Hove: Routledge, 2013); recently Damion Searls, *The Inkblots: Hermann Rorschach, His Iconic Test, and the Power of Seeing* (New York: Crown, 2017).
15. Balmer, 'Walter Morgenthaler', 229–30.
16. Wilhelm Weygandt, 'Psychohygienische Tagung und Ausstellung in der Schweiz', *Zeitschrift für psychische Hygiene* 4, no. 6 (1931): 182; a reproduction of the frieze by the artist Dora Lauterburg can be found in Walter Morgenthaler, 'Über seelische Hygiene', in *Seelische Hygiene* (Berne: Stämpfli & Cie., 1931), 37–59.
17. Erwin Stransky, *Psychopathologie der Ausnahmezustände und Psychopathologie des Alltags*, Arbeiten zur angewandten Psychiatrie 3 (Berne and Leipzig: Bircher, 1921).
18. Gaston Roffenstein, *Zur Psychologie und Psychopathologie der Gegenwartsgeschichte*, Arbeiten zur angewandten Psychiatrie 4 (Berne and Leipzig: Bircher, 1921).
19. Karl Jaspers, *Strindberg und Van Gogh: Versuch einer pathographischen Analyse unter vergleichender Heranziehung von Swedenborg und Hölderlin*, Arbeiten zur angewandten Psychiatrie 5 (Berne and Leipzig: Bircher,

1922); Matthias Bormuth, 'Karl Jaspers the Pathographer', in *One Century of Karl Jaspers' General Psychopathology*, ed. Giovanni Stanghelleni and Thomas Fuchs (Oxford: Oxford University Press, 2013), 133–49.

20. Hans Zulliger, *Einführung in den Behn-Rorschach-Test*, 2 vols, Arbeiten zur angewandten Psychiatrie 6 (Berne: Huber, 1941).
21. Morgenthaler, *Ein Geisteskranker als Künstler*, unpaginated preface.
22. Karl Jaspers to Walter Morgenthaler, 31 January 1921, Walter Morgenthaler papers.
23. Walter Morgenthaler to Erwin Stransky, 7 February 1921, Walter Morgenthaler papers.
24. Morgenthaler, 'Der Kampf um das Erscheinen der Psychodiagnostik', 256–57.
25. J.-D. Zbinden, 'L'organisateur: André Repond (1886–1973)', in *Portraits de psychiatres romands*, ed. Christian Müller (Lausanne: Éditions Payot, 1995), 21.
26. For example, Walter Morgenthaler to Erwin Stransky, 28 January 1921, Walter Morgenthaler papers.
27. Walter Morgenthaler, 'Zur Psychologie der Orientierung nach unten', *Sozialärztliche Rundschau* 2 (1930).
28. Walter Morgenthaler, 'Psychotherapie und Politik', in *I. Internationale Tagung für angewandte Psychopathologie und Psychologie, Wien, 5.-7. Juni 1930: Referate und Vorträge*, ed. Heinz Hartmann, Martin Pappenheim, and Erwin Stransky (Berlin: S. Karger, 1931), 234.
29. Ibid., 235.
30. Geoffrey Cocks, *Psychotherapy in the Third Reich: The Göring Institute*, 2nd ed. (New Brunswick and London: Transaction, 1997), 75–76.
31. Walter Morgenthaler, 'Neurologie, Psychiatrie, Psychotherapie', *Zentralblatt für Psychotherapie* 9, no. 1 (1935): 35–36.
32. Walter Morgenthaler, *Persönliche Neutralität und Geistige Wehrkraft* (Berne: Hans Huber, 1941).
33. Walter Morgenthaler, 'Zur Psychologie des Zeitgeschehens: Über Hitler und Mussolini', *Schweizerische Zeitschrift für Psychologie und ihre Anwendungen* 4, no. 2 (1945): 137–48.
34. Walter Morgenthaler, *Der Mensch Karl Marx* (Berne: Schweizerisches Ost-Institut, 1962).
35. Ibid., 79–80.
36. Ibid., 6–8.
37. Martin Pappenheim, Erwin Stransky, and Heinz Hartmann, 'Zum Geleit', in *I. Internationale Tagung für angewandte Psychopathologie und Psychologie, Wien, 5.-7. Juni 1930: Referate und Vorträge*, ed. Heinz Hartmann, Martin Pappenheim, and Erwin Stransky (Berlin: S. Karger, 1931), III.
38. Susan D. Lamb, *Pathologist of the Mind: Adolf Meyer and the Origins of American Psychiatry* (Baltimore: Johns Hopkins University Press, 2014).

39. Walter Morgenthaler to Erwin Stransky, 30 January 1920, Walter Morgenthaler papers.
40. Walter Morgenthaler to Karl Jaspers, 7 March 1920, Walter Morgenthaler papers.
41. Erwin Stransky to Walter Morgenthaler, 11 February 1920, Walter Morgenthaler papers. Notably, Stransky mentioned the writer Romain Rolland (1866–1944) and the socialist leader Jean Jaurès (1859–1914) as two examples for Frenchmen 'who in the German see the man, and not the animal'.
42. See also Erwin Stransky, 'Curriculum Vitae' (Autographensammlung, Josephinium Wien, no. 2064), 3.
43. Karl Jaspers to Walter Morgenthaler, 3 February 1920, Walter Morgenthaler papers.
44. Walter Morgenthaler to Karl Jaspers, 7 March 1920, Walter Morgenthaler papers.
45. Zbinden, 'André Repond', 17–22; Hans Jakob Ritter, *Psychiatrie und Eugenik: Zur Ausprägung eugenischer Denk- und Handlungsmuster in der schweizerischen Psychiatrie 1850–1950* (Zurich: Chronos, 2009), 161–63.
46. Heinrich Meng and André Repond, 'Vorwort', in *Eine Seele die sich wiederfand: Autobiographie des Begründers der 'Geistigen Hygiene'*, ed. Clifford W. Beers (Basel: Benno Schwabe & Co., 1941). A publication in Germany had been planned earlier, but no publisher was willing to print the book in Germany because the translator, Otto Reuter, was Jewish, Norman Dain, *Clifford W. Beers: Advocate of the Insane* (Pittsburgh: University of Pittsburgh Press, 1980), 278.
47. P.-B. Schneider, O. Riggenbach, and R. Egli, 'Au Docteur André Repond, Directeur de la Maison de Santé de Malévoz, Monthey', *Zeitschrift für Präventivmedizin* 1 (1956): 430.
48. Hans Hoff, 'In Memoriam: Univ.-Professor Dr. Erwin Stransky', *Wiener Medizinische Wochenschrift* 112, no. 9 (1962): 181.
49. Wolfgang Huber, *Psychoanalyse in Österreich seit 1933* (Vienna and Salzburg: Geyer-Edition, 1977), 131. Huber mostly refers to one of Stransky's last talks, published posthumously, Erwin Stransky, 'Auswirkungen der Psychopathologie auf das Gegenwartsdenken', *Wissenschaft und Weltbild* 15 (1962): 1–18.
50. Erwin Stransky, 'Remarks Concerning the Development of Applied Psychopathology', *American Journal of Psychiatry* 92 (1936): 1043.
51. Hoff, 'In Memoriam', 181; Norbert Leser, *Skurille Begegnungen: Mosaike zur österreichischen Geistesgeschichte* (Vienna: Böhlau, 2011), 108.
52. Huber, *Psychoanalyse in Österreich*, 8–10.
53. Anthony D. Kauders, 'Psychoanalysis Is Good, Synthesis Is Better: The German Reception of Freud, 1930 and 1956', *Journal of the History of*

the Behavioral Sciences 47 (2011): 382; Hannah S. Decker, *Freud in Germany: Revolution and Reaction in Science, 1893–1907* (New York: International Universities Press, 1977), 172–73, 253; Anthony D. Kauders, 'Truth, Truthfulness, and Psychoanalysis: The Reception of Freud in Wilhelmine Germany', *German History* 31, no. 1 (2013): 1–22.

54. Decker, *Freud in Germany*, 253.
55. Huber, *Psychoanalyse in Österreich*, 10.
56. Kauders, 'Psychoanalysis Is Good', 381; Paul Lerner, *Hysterical Men: War, Psychiatry, and the Politics of Trauma in Germany, 1890–1930* (Ithaca: Cornell University Press, 2003), 163–89.
57. Huber, *Psychoanalyse in Österreich*, 9.
58. Theodor Meißel, 'Freud und die österreichische Psychiatrie seiner Zeit', in *Psychoanalyse und Psychiatrie*, ed. Heinz Böker (Heidelberg: Springer, 2006), 67.
59. Helmut Weihsmann, *Das Rote Wien: Sozialdemokratische Architektur und Kommunalpolitik 1919–1934* (Vienna: Promedia, 2002); Gerhardt Kapner, 'Der Wiener kommunale Wohnungsbau', in *Aufbruch und Untergang: Österreichische Kultur zwischen 1918 und 1938*, ed. Franz Kadrnoska (Vienna, Munich, and Zurich: Europaverlag, 1981), 135–66.
60. Elizabeth Ann Danto, *Freud's Free Clinics: Psychoanalysis and Social Justice, 1918–1938* (New York: Columbia University Press, 2005), 5–6; Michael Hubenstorf, 'Sozialmedizin, Menschenökonomie, Volksgesundheit', in *Aufbruch und Untergang: Österreichische Kultur zwischen 1918 und 1938*, ed. Franz Kadrnoska (Vienna, Munich, and Zurich: Europaverlag, 1981), 247–66; Karl Sablik, *Julius Tandler: Mediziner und Sozialreformer* (Frankfurt am Main: Peter Lang, 2010); Monika Löscher, 'Zur Umsetzung und Verbreitung von eugenischem/rassenhygienischen Gedankengut in Österreich bis 1934 unter besonderer Berücksichtigung Wiens', in *Medizin im Nationalsozialismus - Wege der Aufarbeitung*, ed. Sonia Horn and Peter Malina, Wiener Gespräche zur Sozialgeschichte der Medizin (Vienna: ÖÄK Verlag, 2001), 99–127; Monika Löscher, 'Zur Popularisierung von Eugenik und Rassenhygiene in Wien', in *Wissenschaft, Politik und Öffentlichkeit: Von der Wiener Moderne bis zur Gegenwart*, ed. Mitchell G. Ash and Christian H. Stifer (Vienna: WUV, 2002), 233–66; Julius Tandler, 'Gefahren der Minderwertigkeit', *Das Wiener Jugendhilfswerk: Jahrbuch*, 1928, 3–22.
61. Johannes Reichmayr and Elisabeth Wiesbauer, 'Das Verhältnis von Sozialdemokratie und Psychoanalyse in Österreich zwischen 1900 und 1938', in *Beiträge zur Geschichte der Psychoanalyse in Österreich*, ed. Wolfgang Huber (Vienna and Salzburg: Geyer-Edition, 1978), 30; Else Pappenheim, 'Politik und Psychoanalyse in Wien vor 1939', *Psyche* 43, no. 2 (1989): 125–26.

62. Reichmayr and Wiesbauer, 'Sozialdemokratie und Psychoanalyse', 29; William M. Johnston, *The Austrian Mind: An Intellectual and Social History 1848–1938* (Berkeley et al.: University of California Press, 1972), 256.
63. Kauders, 'Truth, Truthfulness, and Psychoanalysis', 16; Otto Gross, 'Zur Ueberwindung der kulturellen Krise', *Die Aktion* 3, no. 14 (1913): 384–87.
64. Bernd Nitzschke, '"Ich muss mich dagegen wehren, still kaltgestellt zu werden." Voraussetzungen, Begleitumstände und Folgen des Ausschlusses Wilhelm Reichs aus der DGP/IPV in den Jahren 1933/34', in *Der 'Fall' Wilhelm Reich: Beiträge zum Verhältnis von Psychoanalyse und Politik*, ed. Karl Fallend and Bernd Nitzschke (Gießen: Psychosozial-Verlag, 2002), 83–133.
65. Paul Federn, *Zur Psychologie der Revolution: Die vaterlose Gesellschaft* (Leipzig and Vienna: Anzengruber, 1919); Elke Mühlleitner, *Biographisches Lexikon der Psychoanalyse: Die Mitglieder der Psychoanalytischen Mittwoch-Gesellschaft und der Wiener Psychoanalytischen Vereinigung 1902–1938* (Tübingen: edition diskord, 1992), 90–92.
66. Huber, *Psychoanalyse in Österreich*, 26–27; Carl E. Schorske, *Fin-de-Siècle Vienna: Politics and Culture* (New York: Vintage Books, 1981); Eli Zaretsky, *Secrets of the Soul: A Social and Cultural History of Psychoanalysis* (New York: Vintage, 2005), 126–32.
67. Huber, *Psychoanalyse in Österreich*, 26; Pappenheim, 'Politik und Psychoanalyse', 127.
68. In 1928, Vienna had more than forty child guidance offices. Twenty-one of these were part of the municipal youth welfare services (*Jugendämter*); one was run by the Psychoanalytic Society; and about twenty by the individual psychologists. Other initiatives of the individual psychologists included counselling offices for suicidal adolescents, Rudolf Dreikurs, 'Die Entwicklung der psychischen Hygiene in Wien: Unter besonderer Berücksichtigung der Alkoholiker- und Psychopathen-(Selbstmörder-)fürsorge', *Allgemeine Zeitschrift für Psychiatrie und psychisch-gerichtliche Medizin* 88, no. 8 (1928): 469–89.
69. Ludwig J. Pongratz, ed., 'Rudolf Dreikurs', in *Psychotherapie in Selbstdarstellungen* (Berne, Stuttgart, and Vienna: Hans Huber, 1973), 125.
70. Ibid., 115.
71. Huber, *Psychoanalyse in Österreich*, 26–27; Johannes Reichmayr and Elke Mühlleitner, 'Psychoanalysis in Austria After 1933–34: History and Historiography', *International Forum of Psychoanalysis* 12, nos. 2/3 (2003): 118–29.
72. Danto, *Freud's Free Clinics*, 70; Karl Fallend, *Sonderlinge, Träumer, Sensitive: Psychoanalyse auf dem Weg zur Institution und Profession. Protokolle der Wiener Psychoanalytischen Vereinigung und biographische Studien* (Vienna: Jugend & Volk, 1995), 107–40.

73. Meißel, 'Freud und die österreichische Psychiatrie', 67.
74. Eduard Hitschmann, 'Zehn Jahre Wiener Psychoanalytisches Ambulatorium: Zur Geschichte des Ambulatoriums', *Internationale Zeitschrift für Psychoanalyse* 38, no. 2 (1932): 167–68; Reichmayr and Wiesbauer, 'Sozialdemokratie und Psychoanalyse', 34.
75. Reichmayr and Wiesbauer, 'Sozialdemokratie und Psychoanalyse', 34.
76. Erwin Stransky, 'Behandlungs- und Beratungsstellen für Psychisch-Nervöse', *Wiener Medizinische Wochenschrift* 69, no. 9 (1919): 435–38; David Freis, 'Vertrauen und Subordination: Das psychotherapeutische Ambulatorium der Universität Wien, 1918–1938', *Schriftenreihe der Deutschen Gesellschaft für Geschichte der Nervenheilkunde* 21 (2015): 557–85; David Freis, '"Subordination, Authority, Psychotherapy:" Psychotherapy and Politics in Inter-War Vienna', *History of the Human Sciences* 30, no. 2 (2017): 34–53.
77. Heinrich Kogerer, 'Organisation des Fürsorgewesens in deutschen Ländern', in *Leitfaden der psychischen Hygiene*, ed. Erwin Stransky (Berlin and Vienna: Urban & Schwarzenberg, 1931), 247. On Kogerer, who later was a staff member of the 'Göring institute' and a Wehrmacht psychiatrist in the Second World War, Ernst Klee, *Das Personenlexikon zum Dritten Reich: Wer war was vor und nach 1945* (Frankfurt am Main: Fischer, 2003), 327–28. In its heyday, the outpatient clinic employed 15 medical assistants, two nurses, and five care workers (*Fürsorgepersonen*), Heinrich Kogerer, *Psychotherapie: Ein Lehrbuch Für Studierende Und Ärzte* (Vienna: Wilhelm Maudrich, 1934), 1; Heinrich Kogerer, 'I. Jahresbericht Des Psychotherapeutischen Ambulatoriums an Der Psychiatrisch-Neurologischen Universitätsklinik in Wien', *Wiener Klinische Wochenschrift* 37, no. 11 (1924): 255–57; Heinrich Kogerer, 'Bericht über die Tätigkeit des Psychotherapeutischen Ambulatoriums an der Psychiatrisch-neurologischen Universitätsklinik in Wien, in den Jahren 1922–1925', *Wiener Klinische Wochenschrift* 39, no. 12 (1926): 330–33.
78. Fallend, *Sonderlinge, Träumer, Sensitive*, 121.
79. Kogerer, 'Organisation des Fürsorgewesens', 247.
80. ÖNB HANNA Cod. Ser. n. 24054 a–c.
81. Heinrich Kogerer, 'Die Psychotherapie des praktischen Arztes', *Wiener Klinische Wochenschrift* 41, no. 5 (1928): 168.
82. Heinrich Kogerer, 'Psychische Hygiene, Neurosenlehre und Psychotherapie', in *Leitfaden der psychischen Hygiene*, ed. Erwin Stransky (Vienna and Berlin: Urban & Schwarzenberg, 1931), 74–75.
83. Alma Kreuter, *Deutschsprachige Neurologen und Psychiater: Ein biographisch-bibliographisches Lexikon von den Vorläufern bis zur Mitte des 20. Jahrhunderts* (Munich: K. G. Saur, 1996), 696–98.
84. Heinrich Kogerer, 'Psychische Hygiene in Österreich', *Zeitschrift für psychische Hygiene* 2, no. 4 (1929): 117–18.

85. Kogerer, 'Organisation des Fürsorgewesens', 247–48.
86. Kogerer, 'Psychische Hygiene in Österreich', 117.
87. 'Tätigkeitsbericht der Österr. Gesellschaft für Volksgesundheit über das 5. Vereinsjahr (Mitte November 1929 bis Mitte November 1930)', *Volksgesundheit: Zeitschrift für soziale Hygiene* 4, nos. 10/11 (1930): 211.
88. 'Vorträge über psychische Hygiene, veranstaltet vom österreichischen Unterausschuss für psychische Hygiene in Wien', *Zentralblatt für Psychotherapie* 5, no. 4 (1932): 193; Erwin Stransky, 'Vorträge für Abiturienten über psychische Hygiene in Wien', *Zeitschrift für psychische Hygiene* 5, no. 6 (1932): 184–85.
89. Stransky, 'Aus einem Gelehrtenleben', 510. See also ÖNB HANNA Cod. Ser. no. 24054 a–c. About Reichel's criticism of Stransky's approach to mental hygiene, see also Thomas Mayer, '"...dasz die eigentliche österreichische Rassenhygiene in der Hauptsache das Werk Reichels ist": Der (Rassen-)Hygieniker Heinrich Reichel (1876–1943) und seine Bedeutung für die eugenische Bewegung in Österreich', in *Vorreiter der Vernichtung? Eugenik, Rassenhygiene und Euthanasie in der österreichischen Diskussion vor 1938*, ed. Heinz Eberhard Gabriel and Wolfgang Neugebauer (Vienna, Cologne, and Weimar: Böhlau, 2005), 85.
90. Kurt R. Eissler, 'Julius Wagner-Jaureggs Gutachten über Sigmund Freud und seine Studien zur Psychoanalyse', *Wiener Klinische Wochenschrift* 70, no. 22 (1958): 401–7; Kurt R. Eissler, *Freud und Wagner-Jauregg vor der Kommission zur Erhebung militärischer Pflichtverletzungen*, 2nd ed. (Vienna: Löcker, 2007); Hans-Georg Hofer, *Nervenschwäche und Krieg: Modernitätskritik und Krisenbewältigung in der österreichischen Psychiatrie (1880–1920)* (Vienna, Cologne, and Weimar: Böhlau, 2004), 284–90; Hans-Georg Hofer, 'Beyond Freud and Wagner-Jauregg: War, Psychiatry and the Habsburg Army', in *War, Trauma and Medicine in Germany and Central Europe (1914–1939)*, ed. Hans-Georg Hofer, Cay-Rüdiger Prüll, and Wolfgang U. Eckart (Freiburg: Centaurus, 2011), 49–71.
91. Eissler, *Freud und Wagner-Jauregg*, 53.
92. Ibid., 75.
93. Huber, *Psychoanalyse in Österreich*, 12.
94. Erwin Stransky, 'Aus einem Gelehrtenleben um die Zeitenwende: Rückschau, Ausblick, Gedanken' n.d., 318–19; Josephinum Wien, Autographensammlung, no. 2065.
95. Mühlleitner, *Biographisches Lexikon der Psychoanalyse*, 286–88.
96. Huber, *Psychoanalyse in Österreich*, 12.
97. H. A. Beckh-Widmanstetter, 'Zur Geschichte der Individualpsychologie: Julius Wagner-Jauregg über Alfred Adler', *Unsere Heimat* 36 (1965): 182–88.
98. Huber, *Psychoanalyse in Österreich*, 12–13.
99. Mühlleitner, *Biographisches Lexikon der Psychoanalyse*, 245–47.

100. Erwin Stransky and Bernard Dattner, *Über Psychoanalyse: Einleitender Vortrag von Rudolf Allers in Wien, mit daranschließender Aussprache im Verein für angewandte Psychopathologie und Psychologie in Wien (S.-S. 1920)* (Berlin: S. Karger, 1922), 89.
101. Heinrich Kogerer, 'Was leistet die Psychoanalyse für die Psychotherapie?', *Wiener Klinische Wochenschrift* 42, no. 32 (1929): 1068.
102. Kogerer referred to the independent psychoanalyst Hans von Hattingberg (1879–1944), who claimed that suicide was exceptionally common among psychoanalysts, see Kogerer, 'Die Psychotherapie des praktischen Arztes', 167–68.
103. Decker, *Freud in Germany*, 179–89.
104. Ibid., 185–88; Huber, *Psychoanalyse in Österreich*, 11.
105. WStLA, 1.3.2.119.A32.1939.5695/1939; 'Verein für angewandte Psychopathologie und Psychologie in Wien: Bericht über die Tätigkeit im Wintersemester 1920', *Wiener Medizinische Wochenschrift* 70, no. 47 (1920): 1981; Elke Mühlleitner, *Medizinische Psychologie und Psychotherapie in Österreich 1900–1950*, 2 vols (Klagenfurt: Institut für Psychologie der Universität Klagenfurt, 1994).
106. Erwin Stransky to Walter Morgenthaler, 4 March 1920, Walter Morgenthaler papers.
107. 'Verein für angewandte Psychopathologie und Psychologie in Wien: Bericht Wintersemester 1920', 1983.
108. Ibid.
109. 'Verein für angewandte Psychopathologie und Psychologie in Wien: Bericht Wintersemester 1920'.
110. Erwin Stransky, 'Angewandte Psychopathologie: Vortrag gehalten im Akademischen Verein für medizinische Psychologie in Wien am 10. Dezember 1931', *Psychiatrisch-Neurologische Wochenschrift* 16 (1932): 197.
111. Mühlleitner, *Biographisches Lexikon der Psychoanalyse*, 64.
112. Stransky, 'Gelehrtenleben', 323.
113. UAW, M 32.7–5.
114. Stransky, 'Gelehrtenleben', 323.
115. Ibid.
116. Ibid., 538; Ernest Wilder Spaulding, *The Quiet Invaders: The Story of the Austrian Impact Upon America* (Vienna: Österreichischer Bundesverlag, 1968), 288.
117. Mühlleitner, *Biographisches Lexikon der Psychoanalyse*, 64.
118. Anna L. Staudacher, *'... meldet den Austritt aus dem mosaischen Glauben:' 18.000 Austritte aus dem Judentum in Wien, 1868–1914: Namen - Quellen - Daten* (Frankfurt am Main: Peter Lang, 2009), 498.
119. Mühlleitner, *Biographisches Lexikon der Psychoanalyse*, 273; Erwin Stransky, 'Gaston Roffenstein', *Wiener Medizinische Wochenschrift* 77, no. 39

(1927): 1330–31; Susanne Blumesberger et al., eds., *Handbuch österreichischer Autorinnen und Autoren jüdischer Herkunft, 18. bis 20. Jahrhundert* (Munich: Saur, 2002), 1146.
120. Stransky, 'Gaston Roffenstein', 1330–31.
121. Mühlleitner, *Biographisches Lexikon der Psychoanalyse*, 273.
122. William McGuire, ed., *The Freud/Jung Letters: The Correspondence between Sigmund Freud and C. G. Jung*, trans. Ralph Manheim and R. F. C. Hull (London: The Hogarth Press and Routledge & Kegan Paul, 1977), 504.
123. Arthur Kronfeld, 'Über die psychologischen Theorien Freuds und verwandte Anschauungen: Systematik und kritische Erörterungen', *Archiv für die gesamte Psychologie* 22, nos. 2/3 (1912): 130–248; Ingo-Wolf Kittel, 'Arthur Kronfeld zur Erinnerung - Schicksal und Werk eines jüdischen Psychiaters in drei deutschen Reichen', in *Arthur Kronfeld (1886–1941): Ein Pionier der Psychologie, Sexualwissenschaft und Psychotherapie*, ed. Ingo-Wolf Kittel (Konstanz: Bibliothek der Universität Konstanz, 1988), 10–11; Kauders, 'Truth, Truthfulness, and Psychoanalysis', 5.
124. McGuire, *The Freud/Jung Letters*, 504–5.
125. Ibid., 504.
126. Gaston Rosenstein, 'Eine Kritik', *Jahrbuch für psychoanalytische und psychopathologische Forschungen* 4, no. 2 (1912): 741–99.
127. McGuire, *The Freud/Jung Letters*, 504–5, 43. Ernest Jones, however, found Roffenstein's paper 'rather diffuse', R. Andrew Paskauskas, *The Complete Correspondence of Sigmund Freud and Ernest Jones, 1908–1939* (Cambridge, MA: Harvard University Press, 1993), 197.
128. Mühlleitner, *Biographisches Lexikon der Psychoanalyse*, 273.
129. Stransky, 'Gaston Roffenstein', 1331.
130. UAW, Phil.Rig.Akt 4783.
131. Stransky, 'Gaston Roffenstein', 1330.
132. In particular, Gaston Roffenstein, 'Das Problem der Ideologie in der materialistischen Geschichtsauffassung und das moderne Parteiwesen', in *Partei und Klasse im Lebensprozeß der Gesellschaft*, ed. Richard Thurnwald (Leipzig: C. L. Hirschfeld, 1926), 45–46.
133. Roffenstein, *Psychologie und Psychopathologie*, unpaginated preface.
134. Walter Morgenthaler to Erwin Stransky, 19 April 1920, Walter Morgenthaler papers.
135. Roffenstein, *Psychologie und Psychopathologie*, unpaginated preface.
136. Gaston Roffenstein, 'Einige grundsätzliche Bemerkungen zum Problem Psychopathologie und Gesellschaft', *Zeitschrift für die gesamte Neurologie und Psychiatrie* 109 (1927): 151.
137. Gaston Roffenstein, *Das Problem des psychologischen Verstehens: Ein Versuch über die Grundlagen von Psychologie, Psychoanalyse und Individualpsychologie* (Stuttgart: Julius Püttmann, 1926), 9; Gaston Roffenstein, *Das Problem des Unbewußten* (Stuttgart: Julius Püttmann, 1923).

138. Stransky and Dattner, *Über Psychoanalyse.*
139. Ibid., 1.
140. Helmut Gröger, 'Josef K. Friedjung', in *Vertriebene Vernunft II: Emigration und Exil österreichischer Wissenschaft. Internationales Symposium, 19. bis 23. Oktober 1987 in Wien*, ed. Friedrich Stadler (Vienna and Munich: Jugend und Volk, 1988), 819–26.
141. Stransky and Dattner, *Über Psychoanalyse*, 15.
142. Alfred Lévy, 'Rudolf Allers - ein katholischer Individualpsychologe', in *Gestalten um Alfred Adler: Pioniere der Individualpsychologie*, ed. Alfred Lévy and Gerald Mackenthun (Würzburg: Königshausen & Neumann, 2002), 27–36; Regine Lockot, *Erinnern und Durcharbeiten: Zur Geschichte der Psychoanalyse und Psychotherapie im Nationalsozialismus* (Gießen: Psychosozial-Verlag, 2002), 335–36.
143. Stransky and Dattner, *Über Psychoanalyse*, 21, 45.
144. Ibid., 65; Eduard Hitschmann, 'R. Allers: Über Psychoanalyse', *Internationale Zeitschrift für Psychoanalyse* 10, no. 4 (1924): 476.
145. Brigitte Hamann, *Hitlers Wien: Lehrjahre eines Diktators*, 3rd ed. (Munich: Piper, 1996), 329–33; cf. Alfred Springer, 'Die Verwirklichung der "geeinten deutschen Seelenkunde" im Nationalsozialistischen Österreich: Ideengeschichtliche Aspekte', in *Gründe der Seele: Die Wiener Psychiatrie im 20. Jahrhundert*, ed. Brigitta Keintzel (Wien: Picus, 1999), 108–11.
146. Stransky and Dattner, *Über Psychoanalyse*, 98–100; Hamann, *Hitlers Wien*, 331.
147. Carl Gustav Jung, 'Zur gegenwärtigen Lage der Psychotherapie', *Zentralblatt für Psychotherapie* 7, no. 1 (1934): 1–16; Erwin Stransky, 'Rasse und Psychotherapie', *Zentralblatt für Psychotherapie* 10 (1937): 9–28; Andrea Adams, *Psychopathologie und 'Rasse': Verhandlungen 'rassischer' Differenz in der Erforschung psychischer Leiden (1890–1933)* (Bielefeld: Transcript, 2013).
148. Stransky and Dattner, *Über Psychoanalyse*, 86.
149. Ibid., 90.
150. Erwin Stransky, 'Die Verhandlung gegen Hofrat Professor Dr. Wagner-Jauregg und Genossen. Oder: Dank vom Hause Österreich. Ein Nachruf', *Wiener Medizinische Wochenschrift* 70, no. 45 (1920): 1901–2.
151. Erwin Stransky, 'Psychoanalyse und Kritik', *Wiener Medizinische Wochenschrift* 71, no. 16 (1921): 716–18; Eduard Hitschmann, 'Prof. Erwin Stransky: Psychoanalyse und Kritik', *Internationale Zeitschrift für Psychoanalyse* 8, no. 2 (1922): 223.
152. Stransky, 'Psychoanalyse und Kritik', 718.
153. Erwin Stransky to Walter Morgenthaler, 26 May 1921, Walter Morgenthaler papers.
154. Stransky, 'Gelehrtenleben', 502.
155. Ibid., 502–3.

156. Ibid., 503. Pappenheim is first mentioned as head of the association in June 1927, 'Verein für angewandte Psychopathologie und Psychologie: Sitzung vom 20. Juni 1927', *Wiener Medizinische Wochenschrift* 77, no. 47 (1927): 1602.
157. Ratko Parenžanin, *Gavrilo Princips Bekenntnisse: Ein geschichtlicher Beitrag zur Vorgeschichte des Attentats von Sarajevo* (Vienna: Rudolf Lechner & Sohn, 1926).
158. Else Pappenheim, *Hölderlin, Feuchtersleben, Freud: Beiträge zur Geschichte der Psychoanalyse, der Psychiatrie und Neurologie*, trans. Wilfried Prantner, Else Pappenheim, and Stephen Frishauf (Graz and Vienna: Nausner & Nausner, 2004), 30.
159. Ibid.
160. Stransky and Dattner, *Über Psychoanalyse*, 58–59.
161. Mühlleitner, *Biographisches Lexikon der Psychoanalyse*, 241–42; Danto, *Freud's Free Clinics*, 6. Martin Pappenheim was not related to the Austro-Jewish feminist Berta Pappenheim.
162. Pappenheim, *Hölderlin, Feuchtersleben, Freud*, 46–47.
163. Stransky, 'Gelehrtenleben', 504.
164. See, for example, Martin Pappenheim to Frieda and Karl Grosz, 30 March 1934, ÖNB HANNA Autogr. 1188/30-6.
165. Else Pappenheim, 'Zeitzeugin', in *Vertriebene Vernunft II: Emigration und Exil österreichischer Wissenschaft. Internationales Symposium, 19. bis 23. Oktober 1987 in Wien*, ed. Friedrich Stadler (Vienna and Munich: Jugend und Volk, 1988), 221.
166. Pappenheim, *Hölderlin, Feuchtersleben, Freud*, 22–23.
167. Ibid., 46–47.
168. Martin Pappenheim, '[Report from Soviet Russia]', *Internationale Zeitschrift für Psychoanalyse* 7, no. 3 (1921): 387–88; Mühlleitner, *Biographisches Lexikon der Psychoanalyse*, 241; Alexander Etkind, *Eros des Unmöglichen: Die Geschichte der Psychoanalyse in Rußland*, trans. Andreas Tretner (Leipzig: Gustav Kiepenheuer, 1996), 219–78.
169. Martin Pappenheim, 'Medizinisches und Aerztliches aus Sowjetrußland', *Wiener Klinische Wochenschrift* 35, no. 8 (1922): 186.
170. Mühlleitner, *Biographisches Lexikon der Psychoanalyse*, 242.
171. Karl Fallend, 'Marie Frischauf-Pappenheim', in *Personenlexikon der Sexualforschung*, ed. Volkmar Sigusch (Frankfurt am Main: Campus, 2009), 204–6.
172. Pappenheim, 'Zeitzeugin', 221. In a 1978 letter to Ernst Federn, Else Pappenheim also mentioned the psychoanalyst Helene Deutsch and the social democrat politician Karl Seitz, see Else Pappenheim to Ernst Federn, 11 March 1978, ÖNB HANNA Autogr. 1497/38(1-4).
173. About the Pappenheim couple's first months in Tel Aviv, see their letters to Frieda and Karl Grosz, ÖNB HANNA Autogr. 1188/30(1-16).

174. Eran Rolnik, *Freud auf Hebräisch: Geschichte der Psychoanalyse im jüdischen Palästina*, trans. David Ajchenrand (Göttingen: Vandenhoeck & Ruprecht, 2013), 140; Pappenheim, 'Zeitzeugin', 221.
175. Rolnik, *Freud auf Hebräisch*, 141.
176. Pappenheim, 'Zeitzeugin', 221.
177. Stransky, 'Gaston Roffenstein'.
178. Rakafet Zalashik, *Das unselige Erbe: Die Geschichte der Psychiatrie in Palästina und Israel*, trans. David Ajchenrand (Frankfurt am Main: Campus, 2012), 56–57.
179. Without mentioning the conference in Washington, DC, Stransky saw applied psychopathology and mental hygiene as two interrelated projects, Erwin Stransky, 'Der Tagung für angewandte Psychopathologie und Psychologie zum Gruße', *Wiener Klinische Wochenschrift* 80, no. 23 (1930): 767.
180. Stransky, 'Gelehrtenleben', 503.
181. 'Internationale Tagung für angewandte Psychopathologie und Psychologie', *Wiener Medizinische Wochenschrift* 80, no. 23 (1930): 768.
182. Mühlleitner, *Biographisches Lexikon der Psychoanalyse*, 131–33.
183. Martin S. Bergmann, *The Hartmann Era* (New York: Other Press, 2000).
184. 'Rückblick auf die I. Internationale Tagung für angewandte Psychopathologie und Psychologie in Wien, 5.-7. Juni 1930', *Wiener Medizinische Wochenschrift* 80, no. 31 (1930): 1036–37.
185. Martin Pappenheim, 'Eröffnungsansprache', in *I. Internationale Tagung für angewandte Psychopathologie und Psychologie, Wien, 5.-7. Juni 1930: Referate und Vorträge*, ed. Heinz Hartmann, Martin Pappenheim, and Erwin Stransky (Berlin: S. Karger, 1931), 2.
186. Ibid., 3.
187. Erwin Stransky, 'Angewandte Psychopathologie und Gegenwartszivilisation', in *I. Internationale Tagung für angewandte Psychopathologie und Psychologie, Wien, 5.-7. Juni 1930: Referate und Vorträge*, ed. Heinz Hartmann, Martin Pappenheim, and Erwin Stransky (Berlin: S. Karger, 1931), 146–61.
188. Ibid., 160–61.
189. Paul Federn, 'Der neurotische Stil', in *I. Internationale Tagung für angewandte Psychopathologie und Psychologie, Wien, 5.-7. Juni 1930: Referate und Vorträge*, ed. Heinz Hartmann, Martin Pappenheim, and Erwin Stransky (Berlin: S. Karger, 1931), 194–201; Hans Luxenburger, 'Psychopathologie und Erblichkeit', in *I. Internationale Tagung für angewandte Psychopathologie und Psychologie, Wien, 5.-7. Juni 1930: Referate und Vorträge*, ed. Heinz Hartmann, Martin Pappenheim, and Erwin Stransky (Berlin: S. Karger, 1931), 77–93.
190. Rudolf Allers, 'Die internationale Tagung für angewandte Psychopathologie und Psychologie', *Zentralblatt für Psychotherapie* 3, no. 7 (1930): 389–94.

191. Ibid., 390.
192. Ibid., 394.
193. Ibid.
194. Stransky, 'Gelehrtenleben', 504.
195. Ekkehardt Kumbier and Kathleen Haack, 'Alfred Hauptmann: Schicksal eines deutsch-jüdischen Neurologen', *Fortschritte der Neurologie, Psychiatrie* 70 (2002): 204–9.
196. 'Verein für angewandte Psychopathologie und Psychologie in Wien', *Wiener Medizinische Wochenschrift* 84, no. 22 (1934): 621; Gerhard Benetka, *Psychologie in Wien: Sozial- und Theoriegeschichte des Wiener Psychologischen Instituts 1922–1938* (Vienna: WUV, 1995), 246–47.
197. 'Verein für angewandte Psychopathologie und Psychologie', *Wiener Medizinische Wochenschrift* 85, no. 37 (1935): 999–1002; 'Verein für angewandte Psychopathologie und Psychologie in Wien', *Wiener Medizinische Wochenschrift* 87, no. 32 (1937): 854–56.
198. Stransky, 'Gelehrtenleben', 504.
199. Martin Sack, *Von der Neuropathologie zur Phänomenologie: Alfred Prinz Auersperg und die Geschichte der Heidelberger Schule* (Würzburg: Königshausen & Neumann, 2005), 25–37.
200. Judith Bauer-Merinsky, 'Die Auswirkungen der Annexion Österreichs durch das Deutsche Reich auf die medizinische Fakultät der Universität Wien im Jahre 1938: Biographien entlassener Professoren und Dozenten' (University of Vienna, 1980), 103–6.
201. WStLA, 1.3.2.119.A32.1939.5695/1939 – Verein für angewandte Psychopathologie und Psychologie.
202. Stransky, 'Gelehrtenleben', 505; Hans Hoff, 'Entwicklung der psychischen Hygiene in Österreich', in *Bericht über die 6. Jahresversammlung der Weltvereinigung für Psychische Hygiene, Wien 16.-22. August 1953*, ed. Österreichische Gesellschaft für Psychische Hygiene (Vienna and Bonn: Wilhelm Maudrich, 1956), 22.

CHAPTER 5

Psychiatric Prophylaxis and the Emergence of Mental Hygiene

In the mid-1920s, mental hygiene arrived in the German-speaking countries. Like no other slogan, *psychische Hygiene* or *Psychohygiene*, encapsulated the promise of a new path for psychiatry. Psychiatry, the protagonists of the movement urged, had to step out of the boundaries of the asylums and university clinics to prevent mental disorder before it was too late, instead of inefficaciously trying to heal it. By using the notion of 'hygiene', the movement aligned itself with a variety of other approaches of the same name that, in the previous decades, had opened many new ways for social and individual prophylaxis; what they had done for the body, mental hygiene promised to do for the mind. As Erwin Stransky, who in following his vision of an applied psychiatry became one of the most zealous proponents of the movement in Austria, wrote in a 1931 textbook, 'mental hygiene in the narrow sense is the epitome of every scientific effort to maintain the health of the soul'.[1]

But mental hygiene was more than that. Its roots in the United States lay not in psychiatric prophylaxis, but in the reform of mental institutions. While obscured by the movement's name, institutional reform was always a part of its agenda, although its importance varied over time. Moreover, in its effort to prevent mental disorders, the mental hygiene movement projected into other emerging fields of mental health care outside of psychiatry's traditional sphere of activity. As Stransky argued in 1931, there were two related aspects of mental hygiene, 'maintaining the health of the healthy,

D. Freis, *Psycho-Politics between the World Wars*,
Mental Health in Historical Perspective,
https://doi.org/10.1007/978-3-030-32702-6_5

and preventing those in risk from getting sick'.[2] Some individuals and groups were more at risk of becoming ill and spreading diseases than others, and in the biologistic paradigm of early twentieth-century psychiatry, this mostly came down to heredity. Eugenics were an integral part of mental hygiene from the beginning on. At the same time, mental hygienists also shifted psychiatry's sphere of activity into the vast grey area between mental health and full-blown mental illness and tried to co-opt adjacent fields like psychotherapy, counselling, and pedagogy for their own vision of a psychiatric approach to public health.

What was already a well-organised and successful movement in the United States, spread to the German-speaking countries in the mid-1920s, when associations and committees for mental hygiene sprung up in rapid succession in Germany, Austria, and Switzerland. Partly, this was the result of a lobbying tour by Clifford W. Beers (1876–1943), the founding figure of mental hygiene in the United States, in 1922. However, as the following two chapters show, telling the story of mental hygiene in Europe as that of a transatlantic import would be overly simplistic. As an international movement, mental hygiene had its origin and its organisational centre in the United States, but the underlying idea of a systematic psychiatric prophylaxis for the entire population had already emerged in the German-speaking countries in the decades before and after the turn of the century. Beers' propaganda for mental hygiene in the inter-war period fell on fertile ground that had been prepared for more than three decades.

This chapter traces the origins of mental hygiene and large-scale psychiatric prophylaxis in the German-speaking countries. As early as the first half of the nineteenth century, psychiatrists began to introduce ideas about how mental illness could be prevented. In the following sections, I examine the three most important advocates of psychiatric prophylaxis in the first quarter of the twentieth century: Auguste Forel, Emil Kraepelin, and Robert Sommer. The latter links the early history of psychiatric prophylaxis to the history of the mental hygiene movement in the inter-war period, as Sommer not only introduced the concept of mental hygiene as early as 1902, but also became the founder and main organiser of the German branch of the movement in the mid-1920s.

The notion that mental illness could and should be prevented was intricately connected to changes in scientific knowledge as well as in political thought. Advances in foundational research in psychiatry and the emergence of new theories about the causation of mental disorders in the decade before the turn of the century were one important influence. While psychiatrists failed to translate these advances into effective therapeutics, they hoped that, by means of large-scale and state-led prophylaxis, the problem of mental illness might yet be solved and the notoriously overcrowded asylums relieved. With the rise of the hereditary paradigm in psychiatry, little difference was made between purging the world from mental illness or the mentally ill, and the most effective way for the prevention of mental illness was often seen in preventing future mental patients from even being born. Although other approaches played a role as well, in the course of the following decades, psychiatric prophylaxis in the German-speaking countries remained on its eugenic trajectory. In 1933, mental hygiene in Germany became virtually indistinguishable from racial hygiene, but the intellectual preconditions for this momentous shift had already been prepared in the first decade of the century. Political, cultural, and economic crises added momentum to eugenics, in the aftermath of the First World War and in the late 1920s in particular.

Eugenics were not the only way in which psychiatric prophylaxis was an inherently political affair. As the examples of Forel, Kraepelin, and Sommer illustrate, their visions of psychiatric prophylaxis were embedded in their reflections about modern society and its discontents and were part of much broader utopian ideas. Moreover, these examples also show that the traditional concepts of political history may fall short when it comes to the conjunction of political and scientific thought. The three protagonists of this chapter stood at very different ends of the political spectrum—Forel called himself a socialist and dreamt of a pacifist world society, Kraepelin was a fervent German nationalist and authoritarian, and Sommer, politically more elusive than the others, may best be described as a conservative liberal. Their psycho-political ideas about the role of psychiatry in the engineering of society were, however, far more similar than their different political alignments would suggest. All three passionately believed that society had to follow the laws of nature, and not the laws of men, and all three were convinced that they, as objective scientists and psychiatrists, had recognised and understood these laws. This mindset could attach and combine itself with other political creeds, but as a pre-political stance, it was a key element of mental hygienists' self-understanding and strategy as emerging public health experts in the inter-war period.

Romantic Ancestors

Multifaceted as it was, the movement for mental hygiene was a distinctly modern movement. Its protagonists saw themselves as the avant-garde of their discipline and presented their agenda as the practical result of the latest research. This self-understanding did not require long lines of intellectual ancestors to lend itself legitimacy. In inter-war Germany, the history of mental hygiene was usually traced back no further than the turn of the twentieth century. This was just old enough to be able to claim a German history predating the emergence of a movement for mental hygiene in the United States following the publication of Clifford Beers's *A Mind That Found Itself* in 1908. Robert Sommer's programmatic article about public resting rooms (*öffentliche Ruhehallen*) was widely acknowledged as the founding moment of mental hygiene in Germany and as a direct precursor of the movement's agenda in the 1920s. Sommer had used the term 'mental hygiene' early on, and the fact that he became the founder and first president of the German Association for Mental Hygiene (*Deutscher Verein für psychische Hygiene*, DVPH) lend this narrative a strong sense of continuity. Wilhelm Weygandt (1870–1939), vice president of the association, also saw Emil Kraepelin as a pioneer of mental hygiene,[3] a claim that was as much tactical as plausible. Kraepelin was indeed among the first to call for state-led prophylaxis of mental illness on a national scale. At the same time, however, putting Kraepelin in their line of ancestors helped German mental hygienists to attach themselves to one of the most prestigious names in contemporary psychiatry. This was as much genealogy as was needed; German mental hygienists rarely looked back beyond the turn of the century.

In Austria, much longer and more local traditions were considered. As Otto Kauders (1893–1949) claimed in the early 1930s, the pedigree of mental hygiene—when understood as the effort to 'improve the psychic state of groups of people'—reached back as far as Socrates, Thomas Aquinas, Jean-Jacques Rousseau, and Johann Wolfgang Goethe.[4] The key figure in the genealogy of the Austrian movement for mental hygiene, however, was Ernst von Feuchtersleben (1806–1849), a Viennese aristocrat, popular philosopher, poet, and physician.[5] Although Feuchtersleben's philosophy effectively had very little influence on the practical outlook of the Austrian movement for mental hygiene, the idea that he was an ancestor of the movement was common among mental hygienists in the inter-war period and persisted even after the Second World War. In 1951, Erwin

Stransky opened a lecture for American medical students in Vienna by claiming that mental hygiene had in fact been invented by Feuchtersleben, and not by Beers—and thus in Austria, and not in the United States.[6] In 1960, the Austrian Society for Mental Hygiene celebrated the World Year for Mental Health with a series of lectures about Feuchtersleben.[7]

The perception of Feuchtersleben as a direct precursor of mental hygiene was mostly based on a book entitled *Zur Diätetik der Seele* ('On the dietetics of the soul').[8] Published in 1838, this early self-help book was an instant bestseller and a staple item in bourgeois households throughout the nineteenth century. As one biographer claimed: 'Since the publication of Goethe's *Werther*, perhaps no other German book was, up to 1850, as widely read'.[9] Over the course of the nineteenth century, Feuchtersleben's *Diätetik* was translated into all major European languages; a fiftieth edition appeared in 1907.[10] But different from what the proponents of the Austrian movement for mental hygiene and others have since claimed, Feuchtersleben's dietetics offered no method for psychiatric prophylaxis.[11] Based on the extensive self-observation fashionable in early romantic psychology, he argued that physical illness might be prevented or mitigated by using specific mental techniques. Anticipating some of the basic ideas of twentieth-century psychosomatic medicine, he postulated that psychological processes could affect functions of the body and that fostering patients' belief in their recovery and their trust in their physician should become part of medical treatment. Only after he became a professor at the University of Vienna, Feuchtersleben laid out some rudimentary ideas about the prophylaxis of mental illness in his *Lehrbuch der Seelenheilkunde* (1845). As he explained, mental illness could be warded off by relying on self-knowledge, self-mastery, and virtue.[12]

In 1838, Feuchtersleben began his treatise on dietetics by stating that 'our times are quick, tumultuous, and careless'. Faced with a hectic and confusing outside world, Feuchtersleben promised his readers to guide them somewhere more soothing, to the 'calm regions of the science of the inner man, to the observations of the self'.[13] Half a century later, this *Biedermeier* retreat into the cosiness of the inner self would not be possible anymore. As many in the late nineteenth century believed, in an ever-accelerating industrial modernity, the nerves and the mind had ceased to be sanctuaries of calm self-reflection and had turned into battlefields themselves. As popular theories of nervousness and neurasthenia explained, the nerves were overloaded with more and more information, rattled by railway accidents, and depleted by the constant strain of the struggle for survival.[14] Against this backdrop, defending the mind against the challenges of the modern world became increasingly relevant. It was in this context that psychiatrists, psychologists, and philosophers began to develop forms of 'hygiene' that applied to the psyche.

One of the first authors to expressly propose a prophylactic 'hygiene of the soul' (*Hygieine der Seele*) was the philosopher Eduard Reich (1836–1919), who later occasionally was mentioned as part of the pedigree of their disciplines by social and mental hygienists.[15] Reich's ideas, published in 1884, were still far away from twentieth-century mental hygiene. Similar to Feuchtersleben his 'hygiene of the soul' was less about medical prophylaxis of mental disorders, and more of an holistic theory of felicity, virtue, and human perfection, embedded in an eclectic vitalistic philosophy that relied on a metaphysical concept of the soul rather than a psychological theory of the mind.[16] The psychiatrist Eugen Hallervorden (1853–1914) from Königsberg who, shortly before the turn of the century, tried to establish a science of 'psycho-hygiene' (*Psychohygiene*), was still part of this philosophical tradition. Although Hallervorden passionately announced that he would lay the foundations for a 'general and special psycho-hygiene, based on physiological principles, as a science' and gave a first lecture on 'psycho-hygiene' in 1897, his efforts remained both vague and fruitless.[17] The same was also true for psychiatrist Leo Hirschlaff's 1911 'hygiene of thinking' (*Hygiene des Denkens*), a set of various techniques of mental and bodily self-discipline that were supposed to prevent nervousness and exhaustion.[18]

Although scholars like Feuchtersleben, Reich, Hallervorden, and Hirschlaff were the first to connect the concept of hygiene to the prevention of mental illness, their ideas had little direct import on the intellectual mainstream of the later mental hygiene movement. There were at least three reasons why these earlier approaches were abandoned. First, the speculative psychology of these approaches was difficult to reconcile with mental hygienists' self-understanding as the most progressive representatives of psychiatry as a part of modern, science-based clinical medicine. Feuchtersleben's psycho-physiological holism hardly produced useful categories for clinical research. Although inter-war psychiatrists often argued in highly normative ways, the metaphysical concepts used by Feuchtersleben and others were clearly incompatible with their self-understanding as objective scientists and physicians, who drew their categories from the observation of nature and their patients, and not from religious or philosophical speculation.

Second, as biological models of illness gained importance in psychiatry in the second half of the nineteenth century and the focus shifted to heredity, the possibilities for individual prophylaxis diminished. The more mental illness was perceived as the result of heredity and constitution, the less a person's lifestyle could influence its development. The exception was alcoholism, which was recognised by psychiatrists as a major threat to mental health and was at the centre of many prophylactic efforts.

Third, since the turn of the century, preventive psychiatry appealed to the state rather than to the individual. Prophylactic self-techniques had little in common with the changes in legislation and the state-run public health interventions that became the method of choice for inter-war mental hygienists in Central Europe. However, while the psycho-philosophical tradition of individual prophylaxis was pushed out of the psychiatric mainstream, it never disappeared entirely. Explicitly or implicitly, it continued to influence those parts of the psy-ences that were more interested in the intra-psychic causation of mental disorders. With the rise of psychoanalysis and other psychotherapeutic schools in the inter-war period, parts of this older tradition resurfaced.[19] Notably, Feuchtersleben's prominence in the Austrian branch of the movement coincided with a particularly strong influence of psychoanalysis in local approaches to mental hygiene.

Instead of these psycho-philosophical traditions, the emerging mental hygiene movement of the inter-war period drew from two other sources. On the one hand, mental hygienists tried to emulate the success of other prophylactic programmes of their time that had already established themselves under the umbrella of the term 'hygiene'. On the other hand, and more importantly, mental hygiene was a direct outcome of psychiatry's transformation into a modern, positivist part of scientific medicine in the last third of the nineteenth century.[20] The introduction of new clinical research methods inspired by experimental psychology, the aggregation, and statistical interpretation of patient files, as well as advances in the microscopic study of the brain and in serology had led to new insights and theories about the causation of mental illness. The inability to translate these nosological advances into effective therapeutics was the main reason for psychiatrists' turn to prevention at the end of the century. Visions of psychiatric prophylaxis did not emerge from the fringes of the discipline, but from its core. As the following sections show, the most influential prophylactic ideas were developed and propagated by some of the leading representatives of clinical psychiatry. Among them, three names stand out: Auguste Forel, Emil Kraepelin, and Robert Sommer.

Ants, Esperanto, and Eugenics: Auguste Forel

The first direct precursor of the mental hygiene movement was the Swiss psychiatrist and myrmecologist Auguste Forel (1848–1931), who proposed a prophylactic 'hygiene of the nerves and the mind' (*Hygiene der Nerven und des Geistes*) in a 1903 treatise.[21] Unlike predecessors such as Eduard Reich, Eugen Hallervorden, or Ernst von Feuchtersleben, Forel's vision of hygiene was firmly rooted in modern medicine and based on a biological understanding of the mind as an organic function of the brain. Although not disinclined to philosophical speculation himself, he drew a clear boundary between earlier 'mystical' concepts of the soul and his scientific perspective based on the insights of the 'brain sciences', which had proven 'the oneness of the soul and the brain matter'.[22] Consequently, his 'hygiene of the nerves' was not supposed to be a philosophy for healthy living, but a form of active medical practice—a part of private and public health care and of social prophylaxis.[23] Forel's psychiatric prophylaxis was just one part of a far broader programme combining visions of socialist utopia, gender equality, and international confraternisation with social Darwinism, eugenics, and overt racism. The first half of this section outlines Forel's biography, his psycho-political thought, and the contemporary reception of his ideas. In the second half, I take a closer look at Forel's notion of preventive psychiatry.

Born in the west of Switzerland in 1848, Forel belonged to an older generation than the psychiatrists who came to lead the mental hygiene movement in the inter-war period. Having completed his medical studies in Zurich, he turned to psychiatry, which at that time was only beginning to gain its scientific and medical reputation. He rose quickly in the ranks of the young discipline and became professor of psychiatry in Zurich and director of the Burghölzli university clinic in 1879.[24] Faced with dismal conditions in the overcrowded hospital and psychiatry's notorious lack of effective therapeutics, he embraced Bénédict Morel's (1809–1873) paradigm of hereditary . Believing that the causes of mental illnesses were hereditary and that the therapeutic options therefore were very limited, Forel soon turned to prophylaxis and the hope that if mental illness could not be cured, it might at least be prevented. In particular, he became a zealous proponent of abstinence, campaigning against the negative effects of alcoholism for most of his life.[25] In later years, eugenics emerged as the second pillar of his socio-medical efforts.

In 1898, aged fifty, Forel surprisingly resigned from his professorship and as director of Burghölzli to fully devote himself to his many activities outside the clinic. His humanitarian commitment led him through a series of organisations and secular creeds. He joined the Good Templars in 1892 and founded their first lodge in Switzerland; in 1906, he signed the founding proclamation of the internationalist and freethinker German Monist Association (*Deutscher Monistenbund*); during the First World War, he declared himself a socialist and pacifist, and in 1920, he converted to the Bahá'í faith.[26]

Among his contemporaries, Forel stood out through his zeal and the width of his activities. As a 1931 obituary summarised, 'we may consider August Forel as a myrmecologist, as a brain histologist, as a leader in the fight against alcoholism recognised in both hemispheres, as a helper in sexual problems, as an undaunted opponent of social wrongs, as a reconciler of nations: we can but admire his superior example of mental and moral strength'.[27] This adulation was not shared by everyone. In a 1935 review of Forel's posthumously published autobiography, Erich Fromm (1900–1980) attacked his visions from a left-wing psychoanalytic perspective, deriding him as an exemplar 'progressive petit bourgeois', for whom 'the main motif of his life is the fight against the human drives'.[28] Generally, however, Forel was celebrated as a pioneering philanthrope and reformer. His internationalist and pacifist views and his advocacy of women's suffrage certainly set him apart from most of his contemporaries and colleagues. It also appealed to future generations, who put his face on the Swiss thousand-franc banknote in the late 1970s.[29]

Only recently has Forel's legacy undergone a critical revision.[30] As historians have shown since the turn of the millennium, eugenic, overtly racist, and social-Darwinist ideas are present throughout his work. These views were neither occasional aberrances nor concessions to the zeitgeist, and they were not marginal. Instead, eugenics and social Darwinism were integral parts of Forel's worldview, intricately connected to the foundations of his social thought. Following his monistic views, Forel believed that the same laws governed nature and human society. Hence, the selection of the unfit was an imperative dictated by the laws of nature, which he as a proponent of an unprejudiced, objective, and progressive world view had to defend against false pity and metaphysical considerations.[31] Forel linked eugenics and socialism and proposed the sterilisation of the unfit as a method of a 'scientific social democracy' for the utopian betterment of the world: 'Then a stupid, ignorant, degenerate mental and physical proletariat, which in its unconscious simplicity reproduces like rabbits and thus fouls our society like a harmful pest, will no longer exist'.[32] In Forel's type of socialism, ridding the world from misery was best achieved by getting rid of the miserable. Moreover, he did not limit himself to theorising about the possibility of eugenic sterilisation but took it on himself to act. As he later proudly remembered: 'In the mid of the [eighteen-] nineties, in the Burghölzli asylum, I even had the audacity to use a medical pretext to castrate two hereditary defective monsters, to prevent their reproduction'.[33]

Forel laid out his ideas in numerous tracts and manifestos. However, his vision of the future of human society was most clearly expressed in a booklet entitled *Mensch und Ameise* ('Man and ant') that he published in 1922.[34] Here, Forel, then seventy-four years old, summarised the results of his biological studies about the social life of ants, which he claimed to have conducted for the last sixty-six years, that is, since the age of eight. In his biologistic world view, his findings were directly translatable into normative postulates for human society. As Forel maintained, the society of ants was ethically superior to human civilisation because 'the ant is simply more social than man, and "social" means "ethical" – ethical towards the community in which one lives'.[35] In the course of a long evolutionary process, ants had created a society in which every member had a productive role, and Forel's list of the different vocations among ants told a lot about which human professions he found beneficial for the greater good:

> [...] weavers, butchers, stockbreeders, masons, papermakers, road builders, bakers, mushroom growers, grain collectors or reapers, various exquisite kinds of wet nurses, gardeners, warriors, pacifists, slavers, thieves, robbers and murderers, and parasites (but nowhere to be found are professors, orators, braggarts, bureaucrats, commanders, rulers, generals, not even corporals, and still less capitalists, speculators, and profiteers).[36]

Despite the lack of military brass, Forel found one important drawback in ant society, which he described both as socialist and as a form of 'organised anarchy'. Unable of imagining a community beyond their people and their hill, ants necessarily were at war with other ants, 'since the mind and the whole soul of the absolutely small, but relatively big brain of an ant are utterly incapable of grasping what the terrestrial globe or what internationalism might be'.[37] The future of mankind, Forel believed, therefore depended on combining the social qualities of ants with the visionary potential of humans and on the answer to one question:

> What can we do to become more like ants, and remain humans all at one? The tragic events of the world war and of the subsequent social war since 1919 are well suited to put one in a contemplative mood, and to prompt us to think about a possible solution for the human social question on the basis of a circumspect scientific consideration.[38]

Auguste Forel's myrmeco-utopian plans for the transformation of human society into an anthill reveal the inherent contradictions in his socio-political thought. On the one hand, Forel found human culture to be determined by biological facts; on the other hand, he called for fundamental social and political changes that were to be achieved through a re-education of the mass of the people. As he argued, human behaviour was grounded in the brain and unlike the social ant, man was 'an egoistic, individualist, passionate, rapacious, domineering, vengeful, and jealous creature'.[39] Human civilisation, despite all its changes in thousands of years and although it was acquired individually, was based on traits hard-wired in the brain. Language and writing allowed culture to be handed down from generation to generation and to develop and flourish, but the human brain as its biological basis remained the same. More so, Forel believed that human biology had deteriorated due to the gradual suspension of natural selection and the dysgenic effects of civilisation. Eugenics, both negative and positive, would have to compensate for the detrimental effects of modern society. Eugenics, however, were only a small part of a larger solution to the problem and Forel believed as much in internationalist idealism and education as in determinist neuro-biologism. Thus, what had begun as a treatise about the social behaviour of ants and had moved on to become a reflection about the hereditary and biological basis of human culture and society, culminated in a seventeen-point programme for the creation of a socialist world society.

Forel's programme could hardly have been any more encompassing. The legislative authority of the nation-states would have to be transferred to a supranational 'council of nations' (*Völkerrat*), national armies, and navies would be delivered to the command of a 'pacifist general', who would gradually repurpose their equipment into museum pieces. The 'council of nations' would be based on free and equal franchise for people of any gender and nation. Alcohol would be prohibited. The socialisation of real property, industry, and the economy, the abolition of castes, estates, and rights of succession would create a society of equals. But as Forel saw it, a utopian world society could not be achieved through these measures alone, it also required a new kind of internationalist education. A common language—Esperanto—would help to overcome national differences and the Bahá'í faith would serve as a 'supra-national scientific religion' without dogma and spirituality. Public health was another part of Forel's agenda. 'Sensitive and effective eugenic reforms' would counteract degeneration and the abolition of prostitution would help to contain venereal diseases. Finally, economic production would be internationalised and the colonies gradually liberated—'through supra-national, educational paternalism towards their uneducated inhabitants and the lower races'.[40] Like the unresolved tension between neuro-biologistic determinism and pedagogical ardour, the clash of a rhetoric of internationalist confraternisation with overt racism that ranged from colonialist paternalism to calls for the elimination of entire races was a recurring theme in Forel's work. His ideas about psychiatric prophylaxis were caught between the same poles.

Like Robert Sommer's notion of mental hygiene, discussed later in this chapter, Forel's approach to psychiatric prophylaxis consisted of two complementary parts, targeted at individual lifestyles as well as societal structures. Individually, Forel believed, mental health could be preserved and supported through both positive and negative measures; by refraining from harmful habits such as the consumption of alcohol and other intoxicants, but also by training the nervous system with lifelong learning, sports, sufficient sleep and rest, and by engaging in a wide and harmonious choice of different activities.[41] Individual measures could, however, only be one part of a broader effort that would also have to include the health of the collective. Anticipating what later became the predominant position of mental hygiene associations in the German-speaking countries, Forel insisted that an efficient psychiatric prophylaxis had, first and foremost, to tackle the hereditary transmission of mental illness. Nevertheless, there was also a notable difference between Forel's concept of racial hygiene and that of most inter-war racial hygienists. For the Esperanto-speaking pacifist, socialist, and internationalist Forel, the notion of race was not a matter of national belonging but—at least on first sight—referred to humankind as a whole:

> Public, or rather, social hygiene, which also must be a racial hygiene, should always be given precedence over the individual one as soon as there is a conflict; and of these, there are many. Therefore, international hygiene precedes national hygiene, and the hygiene of the nation precedes that of the family.[42]

However, while Forel emphatically rejected racial nationalism and saw the modern nation as an 'utterly artificial product, created by wars and what the conquerors imposed on the conquered', his cosmopolitanism was far from universal.[43] His social-Darwinist ideas of natural selection extended to the existence of entire races. When Forel summarised the main issues driving his political vision in his autobiography, he named three: women's rights, the need for a common world language, and finally, 'the question of the human race itself. Which races are useful for the continuation of humankind and which are not? And if these lowest races are useless, how we should gradually eliminate them'.[44] While Forel found some peoples to be so inferior that they would disappear by themselves, he saw others as a threat. The 'negroes', which he considered as 'physically strong and robust, extraordinarily fertile, but mentally inferior', seemed particularly dangerous. As Forel stated in a 1910 talk at a neo-Malthusian meeting in the Netherlands, 'when they have adapted to our culture they corrupt it and our race through sloth, lack of ability and by creating such awful, mixed races as the mulatto'.[45] In the end, Forel's famed cosmopolitanism was for whites only.[46]

Throughout his life, Forel tirelessly advertised his vision of social reform, psychiatric prophylaxis, and eugenics to scientific and lay audiences. His most successful publication was an educational book about the 'sexual question' (*Die sexuelle Frage*) in 1905, which became an outright bestseller.[47] It was reprinted in sixteen editions until 1931; in addition, a shortened popular edition reached a similar circulation. His prophylactic ideas were most clearly summarised in another bestseller, *Hygiene der Nerven und des Geistes* ('Hygiene of the nerves and the soul'), that appeared in seven editions between 1903 and 1922. This popular treatise contained almost all of the ideas that became part of the agenda of mental hygiene associations in the second half of the 1920s, including heredity and eugenics, pedagogical interventions targeting children and adolescents, as well as the education of adults about sexuality, reproduction, and substance abuse.[48] Taken together, Forel had sketched the outlines of a socio-psychiatric approach that encompassed not only the entire lifespan of individuals who were healthy but threatened by the demands of modern life and society, but also connected eugenic hygiene of sexuality and reproduction, an individual hygiene of mental health, as well as racial and social hygiene.[49]

As the eight concluding 'postulates for a public and social hygiene of the nerves' show, Forel's vision was neither limited to the reform of existing psychiatric institutions through the implementation of psychotherapy and occupational therapy nor to the creation of new institutions for the confinement of dangerous borderline cases and agricultural colonies for nervous individuals. Forel also envisioned far-reaching social interventions targeting the mental health of the general population through the reform of housing, consumption, education, and sexual reproduction.[50] As Forel later wrote in his memoirs, it was this understanding of the social responsibility of medicine that had led him to give up his professorship in Zurich and to retire from his position as director of the Burghölzli in 1898:

> There was a voice yelling loudly in me, which told the psychiatrist: 'Leave your walls, off to the proclamation of these truths to the public, and to the study of mental abnormalities outside the asylums. You have to become an apostle of truth. Of what use is it to remain eternally there to care for the lost victims of the ignorance (*Unverstand*) of mankind as ruins in closed-off asylums, and thereby to quietly allow the causes of this misery to continue to exist. That is cowardice!'[51]

Despite his prominence in Swiss psychiatry and his anticipation of many of the dominant ideas of the movement, Auguste Forel played only a small role when mental hygiene arrived in Europe during the 1920s. There were several reasons for this: apart from Forel's old age and declining health, which prevented him from being an active part of the fledgling mental hygiene associations, one important factor was that, despite his role in the legitimisation and popularisation of eugenics, Forel was not considered an important scientific authority in this field. Despite his firm advocacy of eugenics, he had not been involved in research in psychiatric genetics and, despite his own forays, remained sceptical about the ethical implications of forced sterilisation.[52] During the inter-war years, eugenics were far more effectively represented by the staff of the Genealogic-Demographic Section of the German Research Institute for Psychiatry in Munich, in particular by Emil Kraepelin's student and colleague Ernst Rüdin.[53] Nevertheless, the name Forel remained part of the history of Swiss mental hygiene. His son Oscar Forel (1891–1982) was a founding member of the Swiss National Committee and became its treasurer and head of 'Commission III', which was tasked with general prophylaxis and, in particular, with the coordination of the committee with the various associations of the temperance movement.[54] At the same time, Oscar Forel also joined the editing board of the Walter Morgenthaler's Studies in Applied Psychiatry.

Moreover, there was another notable connection between the ideas of Auguste Forel and the international movement for mental hygiene. Adolf Meyer (1866–1950), the eminent American psychiatrist who had a crucial part in the early development of Clifford Beers's ideas into the US-based National Committee for Mental Hygiene (NCMH), was originally from Switzerland, where he had been a student of Auguste Forel.[55] When in 1908 Beers began to enlist allies for his efforts to create a movement for the betterment of the situation of the mental ill, Meyer was among his first and subsequently most important supporters. Not only did he recognise the potential of Beers's initiative for the psychiatric profession, he was also the one who came up with the term 'mental hygiene'.[56] The English translation of Forel's *Hygiene der Nerven und des Geistes* was published in the previous year and will not have gone unnoticed by his former student Meyer.[57] Some aspects of mental hygiene were not imported to Europe, but rather re-imported, after having undergone a process of double translation. Auguste Forel's psycho-political utopianism was one of the often-unrecognised roots of the idea of mental hygiene.

From Classification to Social Darwinism: Emil Kraepelin

Born in 1856, Emil Kraepelin was part of a generation of psychiatrists who in the course of their careers experienced rapid and profound changes in their discipline. From the early 1880s onwards, psychiatry established itself as a medical speciality at German universities, developed a scientific self-understanding and methodology based on the ideal of empirical, laboratory- and clinic-based research, and entered an increasingly close cooperation with the state.[58] Kraepelin was not a passive bystander in this transformation; he is widely considered as one of its driving forces. His influence still shapes the field today. Present-day classifications of psychiatric diseases like the DSM-5 (*Diagnostic and Statistical Manual of Mental Disorders, Fifth Edition*, 2013) are, at least to some extent, based on Kraepelin's nosology of psychoses and his notion of clinical, foundational research in psychiatry is still the groundwork of the discipline's scientific self-understanding.[59] Kraepelin, however, was also one of the first and most radical advocates of a systematic approach to psychiatric prophylaxis and many of his ideas had a lasting influence on the German mental hygiene movement emerging around the time of his death in 1926. In this section, I give a concise overview of Kraepelin's biography, scientific formation, and legacy, before discussing in more detail his understanding of the socio-medical duties of psychiatry and his socio-political views.

From the beginning of his medical studies in the mid-1870s on, Kraepelin pursued a career in psychiatry. After completing his studies in Wurzburg in 1878, he spent short periods as an assistant to Bernhard von Gudden (1824–1886) in Munich and Paul Flechsig (1847–1929) in Leipzig.[60] More important for his scientific trajectory was the time he spends in Wilhelm Wundt's (1832–1920) psychological laboratory in Leipzig, which had a crucial and lasting influence on Kraepelin's concept of psychiatric research.[61] His career almost ended early in 1882, when he was fired from his position as an assistant in the psychiatric university clinic of Leipzig after a heated dispute with director Flechsig. After a period of uncertainty, however, Kraepelin's career was on track again when he became chair of psychiatry at the university of Dorpat/Jurjew in Russia (today Tartu in Estonia) in 1886, aged thirty.[62]

As Wolfgang Burgmair, Eric Engstrom, and Matthias Weber, editors of a comprehensive seven-volume edition of Kraepelin's works, have argued, his years in Dorpat were formative for the staunch German nationalism that was a pivotal aspect of his world view for the remainder of his life.[63] The University of Dorpat at that time was formally Russian, but its ethnic make-up was reflective of the more complex realities in the Baltics. While the students mainly were Livonian, Russian, Polish, Estonian, or from Courland, the faculty was predominantly German.[64] On the eastern periphery of German academic life and amidst growing tensions between German professors and Russian authorities, Kraepelin came to consider himself as a forward post of the German nation and civilisation. This feeling was reinforced when, in an attempt to enforce the Russianisation of the Baltics, the authorities restricted the use of German as a teaching language, thereby creating considerable difficulties for the German professors. Increasingly, Kraepelin saw his research as a contribution to German cultural life and, as the next decades would show, the German nation eventually superseded the individual patient as the focal point of his medical efforts.

In 1891, Kraepelin returned to Germany to accept the chair of psychiatry in Heidelberg. Continuing the research programme begun in Dorpat, he reformed the university clinic into a vanguard research and teaching facility.[65] The scientific methods advanced by Kraepelin in Heidelberg became a model for the future development of German, and international, psychiatry. The essential part of Kraepelin's vision of the university clinic was a newly constructed surveillance ward (*Wachabteilung*), a clinical space dedicated to the meticulous observation of selected parts of the clinic's patient population. The introduction of psychiatric surveillance wards in Germany in the late 1880s, pioneered not only by Kraepelin in Heidelberg but also by Robert Sommer in Giessen, and marks a profound epistemological shift. The 'clinical gaze' became an integral part of the psychiatric institution and the university clinic replaced the asylum as the privileged space of psychiatric knowledge production.

Surveillance was, however, only one aspect of the innovation spearheaded by Kraepelin's clinic in Heidelberg; recording, collecting, and comparing patient files were the other. To borrow a notion introduced by Paul Flechsig's patient Daniel Paul Schreber (1842–1911) and later picked up by media theorist Friedrich Kittler (1943–2011), the newly created surveillance wards were the core of an elaborate *Aufschreibesystem*—a 'system of writing-up', or as Kittler defined it, 'a network of techniques and institutions [...] which allow to address, store, and process relevant data'.[66] Around the same time when the psychiatric inmate Schreber experienced himself as the object of a divine apparatus recording his every move and utterance, the psychiatric wards of German university clinics developed similar methods. Probably based on his experiences with the statistical techniques of the Bavarian census in the late 1870s, Kraepelin devised a system of diagnostic cards (*Zählkarten*) to register excerpts from patient histories, diagnoses, and the course of the disease. Notably, what played only a minor role in Kraepelin's conception of scientific psychiatry were the subjective experiences of patients and the content of their delusions.[67] The diagnostic cards would be updated even after a patient had left the clinic, so that the progression of a disease could be followed.[68] Based on this large and growing corpus of quantitative data and the underlying assumption that different mental illnesses could be distinguished as naturally distinct entities, Kraepelin proceeded to construct nosological groups of psychopathologies, differentiating between diseases according to their assumed aetiology, their course, and their final state.[69]

The Kraepelinian nosology, as laid out in the fifth and sixth editions of his textbook in 1896 and 1899, respectively, quickly became the dominant paradigm in German-speaking psychiatry.[70] It gave the ascending discipline a common diagnostic language and provided it with an ambitious empirical research agenda that was based on the prestige of the laboratory sciences.[71] Psychiatry, Kraepelin wrote, now finally had the 'same weapons at its disposal that have served other fields of medicine so well: clinical observation, the microscope, and experimentation'.[72] However, as historians of psychiatry have shown, it would be wrong to reduce Kraepelin's success to the simplistic narrative of a great man, his invention, and the triumph of scientific objectivity. Kraepelin's classification system appeared just at the right moment when psychiatry found itself in a 'nosological limbo' after previous approaches had lost their cogency. Moreover, the publication of the two editions of his textbook coincided with the issuing of new regulations for medical examinations at the universities and thus answered to a 'heightened demand for a teachable psychiatry with clear, concise disease categories'.[73] Although his system quickly found many supporters, it never became an uncontested consensus among psychiatrists; then and now, the details as well as the basis premises of Kraepelin's nosology are continuously discussed and challenged.

The classification of mental diseases according to their assumed cause and progression was directly connected to the prophylactic perspectives that came to dominate Kraepelin's professional activities after the turn of the century. In the preface to the 1899 edition of his textbook Kraepelin conceded that, even with new insights into mental illness, psychiatry's therapeutic options were limited. Instead, recent advances in the aetiology of mental illness would create another way out of the psychiatric stalemate: 'The scientific understanding of mental disorders is the indispensable foundation for the solution of the vitally important practical problems that psychiatry has to solve. Primarily, this will be the prevention of mental illness'.[74] On the one hand, Kraepelin's promise to leave behind the 'therapeutic nihilism' of the nineteenth century was an answer to public and state expectations in the discipline—while previous decades had seen the number of inmates in psychiatric asylums, and hence also the costs of the system, multiply.[75] On the other hand, the consolidation of a common nosology and the promise of a new field for medical action also reflected and bolstered psychiatrists' self-confidence.

Emil Kraepelin's 1899 talk about 'the psychiatric duties of the state' was a striking expression of this new-found confidence.[76] In the nineteenth century, psychiatry had emerged as an institution maintaining social order for the state; now, Kraepelin demanded that the state help fulfil the functions of psychiatry:

> When the mentally ill are a menace or burden to the state, the state must under all circumstances try to reach a decrease of their numbers, or at least a slowdown of the increase. Like with all other diseases, prophylaxis is more promising than the therapy of those who are already ill. Thus, it is necessary for the state to search for the sources of mental illness and, if possible, to clog them.[77]

Different from what this mission statement suggests, Kraepelin's list of demands was only partly concerned with the actual prophylaxis of mental illness. In fact, he named only two causes of disease against which the state might be able to effectively implement preventive measures: substance abuse and syphilis, which together accounted for more than one-third of psychiatric admissions. By far the greater part of Kraepelin's demands to the state had to do with the organisation of psychiatry and the legal framework in which it operated, including the socialisation and expansion of the asylum system, the reform of penal law, the legal regulations for the confinement of the insane, the establishment of additional psychiatric university clinics, the inclusion of psychiatry into the curriculum of medical schools, and, finally, the improvement of psychiatrists' conditions for work and research. Notably, eugenics were still absent in 1899, and the concept of prevention proposed by Kraepelin was limited to those mental diseases that the sixth edition of his textbook in the same year attributed to exterior causes. The textbook itself was slightly more comprehensive; in a short section about prophylaxis Kraepelin already considered marriage restrictions for the mentally ill as a means of preventing the transmission of hereditary disorders.[78] But only over the course of the next decade would fears of degeneration and calls for eugenic interventions move to the fore of Kraepelin's prophylactic agenda.

The shift towards prophylaxis and racial hygiene coincided with Kraepelin's move to Munich in 1903. After Dorpat and Heidelberg, the appointment as professor of psychiatry and head of the university clinic of the Bavarian capital marked the zenith of Kraepelin's academic career and the beginning of a third phase in his scientific trajectory. While the tenure in Dorpat was characterised by Wundtian experimental psychology and Heidelberg by clinical observation and documentation, in Munich Kraepelin's attention turned towards large-scale prophylaxis and the preservation of the health of the German nation as an organic whole.[79] This shift towards socio-medical interventions was a reaction to the discrepancy between the impressive scientific advances that psychiatry had experienced in the last decade of the century and the meagre therapeutic outcome. In this impasse, prophylaxis offered the only auspicious way to capitalise on recent advances in foundational research. Despite recurring waves of therapeutic optimism—like the suggestive treatment of war neurotics, the 'heroic therapies' of the inter-war period,[80] or the rise of psychopharmacology since the 1950s[81]—the idea that individual and large-scale prophylaxis might have to substitute for therapeutic shortcomings remained pertinent throughout the twentieth century.

The 1908 article 'On the Question of Degeneration' (*Zur Entartungsfrage*) summarised Kraepelin's views about the relation between mental illness and society in the first decade of the twentieth century.[82] The article contained many topics that he had already referred to earlier, such as the increasing number of psychiatric patients and the role of alcohol and syphilis as causal factors for mental illness, but integrated them in a broader conceptual and theoretical framework. As Kraepelin claimed, these were only symptoms of a much larger problem: the pathogenic and degenerative influence of modern civilisation. The most obvious sign of this crisis in collective health was the dramatic increase in the percentage of psychiatric inmates compared to the general population in the last decades of the twentieth century. Kraepelin, who had travelled to Java in 1904, believed that this problem was geographically located. It pertained to inhabitants of European countries, but not to natives; a similar imbalance could be found between morbid city dwellers and the healthy rural population.[83] Hence, the increase in mental illness was a result of the living conditions in big cities and of urban modernity in general. That the two 'epidemic toxins' (*Volksgifte*) of alcoholism and syphilis were particularly rampant in urban environments was only one part of Kraepelin's explanation. More important was that he found the progress of civilisation itself 'able to inflict damage on the deepest roots of our mental health'.[84]

Kraepelin named several ways in which modern civilisation exerted its degenerative effect. Drawing on contemporary ideas of nervousness and neurasthenia, he believed that by enmeshing people in a complex web of social relations and responsibilities, civilisation robbed them of their freedom, severed their 'relationship with nature', and created mental strains leading to 'degenerative psychosis' (*Entartungsirresein*).[85] But this was not the end of Kraepelin's broadside critique. He also accused modern civilisation of 'domesticising' people so that, like overbred household pets, they would lose their powers of resistance, of creating pathogenic conditions of 'proletarisation' and urban poverty, of neglecting physical education in favour of a 'one-sided cultivation of intellectual facilities', and finally, of 'weakening the natural drives'.[86] All this would lead to a state of degeneration that would not manifest as a single symptomatic illness, but as a diffuse state of overall morbidity and vulnerability. This process was not limited to individuals but would lead to a progressive 'degeneration of the race'.

Kraepelin's notion of degeneration was both Darwinist and Lamarckian. On the one hand, he decried the corrosive influence of modern civilisation on individuals' fitness in the 'struggle for survival'; on the other, he also claimed that the 'germs' of future generations could not only be damaged by toxins or physical disease, but that 'life-experiences [...] do not leave developing germ cells untouched, but can somehow impinge upon the properties governing the lives of future generations'—a view echoed by present-day epigenetics.[87] Moreover, Kraepelin also departed from Bénédict Morel's hypothesis that degeneration would negatively affect fertility and therefore was a self-limiting process affecting individual families, as illustrated in a classic example of 'decadent' fin de siècle literature, Thomas Mann's history of the ascent and decline of the fictional Buddenbrook family.[88] By contrast, in Kraepelin's view, degeneration could spread and worsen from generation to generation and eventually corrupt entire races. The example of the Jews, he believed, showed where this process was headed, their 'strong disposition to nervous and mental diseases' being a direct outcome of their advanced 'domestication'.

Kraepelin's Lamarckian argument about the influence of 'life-experiences' on 'germ cells' conflated social and cultural processes causing individual mental illness with biological processes threatening the future of the body politic. It elevated common fin de siècle concerns about the diseases of civilisation to an existential question 'of *utmost importance* to our existence as a people'.[89] To save the nation, Kraepelin insisted, large-scale, state-led research into the process of degeneration was urgently needed. Decades-long, meticulous studies of entire cities and districts would have to be 'undertaken by specially trained commissions comprised of physicians and statisticians whose attention is devoted solely to the task of investigating the question of degeneration'.[90] Less than a decade later, this ambitious programme formulated in 1908 was tackled by the newly created German Research Institute for Psychiatry (*Deutsche Forschungsanstalt für Psychiatrie*, DFA). Kraepelin's treatise was widely read and controversially discussed among psychiatrists in pre-war Germany and, like few other sources, marks the ingress of racial hygiene into the mainstream of German psychiatry in the first decade of the twentieth century. There was, however, no consensus about Kraepelin's statist approach even among fellow racial hygienists. Even Kraepelin's assistant Ernst Rüdin, who later personified the eugenic alliance of science and state like few others, was sceptical about the focus on state-led programmes. In an otherwise adulatory review of his superior's article, he questioned whether the state and the *Reich* at this time would be of any help in the struggle against degeneration.[91]

Even though they found themselves in opposite political camps, Auguste Forel and Emil Kraepelin's psycho-political outlooks were strikingly similar. Both Forel and Kraepelin avidly admired Darwin and believed that his ideas had to be applied to human society. They saw themselves as advocates of an objective and unprejudiced science whose uneasy truths had to be asserted against the naïve moralism of society. While such social-Darwinist views were far from uncommon among members of their class, generation, and profession, Forel and Kraepelin were particularly outspoken and zealous and the first psychiatrists to systematically integrate these views into their theories.[92] The same also pertained to the reception of Morel's concept of degeneration. The view that civilisation had a negative, 'degenerative' effect on individuals and groups had already been popularised earlier by Max Nordau and other writers and was among the most influential tropes in fin de siècle scientific and literary debates.[93] For Forel and Kraepelin, however, social Darwinism and the concept of degeneration became starting points for a systematic extension of psychiatry's professional sphere of activity beyond the asylum walls. They both passionately believed that as psychiatrists, they had to become educators and saviours of humanity in its existential struggle against the threat of alcohol, degeneration, and the suspension of the laws of natural selection in modern civilisation.

The main difference was that Kraepelin was far more pragmatic and effective than his Swiss counterpart. The utopian Forel tried to achieve his goal of a eugenic 'scientific social democracy' by drafting a constitution for the 'United States of the Earth'.[94] Kraepelin, by contrast, tried to tap the resources of the existing state authorities for his professional goals. Instead of envisioning a global social-Darwinist scientocracy, he lobbied for a research institute that would conduct foundational research in psychiatric heredity. Unsurprisingly, Kraepelin's strategy proved to be more successful.

Plans for a new kind of psychiatric research institution had already been floated before Kraepelin adopted this idea. In 1910, Robert Sommer had published a memorandum for the creation of a psychiatric department of the *Reich* health office (*Reichsgesundheitsamt*) that would have tackled similar tasks as Kraepelin's future institute. Sommer's psychiatric department was projected as an institute of foundational research, providing psychiatric researchers with the necessary resources and working conditions and freeing them from the distracting and time-consuming everyday routine of hospitals and asylums. Apart from a centralised data collection about psychiatric institutions in Germany and foundational research, its task would have been to create the psychiatric expertise needed to counter the perceived threat of degeneration.[95] Despite some support from within the psychiatric profession, however, Sommer's ambitious programme never even came close to being realised.[96]

After Sommer's plans had been scrapped the German Psychiatric Association (*Deutscher Verein für Psychiatrie*, DVP) asked Kraepelin in 1912 to prepare a second memorandum for a psychiatric research institute.[97] Like Sommer, the DVP's board had initially envisioned an institution that would have been at least partially state-funded and had hoped to obtain funding from the Kaiser Wilhelm Society for the Advancement of Science (*Kaiser-Wilhelm-Gesellschaft zur Förderung der Wissenschaften*, KWG). In a 1916 memorandum, Kraepelin opted for the same approach, arguing that a request for 'vigorous help' by the KWG was the 'natural way' to proceed.[98] At the time of the publication, the KWG had, however, already rejected the funding of a psychiatric research institute, because there was no consensus inside the society about the status of clinical research in its programme and because they feared rivalry with the Kaiser Wilhelm Institute for Brain Research (*Kaiser-Wilhelm-Institut für Hirnforschung*) that had been established in Berlin in 1914.[99] Without available state funding, Kraepelin turned to an approach that he considered a 'last resort': enlisting wealthy patrons to realise the research institute as an independent foundation.[100]

Despite these inauspicious beginnings, the German Research Institute for Psychiatry (*Deutsche Forschungsanstalt für Psychiatrie*) was successfully established during the war. That this founding took place despite the lack of state funding and under wartime conditions was mainly due to Kraepelin's prestige and prominence. But it was also the outcome of a momentous coincidence. In late 1915, Kraepelin had met an 'American gentleman' willing to support his project with a substantial donation. This was James Loeb (1867–1933), a German-born philanthropist, who had made his fortune as a banker in the United States.[101] After retiring in 1902, Loeb devoted himself and his wealth to the arts and charity. As the anecdote has it, he had seen Sigmund Freud after a mental breakdown and, when psychoanalysis was unable to provide help, had consulted Kraepelin.[102] Be that as it may, in January 1916 he agreed to a huge donation of 500,000 marks, provided that other donors would cover the rest of the funds required for the research institute. Bolstered by Loeb's support, Kraepelin successfully convinced numerous other patrons and eventually secured a total of 1,700,000 marks. The German Research Institute for Psychiatry was formally established on 13 February 1917.

On 1 April 1918, while the world war was still raging, research activities at the institute began. At this time, the institute had five departments, representing key areas in Kraepelin's understanding of psychiatry as a science: histopathology I and II, headed by Franz Nissl and Walther Spielmeyer, respectively; histotopography, headed by Korbinian Brodman; serology, Felix Plaut; experimental psychology, headed by Johannes Lange and Kraepelin; and finally, Ernst Rüdin's demographic-genealogical department.[103] Due to a lack of suitable rooms, a planned chemistry department could initially not be set up.[104]

The structure of the research institute was reflective of the major trends in contemporary psychiatric research, which focused on laboratory research, the natural sciences, and biology in particular.[105] To Kraepelin, however, the institute was more than a facility for cutting-edge foundational research. It was also the basis for the salvation of the German nation in a time of existential crisis. 'The devastations that the world war has caused just among our best and healthiest urge us in the strongest manner to do whatever is possible to avert the dangers to our future that arise from this heavy loss of the noblest forces', Kraepelin wrote in the last months of the war: 'Among the many enemies that we must fight, *mental diseases* stand in the front line'.[106]

This bellicose rhetoric echoed political and public language in wartime Germany. To some extent, this alarmism may have been part of a strategy to advertise and legitimise an institution that would pay its director a stately salary of 20,000 marks per year.[107] But more importantly, Kraepelin's concern for the survival of the nation connected his vision of prophylaxis to his nationalism. This idea did not emerge during the war but had already been part of this thinking when he was still in Dorpat in the late 1880s. The experience of the war, however, radicalised Kraepelin's outlook. In 1916, he joined a People's Committee for the Prompt Subjugation of England (*Volksausschuß für die rasche Niederkämpfung Englands*), a right-wing group organising lectures and drawing up guidelines to support all-out submarine warfare and the annexation of vast territories. When Kraepelin soon withdrew from this kind of political activity, it was not because of a change on conviction, but because the inherent squabbling of political organisations went against his impatient activism.[108] After the war, he became an outspoken opponent of the fledgling Weimar Republic in particular and of democracy in general. However, after his brief foray into party politics during the war, he returned to the view that he could better serve his nation as a scientist and physician. The struggle against mental illness as an internal enemy became a continuation of the national fight against external enemies:[109] 'The enormous war we have experienced has shown us what victorious weapons science was able to forge for our fight against a world of enemies – should it be any different in the struggle against an internal enemy seeking to destroy the basis of our existence?'[110]

Rather than the sick individual, the target of Kraepelin's research efforts was the health of the body politic. As he argued, mental illness was among the worst diseases that could afflict an individual but it was also a major threat to the health and well-being of the nation itself. The mentally ill were an almost unbearable burden to families and welfare institutions and the hereditary propagation of mental illness would have a most destructive effect on future generations. Kraepelin was not only worried about the social burden of 'more than a quarter of a million of people who are mentally more or less crippled or destroyed'.[111] Even more he was concerned about an enormous number of borderline cases, who were not mentally ill in the narrower sense, but a menace to society nevertheless:

> [...] those whom we describe as 'nervous', eccentrics, psychopaths, or as feebleminded and inferior, or as degenerates and enemies of society. Many of the former wear themselves out in inner struggles and troubles, and due to their mental deficiencies cause misery and confusion on countless occasions. The latter, however, are born criminals and become a scourge for their environment, or as vagabonds become an epidemic plague (*Volksplage*) against which we are almost powerless.[112]

Kraepelin's concern about borderline cases was not entirely new. In the seventh edition of his textbook, published in 1904, he had spent an entire chapter on 'psychopathic personalities'. The classification of four types of borderline cases introduced then—born criminals, pathological liars, querulous persons, and individuals driven by primitive instincts—remained an important reference for the understanding of deviant behaviour well into the mid-1920s.[113] In the years prior to the war, 'psychopathic personalities' had mainly occupied forensic psychiatrists and criminologists, who often used the concept to argue for an extension of the role of medical expert testimonies in penal law and the introduction of more subtle categories for the assessment of criminal responsibility.[114] After the war however, psychopaths became a primary concern for psychiatrists and lawmakers. The epidemic of 'war neuroses' seemed to have uncovered a vast reservoir of 'inferiors' among the general population, individuals who under normal circumstances were inconspicuous, but whose inherited mental deficiencies made them susceptible to exceptional mental states and suggestive influences and conditions of stress. To conservative psychiatrists, the 1918/1919 revolution was a confirmation of their apprehensions and in numerous diagnoses of current events, participants, and leaders of the revolution were identified as dangerous psychopaths.

Some of the most acrimonious psycho-political diagnoses came from the staff of the recently founded German Research Institute for Psychiatry.[115] Kraepelin explained that the deprivations and mental strain of the wartime had left the German 'national soul' (*Volksseele*) in a state of hysterical weakness that had led to the military collapse and the ensuing civil war.[116] Just like his former student Robert Gaupp and his assistant Eugen Kahn, Kraepelin was convinced that mass hysteria had delivered the masses to the suggestive influence of dangerous psychopaths, who had incited and steered the revolutionary upheaval.[117] Even more than his colleagues, Kraepelin proposed a social-Darwinist interpretation of the revolution when he claimed that the short-lived rule of the Bavarian Soviet with its belief in equality and direct democracy had inversed the natural hierarchy and led to a rule of the irrational masses and mentally defectives known as the 'proletariat'.[118] To save the nation, Kraepelin called for far-reaching socio-medical interventions, including public hygiene, the abolition of many social ills, the re-education of the people, and, most of all, the systematic eugenic breeding of Germany's future leaders and elites.

Kraepelin's views in 1919 were not an exceptional and emotional reaction by an aging scholar overwhelmed by the experience of the post-war turmoil in Munich, they were merely a tapered expression of positions that he had held since long before the war. Since the turn of the century, Kraepelin had positioned himself as the most prominent and outspoken advocate of a form of psychiatry that did not limit itself to caring for the mentally ill, but actively intervened in society. From the onset, the German Research Institute for Psychiatry was part of this agenda. At the opening ceremony of the institute in 1917 Kraepelin declared that in times of war and national crisis, no distinction could be made between foundational research and national interests. Comparing psychiatry to the sciences that had provided the German military with poison gas and explosives, Kraepelin asked whether it 'should it be any different in the fight against an internal foe which aspires to destroy the foundations of our existence?'[119]

Unlike the army, the scientific centre of German psychiatry was not demobilised in late 1918. As Kraepelin wrote about three years after the end of the war, the institute should be 'the home of rigorous science' but its ultimate goal was 'to serve the nation's health and to work toward healing the deep wounds which bitter fate has inflicted upon our fatherland'.[120] As Eric Engstrom has pointed out, an inherent contradiction between scientific universalism and political nationalism permeated the activities of the institute. On the one hand, the aim of its research was to uncover the basic principles of mental illness; a research agenda that could easily transcend national borders. As a centre of foundational research, the institute enjoyed considerable international prestige and attracted many scholars from abroad. On the other hand, however, its scientific legitimacy was based on nationalism, as the institute was to represent the prowess of German science on the international stage and to improve public health as part of the nation's 'struggle for survival'.

Visions of a psycho-political regeneration of the German nation continued to occupy Kraepelin for years after the revolution. Exactly two years after the double proclamation of a German Republic in Berlin, he gave a talk with the telling title 'On uprootedness' (*Über Entwurzelung).*[121] In early 1919, Kraepelin had used the common, but elusive and speculative notion of a 'collective soul' (*Volksseele*) to construe a connection between psychopathological states and socio-political phenomena; in the 1920 lecture, he revisited the topic and tried to explain the relation between individual mental illness and the community more systematically. While the lecture was no departure from his earlier views, it shifted the focus away from biology and heredity to the psycho-social dynamics of mental disorder. Kraepelin began the lecture with a programmatic statement: 'Man is a gregarious animal (*Herdentier*)'.[122] As he argued, human personality was decisively shaped by an individual's relations with his or her social environment, 'primarily by his family, as well as by his companions and friends, and finally by his compatriots (*Volksgenossen*)'. These bonds gave an individual mental support and stability, provided direction in volition and action, and offered refuge in times of crisis. The severing of these social relations, which Kraepelin likened to being 'uprooted' like a plant from the soil, could be a consequence of a pre-existing mental disorder, but it could also be a cause.

Even as Kraepelin focused on the family, the analogy to the nation was obvious to anyone in the audience in 1920 Germany. The war had in fact shattered many families, but in the eyes of conservative nationalists like Kraepelin, 'uprootedness' and the breakdown of social bonds were an apt description of the general state of the German nation. The revolution had replaced the mythologised national unity of August 1914 with political struggle and disorientation. In the second half of his lecture, Kraepelin turned to national politics and extended his notion of the social integration of the individual from the immediate social environment to the nation as a community: 'Furthermore, we all are, by lineage, upbringing, and fate, members of a nation (*Volk*), whose whole development is the primal ground (*Urgrund*) of our existence. It is here where our mental life is firmly grounded; it is here where, as the poet says, the strong roots of our power are'. As he had already done in earlier writings, Kraepelin used the Jews as an example to illustrate where he saw this process going and to construe a connection between psychopathologies and alleged racial traits when he claimed that 'the unpleasant internationalism of the Jewish people was brought up by the national uprootedness that was imposed on them'.[123] The loss of rootedness that, as Kraepelin believed, had already befallen the Jewish people, was now threatening the Germans. As he warned, Germans were increasingly marrying foreigners and gradually losing their native language, which was becoming increasingly interspersed with words of Latin origin.[124]

Kraepelin's lecture followed the usual script of the psycho-political tracts of the post-war period. After vividly portraying the looming threats to the very existence of the nation and the body politic, a programme for national salvation was laid out. First, Kraepelin proposed, the connection between mental disorder and uprootedness had to be thoroughly researched. If, as he believed certain, a link between the two were to be established, resolute socio-medical actions would have to be taken. Different from his earlier writings on degeneration, Kraepelin refrained from any reference to eugenics and racial hygiene and focused on living conditions and the restoration of the internal cohesion of the national community instead. Two years after Germany had lost its colonies abroad, Kraepelin advocated a programme of 'internal colonisation' to

> strengthen the cohesion of the families, [create] the possibility to settle on one's own land, foster family research and the creation of families, the facilitation of early marriage and child-rearing, to prevent the scattering of the

> families, [and work towards] a prohibition of child labour and restrictions for taverns, and finally, [to promote] all measures that put a stop to the subversive influence of internationalism, and invigorate the inner cohesion among all compatriots.[125]

This was a particularly reactionary variation on a motive of national regeneration that was ubiquitous in post-war Germany. Against the corrosive effects of urban modernity and the international circulation of people and ideas, Kraepelin advocated a return to blood relations and soil-bound rural life, and as the key concepts indicate, his ideas were at least compatible with the Nazi ideology that took shape during the same time and in Munich as well.

However, Kraepelin's 1920 lecture was also notable for introducing a notion that would gain importance during the following decade and again after the Second World War: 'social psychiatry', described by Kraepelin as a new 'science, which we today rather conjecture than know'.[126] In the second half of the century, social psychiatry emerged as a movement for the reform of psychiatric institutions, for a move away from biologism to an understanding of the patient in his or her social context, as well as for treatment methods questioning the hierarchies of the traditional doctor—patient relationship.[127] While Kraepelin ventured beyond a purely biological understanding of mental illness and into the field of the psycho-social, his notion of 'social psychiatry' had little in common with this. His social psychiatry was not interested in the individual patient or in challenging hierarchies in psychiatric treatment. Instead, Kraepelin's plan was for psychiatry to leave the asylum behind and devote its resources to prophylaxis on a national scale and to the paternalist re-education of the nation.

Kraepelin's 'social psychiatry' never became a reality. After retiring from his professorship in 1922, he devoted himself to the German Research Institute for Psychiatry until his death in 1926. As one of the earliest and most influential proponents of a systematic approach to psychiatric prophylaxis, he was a direct and important precursor for many ideas that would later become part of the agenda of the German mental hygiene movement. His social-Darwinist views directly or indirectly influenced most of the protagonists of the movement. A few years after this death, Kraepelin's ideas, however, also spelled the end of the pluralist approach to mental hygiene in Germany, when racial hygiene, bolstered by its new-found political leverage, supplanted other, less biologistic methods of psychiatric prophylaxis.

Sleep, Heredity, and the Invention of Mental Hygiene: Robert Sommer

That an organised movement for mental hygiene emerged in Germany in the second half of the 1920s was a result of the activities of Robert Sommer. He was the founder and the first chairman of the German Association for Mental Hygiene (*Deutscher Verband für psychische Hygiene*, DVPH), as well as the co-founder and president of another association occupied with questions of mental hygiene, the General Medical Society for Psychotherapy (*Allgemeine Ärztliche Gesellschaft für Psychotherapie*, AÄGP). Sommer only began to lobby for the founding of a mental hygiene association after Clifford Beers's voyage to Europe in 1923. However, his pursuit of mental hygiene and, more generally, the idea psychiatric prophylaxis, went back to the turn of the century, antedating even the founding of the first mental hygiene association in the United States in 1908 by almost a decade. Protagonists of mental hygiene in Germany saw Sommer as the leader and founder of their movement and credited him with having introduced the term 'mental hygiene' (*psychische Hygiene*) as early as 1901.[128]

Nevertheless, the life and work of Robert Sommer have received little scholarly attention. In this section, I give an overview of the biography of the 'founding father' of German mental hygiene and assess his contribution to the extension of psychiatry's sphere of activity before and after the First World War. In particular, Sommer's life shows how the mental hygiene ideas of the inter-war period were rooted in fin de siècle debates about nervousness, neurasthenia, and the psychiatric challenges of urban modernity, as well as to Sommer's specific notion of heredity. Following this sketch of Sommer's career, I discuss his approach to psychiatric prophylaxis, examining the two major strands: the prevention of exogenous neuroses through the establishment of public resting rooms and related measures, and the prevention of endogenous neuroses through family studies, research in heredity, and eugenics.

Born in 1864 as son of a Protestant lawyer in the Silesian town of Grottkau (today Grotków in Poland), Sommer studied philosophy and medicine in Leipzig.[129] He completed his studies with a doctorate in philosophy in 1887 with a thesis about John Locke and René Descartes and passed his state examination in medicine in the following year. Subsequently, he joined Wilhelm Wundt's psycho-physiological laboratory in Leipzig for a brief period. Wundt's laboratory was then the undisputed world centre of experimental psychology, attracting leading German psychologists and psychiatrists as well as many foreign scholars. Among others, Emil Kraepelin, eight years Sommer's senior, had worked there a decade earlier. Although Sommer only spent little time in Leipzig, his studies with Wundt and the encounter with the methods of experimental psychological shaped his scientific outlook for the following decades. After subsequent assistantships in Rybnik and Wurzburg, Sommer completed a second, medical doctorate in 1891 with a thesis about Samuel Thomas von Soemmering's (1755–1830) theory on the localisation of the soul. In May 1895, aged thirty, he was appointed as professor of psychiatry at the University of Giessen and became head of the new psychiatric clinic, still under construction.[130] Until his death in 1937, Sommer spent his entire career and most of his life in Giessen.

Economically secure and scientifically independent, Sommer used the possibilities that came with his tenure to follow an exceptionally broad range of research interests. Almost all fields of contemporary psychology and psychiatry were part of his research at one time or another: criminal psychology and forensic psychiatry, the new examination methods of experimental psychology, family studies and psychiatric heredity research, the psychology of genius, animal psychology, as well as psychotherapy and different approaches to psychiatric prophylaxis. After the turn of the century, Sommer began a remarkable organisational activity, hosting a series of conferences and seminars in Giessen. Following a 1904 congress on experimental psychology and a 1906 seminar on the treatment and education of the feebleminded, Sommer set up two seminars about criminal psychology and forensic psychiatry in 1907 and 1909. Two more seminars on 'family research and the study of heredity and regeneration' in 1908 and 1912 were crucial for the development of Sommer's prophylactic and eugenic ideas. A quarter-century later, these seminars were one reason why Sommer was lauded as an early advocate and pioneer of the Nazis' concept of racial hygiene—a questionable and undeserved praise.[131]

As Sommer claimed in 1912, his shifting interests were no mere eclecticism, but together formed a more encompassing programme, as the seminars were 'a coherent series of efforts to methodologically represent the hereditary disposition and whole personality of individual humans, and the natural character of specific groups of humans on the basis of an observing psychology and the natural sciences'.[132] In like manner, a biographer of Sommer has claimed that his scientific oeuvre followed the unifying idea of a holistic 'extended psychiatry', derived from Wundt's psycho-physiological school.[133] Even as Sommer employed the notion of 'extended psychiatry' this seems more like a post hoc rationalisation of his eclecticism, in which, despite some recurring themes, a consciously defined and encompassing research agenda is difficult to discern. Notably, even close collaborators like Wilhelm Weygandt (1870–1939) complained about the missing coherence and scientificity of some of Sommer's work.[134] There were few fields in contemporary psychiatry and psychology that did not attract his interest at some point, but not always did his reflections produce viable results.

Sommer's bustling activity went beyond the medical field. He was a local politician and served as a member of Giessen's city council from 1910 to 1922; he published on the ancient history of the region and authored poetry and comedic plays of questionable quality. Moreover, Sommer also considered himself an inventor—his most remarkable contraption being a pair of clunky water-walking shoes that he used to hike the local river Lahn and for which he had filed a patent application. During the war, he tried to put his inventive mind into the service of the nation by drafting flying machines for the army; in the early 1930s, he delved into another idea that would only come to realise its potentials several decades later: electronic music. An assiduous organiser as much as an inventor, Sommer would not limit himself to designing his own gadgets, but also lobbied for the creation of a national institute for inventors in the early 1930s.[135] There were also connections between his inventing activities and his professional interests. For his psychological research, Sommer devised equipment to measure the physical expressions of psychological processes. At the same time, he also pondered the psychological aspects of being an inventor and his observations about the inventor's psychology provide us with a clear expression of how he saw himself and his motivations:

> The true inventor, with his mind set on the shaping of a future, often unwillingly and through an organic pressure occupies a special place in relation to his environment. From this side, this often asserts itself as rejection, scorn, if not in doubting the normal mental constitution of the inventor, while he, if life does not provide him with spiritually related people, becomes increasingly self-reliant, retracts, and works on his ideas as an eccentric character. Only if his invention leads to exterior success, this tension between the inventor and his environment becomes balanced.[136]

Throughout his career, Robert Sommer's political, societal, and medical ideas frequently intertwined. The promotion and preservation of public health was one important concern for his political activities as city council member and his medical reflections about individual and collective pathologies were pivotal for Sommer's ideas about political, social, and economic reform; a connection that eventually led him to become a central figure in the formation of mental hygiene in Germany. There are, however, good reasons not to adopt the movement's own teleological narrative according to which Sommer's turn-of-the-century ideas led directly to the inter-war period movement.[137] Doing so would mean to understate the role that the US-based NCMH played in the global founding of mental hygiene associations in the 1920s, and it would also mean to overlook that the ideas that Sommer associated with the notion of 'mental hygiene' in 1902 were still far apart from the international movement in the inter-war period. Instead, Sommer introduced the term 'mental hygiene' as part of the pervasive debate about nervousness and neurasthenia that reached its peak around the turn of the century.[138]

What the example of Sommer shows, is that the emergence of psychiatric prophylaxis was part of a broader debate about the detriments of modernity. The debate about neurasthenia was, first and foremost, about managing and balancing the energy inside the nervous system in a rapidly modernising environment, in which the increasing acceleration of social and economic life, new technologies and new and intense stimuli put the mind in a state of constant stress. It was in this context that Robert Sommer first employed the notion of 'mental hygiene'. As he wrote in 1902, one of the most serious challenges to mental health was the increasing lack of sleep. Insufficient sleep, he argued, was not only be a potential symptom of mental illness, but could also be its cause, as only sufficient rest could ensure the necessary restoration of nervous energy: 'Only sleep can be a corrective against the damage caused by the haste of present-day traffic'.[139] Hence, insufficient rest and sleep were an important problem that had to be tackled by public health initiatives: 'If one finally wants to take serious the idea of mental hygiene and the preservation of nervous energy, then the public organisation of rest will be one of the first and, to a certain degree, solvable tasks'.[140]

Mental hygiene in this sense meant the 'preservation of nervous energy' against the strains of accelerating urban modernity. For Sommer, two groups of people were particularly prone to nervous exhaustion: big city dwellers and the visitors of trade fairs and exhibitions who were overwhelmed by new and unfamiliar impressions for hours on end. He proposed a simple solution: the establishment of 'public resting rooms' (*öffentliche*

Ruhehallen), where one could sleep and relax for an hour or a half.[141] And Sommer did not only formulate a general idea, he was also concerned about the details of the implementation. His article not only included detailed plans for a model *Ruhehalle* and its furnishings, but also financial estimates of building expenses and cost return.

Public resting rooms were not just a passing fad of Sommer's, but a project for which he persistently continued to lobby for several decades. A prototype *Ruhehalle* was built for the 1911 hygiene exhibition in Dresden; in the following year, the proposal received an award at the International Exhibition for Social Hygiene (*Esposizione Internazionale d'Igiene Sociale*) in Rome.[142] Spurred by the prize and the fact that the model in Dresden had been well received by colleagues and visitors, Sommer intensified his efforts. He distributed reprints of his plans, published additional articles, and sent a memorandum to the administrations of numerous big cities, both in Germany and abroad—yet, to no avail.[143]

The world war brought Sommer's efforts to a halt. Some years later, however, the founding of the German Society for Mental Hygiene provided Sommer with new platform for his idea. The public resting rooms appeared in the society's programme, as Sommer optimistically hoped that the fledgling society in cooperation with the Reich Ministry of the Interior would now push German city administrations to realise his plans.[144] However, his fellow mental hygienists did not share this enthusiasm, and neither did the city administrations.[145] Only on two occasions was Sommer's plan actually translated into built architecture in inter-war Germany; in 1928 for the International Press Exhibition ('Pressa') in Cologne[146] and in 1930 at the II. International Hygiene Exhibition in Dresden, where both a room and a marquee were designated as rest areas.[147]

In the east, the idea that occasional public rest and sleep might have a beneficial effect on the mental health of the population was apparently received more positively. As the Russian neurologist Johann Susmann Galant reported in 1928, the Soviet authorities had begun to set up similar facilities in the 'houses of culture' (*doma kul'tury*) in Leningrad and Moscow as part of broader efforts for psychiatric prophylaxis. It is, however, doubtful if there was any direct connection between Sommer's ideas and the Soviet initiative, as Galant implied.[148]

In the 1920s and 1930s, Robert Sommer's approach to psychiatric prophylaxis was still shaped by a turn-of-the-century concept of nervousness. But his concerns were not limited to the psychiatric effects of insufficient sleep. For Sommer, the mind of modern humans was under constant attack from an increasingly stressful and demanding environment; if not counteracted by rest, relaxation, temperance, and self-discipline, the relentless bombardment by affects and impressions would invariably produce a mental strain that could lead to exhaustion, nervousness, and neuroses. Even small everyday annoyances could build up until they became a threat to the mental health of the individual and even to public health. In a manuscript for an 'international manual of mental hygiene', which eventually went unpublished due to the earlier release of a handbook edited by Oswald Bumke and others in 1930, Sommer declared: 'Doubtlessly, the preservation of the peace of mind of both the individual and the whole of the nation is one of the objectives of mental hygiene'.[149]

Consequently, mental hygiene had a role to play in even the most mundane aspects of everyday life. By ensuring a smooth functioning of the household, public events, and buildings, Sommer was convinced, anger, and frustration could be avoided and the peace of mind preserved. One of the educational tasks of mental hygiene would be to propagate healthy forms of recreation. In a paper for the 1930 First International Congress, Sommer recommended moderate physical activity, the appreciation of art, and soothing hobbies, such as collecting things. The new medium of radio revealed Sommer's hopes in technological improvements as well as his deep-rooted reservations against what he considered the excesses of modernity:

> And we must take a stand regarding the modern invention of the radio, which allows the individual to expose himself to a great number of impressions. [...] But if these technical achievements are sensibly used, if people are temperate in listening to music and lectures, and do not, as often occurs, try to take in in a short time an international mixture from all sorts of cities, the radio can be used for the problems of mental hygiene.[150]

Most other members of the mental hygiene movement would not share Sommer's broadly defined approach that included the 'prophylaxis of anger' and other intrusions into everyday life. And yet, his concerns about the small nuisances of modern life were more than a personal quirk. They overlapped with views propagated by a Wilhelmine 'anti-noise' movement that had begun its crusade against the pathogenic effects of noise shortly before the turn of the century.[151] Sommer proposed a 'mental hygiene of noise' against the racket of road traffic and, as he emphatically stressed, of motorcycles in particular.[152] Despite Sommer's continuing efforts, this topic remained marginal in the debates of the German mental hygiene movement. Nevertheless, Sommer's concerns about noise were symptomatic of his ambiguous stance towards urban modernity. Rather than an outspoken anti-modernist, he was cautious about what he perceived as mental effects of an accelerating modernity. As a moderate liberal conservative, Sommer did not share Auguste Forel's or Emil Kraepelin's socio-medical fervour. His vision was not to fundamentally reshape society, but to blunt the harmful impact of modernity, using the potential of new technologies without disturbing the status quo too much. While Forel and Kraepelin called for top-down, state-led social engineering, Sommer found society and the public to be where societal change had to begin.

The idea of public *Ruhehallen* was not the only reason Robert Sommer became the founder and leader of the mental hygiene movement in Germany. Even before the First World War, he had persistently stressed the role of hereditary factors for mental illness and positioned himself as a staunch supporter of eugenics in the name of psychiatric prophylaxis. At first glance, his advocacy of socio-medical interventions aimed at the reproductive behaviour of the population may seem in sharp contrast to his rather thin-skinned attempts to defend peoples' minds against the mental dangers of everyday nuisances such like noise, insufficient sleep, and the mind-boggling diversity of international radio broadcasts. For Sommer, however, these approaches complemented each other. As he summarised in 1930, psychiatric prophylaxis could only be successful when both kinds of causative factors of mental illness—exogenous and endogenous—were addressed.[153] *Ruhehallen* and eugenics were two sides of the same coin named mental hygiene.

Unlike many other eugenicists, Robert Sommer was no unconditional adherent of the theory of degeneration. In 1901, at the height of the public interest in degeneration, Sommer forcibly positioned himself against the widespread simplistic and inflationary use of the concept. Mental illness could be hereditary, Sommer argued, but this alone could not support the pessimistic world view of degeneration and *décadence*, for heredity was neither a necessary cause for mental illness nor a unidirectional process: 'Against the fact of degeneration, which for the literature of the last decades has been the scientific background for its pessimism, one must set the equally assured fact of the regeneration of families'.[154]

Moreover, Sommer also questioned psychiatrists' and criminal anthropologists' obsession with small morphological oddities and deformations as 'signs of degeneration'. A deviance from a morphological norm without functional impairment could hardly be considered pathological, he pointed out, and even significant physical deformations were not necessarily connected to any mental abnormality.[155] By challenging the reach of the degeneration paradigm, he also rejected the corresponding concepts and research methods. In direct opposition to Kraepelin, Sommer dismissed the use of conflating diverse symptoms into a common category of 'degenerative madness' (*Entartungsirresein*). He also doubted the use of statistical methods for understanding the role of heredity for mental disorders: 'It would be better to break with the statistical method in this complex area of organic phenomena, and to replace the statistical pooling of incongruent cases with a thorough analysis of the individual case from the perspective of its pathogenesis'.[156]

As spokesman of the German mental hygiene association from the second half of the 1920s, Sommer repeatedly stressed his two-pronged approach to mental hygiene, aimed at the prevention of both endogenous and exogenous mental illness.[157] In his own work, however, these two approaches had not appeared simultaneously. When laying out his plans for the *Ruhehallen* in 1902, he had vehemently argued against the exaggerated and ubiquitous talk of degeneration and advertised relaxation and sleep as the method of choice for the prevention of mental disorder instead.[158] Only a few years later, his notion of psychiatric prophylaxis extended to endogenous factors.

Sommer developed and systematised his ideas for a prophylaxis of hereditary mental disorder in his 1907 book *Familienforschung und Vererbungslehre* ('Family research and genetics'). In keeping with his earlier statements about the futility of the statistical method, his studies in heredity were not based on the aggregation of mass data but relied heavily on the in-depth analysis of a single family history reaching from the fourteenth to the early twentieth century. Instead of gathering morphological signs of degeneration, Sommer traced biographies, careers, literary works, and the changes in family crests. This methodology, he claimed, offered a unique long-term perspective unavailable to quantitative approaches.[159] Despite his idiosyncratic method, Sommer reached the same conclusions as many of his more clinically oriented colleagues: on the one hand, heredity was a major cause for various forms of mental illness, on the other, exogenous pathogens such as alcohol and syphilis could damage the 'germs' and thus cause endogenous mental illness in future generations.[160] Like Kraepelin, he believed that these insights into the causation of mental illness would reshape psychiatry, providing it with novel possibilities for prevention, and shifting its focus from the clinic to the social sphere:

> Just like analytical psychopathology is the foundation of psychiatry as a science, the knowledge about hereditary characteristics and the causes of degeneration is the foundation for the methodical advancement of regeneration, which is the goal of social psychiatry.[161]

Sommer's programme for 'regeneration' became the basis of his definition of mental hygiene. As far as exogenous factors were concerned, his demands were hardly distinguishable from those of the other protagonists of psychiatric prophylaxis; he called for an improvement of unhealthy living conditions and the fight against alcoholism, morphinism, and the spread of syphilis.[162] When it came to hereditary mental illness, however, the differences were more pronounced. Sommer agreed with other eugenicists that the only way to prevent endogenous mental illness was to actively influence reproductive behaviour. But this was where the similarities ended. Despite all the talk of race, heredity, and degeneration, Sommer's 1907 eugenic musings were largely free from the social-Darwinist jargon that was rampant in Forel and Kraepelin's contemporary writings. Sommer did not believe that state-led socio-medical coercion was the method of choice. Marriage restrictions for people suffering from hereditary diseases would be 'an extraordinary violation of personal liberties'. Sommer was appalled by the more radical measures proposed by some his colleagues; to him, calls for the castration of the mentally ill were nothing but ideas 'of brutal natures, who thereby betray their own share in the moral degeneration of our times'. Even more resolutely, he rejected any notion of restoring the health of the body politic by killing people suffering from hereditary mental illness:

> The notion of preventing degeneration by brutally annihilating weaker beings is nothing but a cultural expression of this degeneration, and has been disproved by history, as, for example, the case of the Spartans shows. The killing of creatures, who were believed by certain people to be harmful in some way, has never helped to rid the world of what it was intended to.[163]

This passage was among the most unambiguous repudiations of coercive eugenics by a German psychiatrist in the first half of the twentieth century. Even as the First World War shifted Sommer's politics to the right, and although he increasingly adopted nationalist and social-Darwinist views after 1914, this passage remained unchanged in two subsequent editions of his book about family research, published in 1922 and 1927, respectively.[164]

Instead, Sommer remained convinced that eugenic regeneration had to be the result of decisions taken voluntarily and without coercion. He believed in timeless inner values and argued against marriage decisions taken for exterior, superficial motives such as money, possessions, degrees, or titles. For the progeny, the quality of their 'germs' was more important than the social status of their parents, and the best way to ensure the reproduction of the 'capable and healthy' was the propagation of love marriages.[165] These voluntaristic eugenics were embedded in a broader, and equally vague notion of a 'natural aristocracy'. The social group that until now had called itself 'aristocracy' had not even been able to prevent its own degeneration, Sommer claimed; what was needed instead, was the permeation of the nation with a novel idea of an aristocracy based on the natural sciences, which would effect a voluntary selection of the healthy and capable and pave the way to regeneration.[166]

Sommer's staunch rejection of coercion set him apart from the eugenic mainstream. While his attempts to introduce the notion of 'natural aristocracy' to the programme of the German Association for Mental Hygiene failed, he continued to argue for the voluntariness of eugenics into the 1930s.[167] Hence, it was not without irony that the German Association for Mental Hygiene, founded on Sommer's initiative in 1925, became a mouthpiece for more radical interpretations of eugenics, and after 1933 a propaganda tool for the racial hygiene policies of the Third Reich. On the occasion of Sommer's death in 1937, Ernst Rüdin and Hans Roemer lauded Sommer as a pioneer of the racial hygiene policies of the Third Reich, claiming that with his research and his lectures on psychiatric heredity, he had 'long beforehand actively contributed to the creation of the scientific and personal preconditions for the hereditary health policies of the Third Reich'.[168] Despite Sommer's temporary shift to the nationalist right after 1914, this kind of praise was undeserved.

In his 1907 book on family research and heredity, Sommer had announced a new kind of 'social psychiatry' and had called for an education of the masses that would teach them the ideal of a 'natural aristocracy' and the importance of voluntary eugenics. At this point in time, however, he said nothing about how these lofty goals were to be achieved. While Sommer had immediately laid out his plans and budgets for his public resting rooms, the reorientation of psychiatry towards prophylaxis was a more complicated project. Only after 1910 he began to ponder the more practical aspects of his ideas. Recognising that they could not be fruitfully realised as an independent initiative, he sought to tap the resources of the state, lobbying for the creation of a psychiatric department of the *Reich* health office as a focal point for psychiatry's socio-medical efforts.[169] In the end Sommer's plans came to nothing, but his efforts are noteworthy nevertheless: they constitute the first attempt to institutionalise a psychiatric prevention as part of state health policy, they were an important step towards the agenda of mental hygiene, and finally, these plans directly led to Emil Kraepelin's initiative for the founding of the German Research Institute for Psychiatry.

Robert Sommer took the decision to lobby for a national state-run psychiatric research institute shortly after attending the Fourth International Congress for the Care of the Insane in Berlin in October 1910.[170] This congress, he wrote, had most clearly revealed to what degree psychiatry had already become a 'social science'.[171] Psychiatrists were now discussing the social role of their discipline and the interplay between mental illness and society—from the reform and extension of institutional care to the relations between psychiatry and penal justice, and the social roots of mental illness and their relation to 'specific widespread illnesses, mores and nuisances, and to civilisation in general'. None of these perspectives was entirely new, but as Sommer saw it, psychiatry's extension into the social sphere now had reached a tipping point. Moreover, the increasing social relevance of psychiatry had changed its relation to the political authorities. Already, representatives of state, province, and city administrations were attending the conference in ceremonial functions. What mattered now was to translate this 'decorative phenomenon' into a more permanent exchange profitable to both sides.[172]

Sommer's attempt to provide the state with valuable public health expertise in exchange for research funding and social leverage was a textbook example of scientific experts and political actors providing 'resources for each other'.[173] However, the alliance between psychiatry and the state was not necessarily a love marriage. Even a right-wing nationalist and alleged representative of 'state psychiatry' like Emil Kraepelin, who considered as his medical duty the preservation and restoration of the body politic and the nation, was ambiguous about the role of the state.[174] In line with his social-Darwinist views, he blamed the state for having introduced a welfare system that suspended natural selection and was therefore responsible for the rampant degeneration. However, as his own attempts to receive state funding for the research institute and its eventual acquisition by the Kaiser Wilhelm Society show, he had no hesitations to exploit the state's resources to advance his scientific and political agenda.

Likewise, Robert Sommer was not overly enthusiastic about the bargain with the state that he himself had proposed in 1910. The reason, however, was entirely different from Kraepelin's social-Darwinist concerns. A staunch believer in scientific internationalism, Sommer's vision of 'social psychiatry' was not limited by state borders, but followed the model of pre-war international organisations like the awkwardly named and short-lived International Commission for the Study of the Causes of Mental Diseases and Their Prophylaxis, founded in Milan in 1906, or the International League against Epilepsy, founded in Budapest in 1910.[175] Cooperating with the state was neither an end in itself, nor was it a retreat into national boundaries. Instead, Sommer was convinced that the integration of psychiatry into established national frameworks of 'social medicine' was the most effective way to ensure the advancement of a project that was inherently international.[176]

With recent developments in clinical psychiatry and a new understanding of the causation of mental illness, Sommer argued, psychiatry was necessarily pushed into the 'social field'. While institutional care would have to remain in its present decentralised form, the newly emerging social psychiatry required a 'common centre for research and organisation'.[177] To represent all aspects of psychiatry as a social science and a part of public health, Sommer's plans prevised four sections for the department. First, a section for asylums and institutional care, which would collect and assess statistics and reports from all German states; second, a clinical section with thirty to fifty beds for the observation of 'scientifically important cases'; third, a section for forensic psychiatry, which would mainly have to defend psychiatry against unjustified charges of abusing its power in the courtrooms; and finally, a fourth section devoted to 'heredity research and mental hygiene'. This was Sommer's second attempt to implement something that he called 'mental hygiene'. However, whereas in 1902 he had defined mental hygiene as methods for the 'preservation of nervous energy', in 1910 the term took on another meaning and became largely identical with psychiatric prophylaxis through eugenics. To illustrate what he meant by mental hygiene, Sommer referred to the *Archiv für Rassen- und Gesellschaftsbiologie*, the main journal of German racial hygienists. In the inter-war period, he would try to reconcile both approaches as complementary parts of a two-pronged strategy of mental hygiene, but an inherent tension remained.

Sommer's call for the creation of a psychiatric department of the *Reich* health office made it to the petition committee of the *Reichstag*, but this was where the project ended. On 25 January 1911, Sommer's foray was rejected for two reasons. First, as the government commissioner in charge pointed out, the *Reich* health office would not be able to support a clinical research department for psychiatry without ignoring similar demands by other disciplines, or fundamentally changing its function as a state agency. Foundational research was to remain in the university clinics. Furthermore, Sommer's plans also were in conflict with the federal structure of German psychiatry, in which the individual German states, and not the *Reich*, would have been responsible for the maintenance of psychiatric institutions.[178] Despite some continued lobbying efforts, which were also supported by the chair of psychiatry in Breslau, Alois Alzheimer (1864–1915), this was the end of Sommer's plans.[179] His subsequent calls for the creation of a *Reich* institute for family research and genetics (*Reichsinsitut für Familienforschung und Vererbungslehre*) in 1914, based on the fourth section of the department in his earlier plans and some reflections from his 1907 book, were equally ineffective.[180]

In his memories of Central Europe before the First World War, written after the beginning of the second, Stefan Zweig remembered an idyllic continent of safety, progress, and international mobility. Careers, morals, and currencies were safe, ideas and people travelled lightly from country to country, and the victory over injustice, sickness, and poverty seemed only a matter of time.[181] There are some obvious reasons not to take this idealised account at face value; it tells as much about the realities of pre-war Europe as about an émigré's nostalgia for a world that he had lost forever. The writings of Robert Sommer, however, confirm Zweig's depiction of the caesura of 1914. But while Zweig helplessly witnessed Europe's shift towards nationalism, Sommer took part in it. A dedicated proponent of scientific internationalism and a liberal believing in the advancement of humanity before the war, Sommer discovered his nationalist leanings in August 1914. Quickly, he abandoned his cosmopolitanism and embraced the preservation of the collective health of a beleaguered German nation.[182] His poetry marks a sharp caesura. In late July, he invoked 'peace' in a poem of the same name: 'Lay down your arms! Do you want to struggle eternally? / Shall all of Europe drown in blood?' By 8 August, he had already penned the first of a series of bellicose patriotic hymns: 'I am a German. Do you know my colours? / The flag that flies ahead of us is black, white, red'.[183]

The beginning of the First World War coincided with Sommer's tenure as chancellor of the University of Giessen. He used this position to help mobilise the university and its medical school for the war effort. A 'war commission' set up and headed by Sommer tried to tackle the many challenges that the war brought to Giessen. Although far removed from the frontlines in the East and West, the university clinic was turned into a military hospital for an increasing number of wounded soldiers. The rising workload was exacerbated by the fact that numerous physicians, nurses, and students were drafted for military service, so that a smaller staff had to deal with a rising number of patients. This was not limited to the university clinic. Numerous general practitioners had also been called to service, so that civilian patients had to frequent the military hospitals. Medical operations at the university had to adapt quickly to the wartime situation and so did teaching and research. With most of the students in military service, the lectures for the remaining few almost entirely dealt with practical aspects of wartime medicine and other war-related topics.[184] At the same time, personal and material resources for research were becoming scarce.[185] It was not only a general change of the political climate, but also a very concrete and pressing organisational, medical, and social crisis that shaped Sommer's wartime activities.[186]

In his chancellor's speech on 1 July 1915, Sommer pondered the psychiatric questions posed by the war from various perspectives. At this point in time, his outlook was still optimistic. The 'mental resilience of the German nation', both of the troops and the civilian population, had turned out to be unexpectedly strong and while the war had caused a serious number of neuroses and other mental disorders, it had also mobilised regenerative forces. Nevertheless, Sommer argued, the systematic regeneration of the German people as envisioned in his earlier writings would have to become a national priority once the fighting was over:

> After this war, the German nation will still be surrounded by enemies and can only persist as a nation and as a polity through its own strength. Together with the enhancement of our state institutions, the efforts for *regeneration* will offer the best guarantee against the decay of our strength.[187]

Sommer verbosely discussed the psychological and psychopathological impact of the war, but he also tried to find practical solutions for the new challenges. Before the war, he had already proposed solving socio-medical problems through architectural means. Instead of a public resting room for the calming of exhausted nerves, Sommer's wartime project was the construction of athletic training grounds for the students of his university.[188] By the summer of 1915, prisoners of war had already prepared an area of 3000 square meters (one-tenth of the projected size of the whole facility). To Sommer, this was an integral part of the German war effort, preparing the student body for the strenuous times that lay ahead:

> Due to the war, this physical education, which at the same time also means strengthening the will and the character, has ceased to be mere play and competition, and has become an urgent national duty. The physical education of the German student body is one of the most important aspects of the regenerative efforts, on which after the end of the war the whole future of our nation will rely.[189]

The construction of the training grounds directly answered to the perceived needs of a nation at war, but they were also a continuation of Sommer's earlier research interests. From the turn of the century, he had been concerned both with methods for the exact measurement of psychophysical processes and the advancement of public health. Apart from the giving the students of Giessen a place to exercise, the newly established training grounds could also be used as a facility to research the effectiveness of different sports and forms of physical education. Previously, he claimed, this kind of research had been entirely focused on improving individual performance at competitive sporting events but had ignored how the relative health and fitness of the general population might be improved. By measuring and calculating individual performance gains, the most effective training for each person could be found, while at the same time contributing to a psycho-physical science of the whole human personality.[190] About a decade later, this idea became part of Sommer's vision of mental hygiene.[191]

The training grounds were not the only way in which Sommer tried to bring his pre-war interests into the service of the nation. His water-walking shoes, previously used for recreational activities, were now reimagined as military equipment for an amphibious invasion of Britain. He also urged Ferdinand von Zeppelin (1838–1917), whose airships were already conducting bombing raids for the German military, to construct airplanes that could hover in the air.[192] While these remained pipe dreams, other ideas were useful to the needs of the military and military medicine in particular. At the height of the psychiatric debate about 'war hysteria' in 1917, Sommer reused an invention from his earlier psychological research as method for the treatment of hysterical deafness and muteness. Unlike some other treatments of 'war hysteria', Sommer's method did not rely on pain and coercion, but used a more subtle approach to convince a patients to give up his symptoms: the patient's forearm would be placed in an apparatus recording the movement of his fingers on a graph. When a bell was suddenly and loudly rung behind the patient's head, the machine would register involuntary hand movements, thus providing visual evidence that the noise had in fact been heard. Like other wartime 'miracle cures', the aim was to remove hysterical symptoms at once by exposing them as psychogenic. In one case, Sommer claimed, a deaf-mute patient had immediately reacted by joyfully uttering 'I can hear again'. After some speech exercises, he was also able to softly sing along the patriotic song and future national anthem, 'Deutschland über alles', symbolically completing the cure.[193]

In Giessen, unlike in Munich or in Berlin, the revolution was bloodless and peaceful. Nevertheless, Robert Sommer was deeply unsettled by the events of November 1918. As has already been discussed in the Chapter 2, he voiced his concerns in a 'medical alarm' (*Ärztlicher Notruf*) in late 1918.[194] As he argued, the German people had suffered a 'profound shock of their nervous system'; the economic hardships imposed by the victors were leading to a 'mass neurosis' manifesting itself as an epidemic of 'nervous depression' and 'political madness'. The prognosis was poor: if the economic conditions would not change in the next two months, the disease would show its most terrible symptoms—a wave of suicides, violent political upheaval, and finally, 'general destruction'. Sommer's diagnosis of the mental state of the nation clearly showed his complete bewilderment when faced with civil unrest and the breakdown of the old political order. However, more clearly than in the agitated 1918 pamphlet, his ideas about the future of society and the socio-political role of the scientist were expressed in a non-scientific text: Sommer's 1921 comedy *Die Goldmacher* ('The Gold-Makers').[195]

Sommer had already dabbled as a playwright before and with some local success. *Die chemische Hexenküche* ('The Chemical Witches' Kitchen') was performed on the stage of the Giessen city theatre on occasion of the opening of the Liebig Museum in 1920.[196] His next play, 'The Gold-Makers', was about the social and political situation during and after the revolution.

In five tableaus of clumsy rimes and clichés, Sommer introduced a variety of stereotypical figures—the worker, the patriot, the critic, the veteran, and plenty of crooks and profiteers—to illustrate his interpretation of recent events. While he had a pinch of scorn for the naïve nationalism of 'the patriot', he had even less sympathy for the revolutionists, whom he portrayed as criminals led by no one else but the devil in guise of a socialist agitator. Contemporary psychiatric debates appear throughout the text—the profiteer had dodged the draft by faking mental illness and the physician, 'Dr. Medicus', explains that the revolution might yield psychoses.[197]

However, Sommer's voice in the play was not that of the physician, who is portrayed as weak and unable to exert any positive influence on the current situation. Instead of the impotent physician, the hero is the 'gold-maker', a modern-day alchemist who uses his scientific knowledge to save society. Unlike historical gold-makers, Sommer's hero is no charlatan but in fact capable of performing his miracle. As the protagonist, and through him the author, argues, it is the greed for material possessions that is the reason for the social and political misery. By chemically creating gold in unlimited quantities, the gold-maker undermines the concept of currency and thus paves the way for a future society based on the principles of work and community.

Finally, Sommer's scientist-saviour banishes the devil and with him 'the stock exchange speculators, profiteers, parasites, and gossipers'.[198] In the final scene of the play, the productive members of society—'men and women of the working class and the strenuous bourgeoisie'—form a circle around their new leader and solemnly pledge to reconstruct the fatherland. Written little more than two years after the end of the war, this scene encapsulates the vision of a national community that had become the centre of Sommer's politics in the previous years. Without overtly anti-Jewish tirades, Sommer used many of the key elements of a contemporary variety of an anti-Semitic critique of capitalism, which revolved around the romanticised vision of an organic national community and productive work. While the envisioned national community would overcome class distinctions, it also relied on a strict separation between productive and non-productive, and hence valuable and invaluable members of society. The emphatic juxtaposition of productive German labour on the one side, and foreign gold and economical abstractions on the other, became a key motive of Sommer's political and economic thought in the aftermath of the First World War.

Consequently, the idea that the social crisis could be overcome by changing the foundation from which the value of money was derived was not just

Sommer's punchline for a comedic play. It was a vision that he continued to seriously entertain and propagate into the 1930s. In three articles, published in a local newspaper at the peak of the 1923 hyper-inflation and re-published as a booklet in 1931 against the backdrop of the world economic crisis, he proposed the introduction of a 'work currency' (*Werk-Währung*).[199] Like the protagonist of his 1921 play, Sommer was convinced that the pressing social and economic problems stemmed from the fact that the value of money was nominally based on gold—a resource that Germany did not possess in sufficient amounts to provide a solid foundation for its currency.

If Germany's wealth was based on work, not gold, then work was the appropriate foundation of its currency. Different from the play, this transvaluation of currency would not have to be effectuated by alchemy or chemistry, but by psycho-physical research. Recent developments in experimental psychology and *Psychotechnik* had created the tools for the objective measurement and quantification of human activity, Sommer claimed, and thus, the possibility to accurately and scientifically define the basic unit of the 'work currency': one 'work' would be defined as the average productivity of a skilled builder in one hour, and equivalent measures for other kinds of physical and intellectual labour could be calculated accordingly.[200] The completion of a certain amount of work would be certified on bills replacing existing paper money and bullion. What the dabbling political economist apparently had not done was reading the classics. Sommer's proposed solution for the problems of a capitalist economy, was what Karl Marx had described as its reality; a system in which the value of every commodity was derived from a quantifiable amount of abstract 'social labour' invested in its creation, represented by a reference commodity that traditionally and arbitrarily was gold.[201]

Sommer's side trip into political economy was not just a result of his intellectual eclecticism but, as he saw it, a direct consequence of him being a psychiatrist and physician. Not only that the methods of experimental psychology would have to play a key role in the creation of the new currency, Sommer described his ideas as based on a thorough examination of political and economic life as a supra-individual 'psycho-physiological organism'. Admitting that the human body had often provided metaphors for the state, Sommer insisted that this analogy was more than that: 'The extraordinary disruption in the exchange of goods and services with its mental after-effects is, in the medical sense, a disorder of the metabolism with mental depression and inhibition'.[202] Hence, the boundaries between medical therapy and political reform were blurry at best.

It was in this troubled post-war situation that Robert Sommer, then in his late fifties, met the American Clifford W. Beers in 1923. Beers had come to Europe to spread the gospel of mental hygiene and to rally supporters abroad for the founding of an International Committee for Mental Hygiene (ICMH). In Sommer, he found one of his most assiduous followers. Sommer's own efforts to establish and institutionalise different forms of psychiatric prophylaxis in the previous two decades had yielded little concrete results and although he had at times been able to gather like-minded physicians and laypeople around his various projects, for most of the time, it had been a solitary pursuit. The emergence of an international movement for mental hygiene promised to change this. It offered Sommer a chance to bring his earlier ideas into a well-organised movement, whose name he could claim to have introduced himself as early as 1902.

Apart from giving his ideas greater clout inside and outside the psychiatric discipline, joining the mental hygiene movement answered to Sommer's needs in various ways. In his reflections about the psychology of the 'true inventor', quoted earlier in this section, he had lamented the scorn, rejection, and isolation that an inventive mind had to endure and had claimed that only 'if his invention leads to exterior success, this tension between the inventor and his environment becomes balanced'.[203] As the inventor of mental hygiene in Germany, Sommer finally found the recognition he had wished for.[204] The charisma of Clifford Beers was probably another reason. In his 1921 play about the gold-making scientist, Sommer had dreamt of a charismatic leader who would solve the social and political crisis. While this was a dream shared by many contemporaries in post-war Germany, Sommer apparently had little interest in political leaders. But as his adulatory review of *A Mind That Found Itself* shows, Beers very much was the ingenious leader that he had waited for and the utopian optimism of the mental hygiene movement was not lost on Sommer.[205] And finally, as an international movement, mental hygiene offered Sommer a way back on the international stage. Like many others, Sommer would never be able to fully shake off wartime nationalism, but being part of European and international committees and preparing the First International Congress on Mental Hygiene offered him a way out of the political and intellectual isolation of German science after the First World War.

Notes

1. Erwin Stransky, 'Wesen und Programmatik der psychischen Hygiene', in *Leitfaden der psychischen Hygiene*, ed. Erwin Stransky (Vienna: Urban & Schwarzenberg, 1931), 1.
2. Ibid.
3. Frankwood E. Williams, ed., 'World View of Mental Hygiene', in *Proceedings of the First International Congress on Mental Hygiene, Held at Washington D.C., U.S.A. May 5th to 10th, 1930*, vol. 1 (New York: The International Committee for Mental Hygiene, 1932), 101.
4. Otto Kauders, 'Geschichte der psychischen Hygiene', in *Leitfaden der psychischen Hygiene*, ed. Erwin Stransky (Vienna: Urban & Schwarzenberg, 1931), 11–12.
5. Wilhelm Bietak, 'Feuchtersleben, Ernst Maria Johann Karl von', in *Neue Deutsche Biographie 5*, 1961, 105–8; Karl Pisa, *Ernst Freiherr von Feuchtersleben: Pionier der Psychosomatik* (Vienna, Cologne, and Weimar: Böhlau, 1998).
6. ÖNB HANNA, Cod. Ser. 24072.
7. Erwin Stransky, 'Geschichtliches zur psychischen Hygiene in aktueller Sicht,' *Wiener Klinische Wochenschrift* 73, no. 13 (1961): 217. There was, however, a reception of Feuchtersleben at Adolf Meyer's clinic in Baltimore, as émigré psychoanalyst Else Pappenheim was astonished to find out in the late 1930s, see Else Pappenheim, "Zeitzeugin", in *Vertriebene Vernunft II: Emigration und Exil österreichischer Wissenschaft. Internationales Symposium, 19. bis 23. Oktober 1987 in Wien*, ed. Friedrich Stadler (Vienna and Munich: Jugend und Volk, 1988), 225.
8. Ernst von Feuchtersleben, *Zur Diätetik der Seele* (Vienna: Carl Armbruster, 1838).
9. Gustav Pollak, *The Hygiene of the Soul: The Memoir of a Physician and Philosopher* (New York: Dodd, Mead and Co., 1910), 18.
10. Bietak, 'Feuchtersleben'; Else Pappenheim, *Hölderlin, Feuchtersleben, Freud: Beiträge zur Geschichte der Psychoanalyse, der Psychiatrie und Neurologie*, trans. Wilfried Prantner, Else Pappenheim, and Stephen Frishauf (Graz and Vienna: Nausner & Nausner, 2004), 315–46; Otto F. Ehrentheil, 'The Almost Forgotten Feuchtersleben: Poet, Essayist, Popular Philosopher and Psychiatrist', *Journal of the History of the Behavioral Sciences* 11, no. 1 (1975): 82–86.
11. Kauders, 'Geschichte', 12.
12. Ernst von Feuchtersleben, *Lehrbuch der ärztlichen Seelenkunde* (Vienna: C. Gerold, 1845).
13. Feuchtersleben, *Diätetik*, IX.

14. Joachim Radkau, *Das Zeitalter der Nervosität: Deutschland zwischen Bismarck und Hitler* (Munich: Hanser, 1998); Hans-Georg Hofer, *Nervenschwäche und Krieg: Modernitätskritik und Krisenbewältigung in der österreichischen Psychiatrie (1880–1920)* (Vienna, Cologne, and Weimar: Böhlau, 2004); Andreas Killen, *Berlin Electropolis: Shock, Nerves, and German Modernity* (Berkeley, Los Angeles, and London: University of California Press, 2006); Esther Fischer-Homberger, *Die traumatische Neurose: Vom somatischen zum sozialen Leiden* (Bern: H. Huber, 1975).
15. Eduard Reich, *Die Geschichte der Seele, die Hygieine des Geisteslebens und die Civilisation* (Minden: J.C.C. Bruns, 1884); Eduard Reich, *Studien über die Volksseele aus dem Gesichtspunkte der Physiologie und Hygieine*, 2nd ed. (Jena: Hermann Costenoble, 1879); Martin Vogel, 'Aufklärung, hygienische und Volksaufklärung: Allgemeines, Grundsätzliches und Geschichtliches', in *Handwörterbuch der psychischen Hygiene und der psychiatrischen Fürsorge*, ed. Oswald Bumke et al. (Berlin and Leipzig: Walter de Gruyter, 1930), 25, 29.
16. Reich, *Die Geschichte der Seele*, 458–60.
17. Eugen Hallervorden, 'Klinische Psychologie, die Vorstufe der Psychohygiene', *Deutsche Medizinische Wochenschrift* 22, no. 41 (1896): 656–59; Eugen Hallervorden, *Arbeit und Wille: Personenkunde oder klinische Psychologie zur Grundlegung der Psychohygiene* (Würzburg: A. Stuber, 1897). One of the few to pick up Hallervorden's ideas was the gymnasium teacher Wilhelm Könnemann, *Über Psychohygiene in Schule und Haus auf Grundlage einer Erörterung über das Verhältnis von Geist und Körper, Seele und Leib* (Posen: Merzbach'sche Buchdruckerei, 1902).On Eugen Hallervorden, see Alma Kreuter, *Deutschsprachige Neurologen und Psychiater: Ein biographisch-bibliographisches Lexikon von den Vorläufern bis zur Mitte des 20. Jahrhunderts* (Munich: K. G. Saur, 1996), 511–12.
18. Leo Hirschlaff, 'Zur Psychologie und Hygiene des Denkens', *Zeitschrift für die gesamte Neurologie und Psychiatrie* 6, no. 1 (1911): 215–41.
19. Paul Federn, 'Schutz vor Nerven- und Geisteskrankheiten', in *Das psychoanalytische Volksbuch*, ed. Paul Federn and Heinrich Meng (Stuttgart: Hippokrates, 1926), 224–30; Ernst Schneider, 'Schutz durch Beratung in Lebensfragen', in *Das psychoanalytische Volksbuch*, ed. Paul Federn and Heinrich Meng (Stuttgart: Hippokrates, 1926), 278–87.
20. Volker Roelcke, 'Die Entwicklung der Psychiatrie zwischen 1880 und 1932: Theoriebildung, Institutionen, Interaktionen mit zeitgenössischer Wissenschafts- und Sozialpolitik', in *Wissenschaften und Wissenschaftspolitik: Bestandsaufnahmen zu Formationen, Brüchen und Kontinuitäten im Deutschland des 20. Jahrhunderts*, ed. Rüdiger vom Bruch and Brigitte Kaderas (Stuttgart: Franz Steiner, 2002), 109–24.
21. Hans Jakob Ritter, *Psychiatrie und Eugenik: Zur Ausprägung eugenischer Denk- und Handlungsmuster in der schweizerischen Psychiatrie 1850–1950*

(Zurich: Chronos, 2009), 160–61; Mirjam Bugmann, *Hypnosepolitik: Der Psychiater August Forel, das Gehirn und die Gesellschaft (1870–1920)* (Vienna, Cologne, and Weimar: Böhlau, 2015).

22. Auguste Forel, *Hygiene der Nerven und des Geistes im gesunden und kranken Zustande*, 4th ed. (Stuttgart: Ernst Heinrich Moritz, 1913), 3; Auguste Forel, *Gehirn und Seele: Ein Vortrag gehalten bei der 66. Versammlung deutscher Naturforscher und Aerzte in Wien am 26. September 1894* (Bonn: Emil Strauss, 1894).
23. Forel, *Hygiene*, 219; Auguste Forel, *Rückblick auf mein Leben* (Zurich: Europa-Verlag, 1935), 211–12.
24. This account of Forel's biography follows Bernhard Kuechenhoff, 'The Psychiatrist Auguste Forel and His Attitude to Eugenics', *History of Psychiatry* 19, no. 2 (2008): 215–23. See also Rolf Meier, *August Forel, 1848–1931: Arzt, Naturforscher, Sozialreformer* (Zurich: Universität Zürich, 1986); Anton Leist, ed., *Auguste Forel: Eugenik und Erinnerungskultur* (Zurich: vdf Hochschulverlag, 2006).
25. Auguste Forel, *Die Trinksitten, ihre hygienische und sociale Bedeutung und ihre Beziehungen zur akademischen Jugend* (Stuttgart: Ferdinand Enke, 1891); Martin Lengwiler, 'Im Zeichen der Degeneration: Psychiatrie und internationale Abstinenzbewegung im ausgehenden 19. Jahrhundert', in *Biopolitik und Sittlichkeitsreform: Kampagnen gegen Alkohol, Drogen und Prostitution 1880–1950*, ed. Judith Große, Francesco Spöring, and Jana Tschurenev (Frankfurt am Main: Campus, 2014), 85–110; Francesco Spöring, '"Du musst Apostel der Wahrheit werden:" Auguste Forel und der sozialhygienische Antialkoholdiskurs, 1886–1931', in *Biopolitik und Sittlichkeitsreform: Kampagnen gegen Alkohol, Drogen und Prostitution 1880–1950*, ed. Judith Große, Francesco Spöring, and Jana Tschurenev (Frankfurt am Main: Campus, 2014), 111–44.
26. Vera Koelbing-Waldis, 'Forel, Auguste', *Historisches Lexikon der Schweiz*, 2005; Annemarie Wettley, 'Forel, August', in *Neue Deutsche Biographie*, vol. 5, 1961, 298–99.
27. Julius Donath, 'August Forel †', *Zeitschrift für die gesamte Neurologie und Psychiatrie*, 136 (1931): 642.
28. Erich Fromm, 'Forel, August: Rückblick auf mein Leben, 1935', *Zeitschrift für Sozialforschung* 4, no. 1 (1935): 113.
29. Jakob Tanner, 'Auguste Forel als Ikone der Wissenschaft: Ein Plädoyer für historische Forschung', in *Auguste Forel: Eugenik und Erinnerungskultur*, ed. Anton Leist (Zurich: vdf Hochschulverlag, 2006), 81–106.
30. Kuechenhoff, 'Auguste Forel'; Leist, *Auguste Forel.*
31. Auguste Forel, 'Der Begriff des Monismus', *Der Monismus* 3, no. 1 (1908): 10–14.
32. Auguste Forel, *Malthusianismus oder Eugenik?* (Munich: E. Reinhardt, 1911); quoted after Kuechenhoff, 'Auguste Forel', 222.

33. Auguste Forel, *Mensch und Ameise: Ein Beitrag zur Frage der Vererbung und Fortschrittsfähigkeit* (Vienna, Berlin, and Leipzig: Rikola, 1922), 49.
34. Ibid.
35. Ibid., 9.
36. Ibid., 20.
37. Ibid., 22.
38. Ibid., 31.
39. Ibid., 29–30.
40. Ibid., 57–70.
41. Forel, *Hygiene*, 221–41.
42. Ibid., 220.
43. Quoted after Kuechenhoff, 'Auguste Forel', 221.
44. Forel, *Rückblick*, 158; quoted after Kuechenhoff, 'Auguste Forel', 218.
45. Forel, *Malthusianismus oder Eugenik?*
46. Stefan Kühl, *Die Internationale der Rassisten: Aufstieg und Niedergang der internationalen eugenischen Bewegung im 20. Jahrhundert*, 2nd ed. (Frankfurt am Main and New York: Campus, 2014), 97; Isabel Miko Iso and Bernhard C. Schär, 'Kolonialer Rassismus, eugenisches Denken und Geschlecht: Auguste Forel und Otto Stoll in der Debatte um die "allgemeine Natur des Menschen" um 1900', in *Gender Scripts: Widerspenstige Aneignungen von Geschlechternormen*, ed. Christa Binswanger et al. (Frankfurt am Main and New York: Campus, 2009), 61–84.
47. Auguste Forel, *Die sexuelle Frage: Eine naturwissenschaftliche, psychologische, hygienische und soziologische Studie für Gebildete* (Munich: Ernst Reinhardt, 1905).
48. Auguste Forel, *Die Gehirnhygiene der Schüler* (Vienna: Manzsche k.u.k. Hof-Verlags- und Universitätsbuchhandlung, 1908).
49. Ritter, *Psychiatrie und Eugenik*, 160.
50. Forel, *Hygiene*, 325–28.
51. Forel, *Rückblick*, 156.
52. Kuechenhoff, 'Auguste Forel', 222; Forel, *Hygiene*, 265.
53. Volker Roelcke, 'Ernst Rüdin: Renommierter Wissenschaftler, radikaler Rassenhygieniker', *Der Nervenarzt* 83, no. 3 (2012): 303–10.
54. André Repond, 'Die Bewegung für psychische Hygiene in der Schweiz', *Zeitschrift für psychische Hygiene* 1, no. 6 (1928): 189.
55. Susan D. Lamb, 'Pathologist of the Mind: Adolf Meyer, Psychobiology and the Phipps Psychiatric Clinic at the Johns Hopkins Hospital, 1908–1917' (PhD thesis, Johns Hopkins University, 2010), 32–26.
56. Hans Pols, 'Managing the Mind: The Culture of American Mental Hygiene, 1910–1950' (PhD thesis, University of Pennsylvania, 1997), 41; Hans Roemer, 'Was will die internationale Bewegung für geistige Hygiene?', *Zeitschrift für psychische Hygiene* 1, no. 2 (1928): 34.

57. Auguste Forel, *Hygiene of Nerves and Mind in Health and Disease*, trans. Herbert Austin Aikins (New York and London: G.P. Putnam's Son, 1907).
58. Roelcke, 'Entwicklung'.
59. Assen Jablensky, 'Living in a Kraepelinian World: Kraepelin's Impact on Modern Psychiatry', *History of Psychiatry* 18, no. 3 (2007): 381–88; Matthias M. Weber, Wolfgang Burgmair, and Eric J. Engstrom, 'Emil Kraepelin: Zwischen klinischen Krankheitsbildern und "psychischer Volkshygiene"', *Deutsches Ärzteblatt* 103, no. 41 (2006): 2685–90; Eric J. Engstrom and Matthias M. Weber, 'Making Kraepelin History: A Great Instauration?', *History of Psychiatry* 18, no. 3 (2007): 267–73.
60. Henry Mapother, 'Emil Kraepelin', *British Journal of Psychiatry* 73, no. 303 (1927): 509–15.
61. Weber, Burgmair, and Engstrom, 'Kraepelin', 2686; Holger Steinberg, *Kraepelin in Leipzig: Eine Begegnung von Psychiatrie und Psychologie* (Bonn: Psychiatrie-Verlag, 2001).
62. Holger Steinberg and Matthias C. Angermeyer, 'Emil Kraepelin's Years at Dorpat as Professor of Psychiatry in Nineteenth-Century Russia', *History of Psychiatry* 12, no. 47 (2001): 297–327.
63. Weber, Burgmair, and Engstrom, 'Kraepelin', 2686; Wolfgang Burgmair, Eric J. Engstrom, and Matthias M. Weber, *Emil Kraepelin*, 7 vols (Munich: belleville, 2000).
64. Steinberg and Angermeyer, 'Emil Kraepelin's Years at Dorpat', 302.
65. Emil Kraepelin, 'Über die Wachabteilung der Heidelberger Irrenklinik', *Allgemeine Zeitschrift für Psychiatrie* 51 (1895): 1–21; Eric J. Engstrom, *Clinical Psychiatry in Imperial Germany* (Ithaca: Cornell University Press, 2003), 121–46; Volker Roelcke, 'Unterwegs zur Psychiatrie als Wissenschaft: Das Projekt einer Irrenstatistik und Emil Kraepelins Neuformulierung der psychiatrischen Klassifikation', in *Psychiatrie im 19. Jahrhundert: Forschungen zur Geschichte von psychiatrischen Institutionen, Debatten und Praktiken im deutschen Sprachraum*, ed. Eric J. Engstrom and Volker Roelcke (Basel: Schwabe, 2003), 189–218.
66. Daniel Paul Schreber, *Denkwürdigkeiten eines Nervenkranken* (Frankfurt am Main: Syndikat, 1985), 84–95; Friedrich Kittler, *Aufschreibesysteme 1800–1900*, 3rd ed. (Munich: Fink, 1995), 519.
67. Volker Roelcke, *Krankheit und Kulturkritik: Psychiatrische Gesellschaftsdeutungen im bürgerlichen Zeitalter (1790–1914)* (Frankfurt am Main: Campus, 1999), 160; Roelcke, *Krankheit und Kulturkritik*, 160.
68. Engstrom, *Clinical Psychiatry*, 140–42.
69. Weber, Burgmair, and Engstrom, 'Kraepelin', 2688; Armin Schäfer, 'Die Archivfunktion der Psychiatrie (Kraepelin, Jaspers)', in *Gewalt der Archive: Studien zur Kulturgeschichte der Wissensspeicherung*, ed. Thomas Weitin and Burkhardt Wolf (Konstanz: Konstanz University Press, 2012), 235–54.

70. Emil Kraepelin, *Psychiatrie: Ein Lehrbuch für Studirende und Aerzte*, 6th ed., 2 vols (Leipzig: Barth, 1899).
71. Roelcke, 'Entwicklung', 112.
72. Kraepelin, *Psychiatrie*, 1899, 11.
73. Engstrom, *Clinical Psychiatry*, 146.
74. Kraepelin, *Psychiatrie*, 1899, 8–9.
75. Roelcke, *Krankheit*, 158; Dirk Blasius, *Einfache Seelenstörung: Geschichte der deutschen Psychiatrie 1800–1945* (Frankfurt am Main: Fischer, 1994), 61–115.
76. Emil Kraepelin, *Die psychiatrischen Aufgaben des Staates* (Jena: Gustav Fischer, 1900); Eric J. Engstrom, 'Organizing Psychiatric Research in Munich (1903–1925): A Psychiatric Zoon Politicon between State Bureaucracy and American Philanthropy', in *International Relations in Psychiatry: Britain, Germany, and the United States to World War II*, ed. Volker Roelcke, Paul Weindling, and Louise Westwood (Rochester: Rochester University Press, 2010), 50–51.
77. Kraepelin, *Aufgaben*, 2.
78. Kraepelin, *Psychiatrie*, 1899, 295–302.
79. Eric J. Engstrom, '"On the Question of Degeneration" by Emil Kraepelin (1908)', *History of Psychiatry* 18, no. 3 (2007): 395–96; Eric J. Engstrom, 'Emil Kraepelin: Psychiatry and Public Affairs in Wilhelmine Germany', *History of Psychiatry* 2, no. 6 (1991): 111–32; Michael Shepherd, 'Two Faces of Emil Kraepelin', *British Journal of Psychiatry* 167, no. 2 (1995): 174–83.
80. Hans-Walter Schmuhl and Volker Roelcke, eds., *'Heroische Therapien:' Die deutsche Psychiatrie im internationalen Vergleich 1918–1945* (Göttingen: Wallstein, 2013).
81. Edward Shorter, *A History of Psychiatry: From the Era of the Asylum to the Age of Prozac* (New York: Wiley, 1997), 246–62.
82. Emil Kraepelin, 'Zur Entartungsfrage', *Zentralblatt für Nervenheilkunde und Psychiatrie* 31 (1908): 745–51; English translation: Emil Kraepelin, 'On the Question of Degeneration (1908)', trans. Eric J. Engstrom, *History of Psychiatry* 18, no. 3 (2007): 399–404.
83. Emil Kraepelin, 'Vergleichende Psychiatrie', *Centralblatt für Nervenheilkunde und Psychiatrie* 27 (1904): 433–37; Kraepelin, 'Degeneration', 392; Eric J. Engstrom and Ivan Crozier, 'Race, Alcohol and General Paralysis: Emil Kraepelin's Comparative Psychiatry and His Trips to Java (1904) and North America (1925)', *History of Psychiatry* 29, no. 3 (2018): 263–81.
84. Kraepelin, 'Degeneration', 400.
85. Ibid., 401.
86. Ibid., 401–2.

87. Ibid., 403; Engstrom, 'Degeneration', 393; Philipp Sarasin, 'Kampf ums Dasein', in *Evolution: Ein interdisziplinäres Handbuch*, ed. Philipp Sarasin and Marianne Sommer (Stuttgart and Weimar: J. B. Metzler, 2010), 33–36.
88. Volker Roelcke, 'Biologizing Social Facts: An Early 20th Century Debate on Kraepelin's Concepts of Culture, Neurasthenia, and Degeneration', *Culture, Medicine, and Psychiatry* 21, no. 4 (1997): 390–91; Daniel Pick, *Faces of Degeneration: A European Disorder, c. 1848–c. 1918* (Cambridge: Cambridge University Press, 1989), 44–59.
89. Kraepelin, 'Degeneration', 403 original emphasis.
90. Ibid.
91. Ernst Rüdin, 'Emil Kraepelin, Zur Entartungsfrage', *Archiv Für Rassen-Und Gesellschaftsbiologie* 6, no. 2 (1909): 256.
92. Roelcke, *Krankheit*, 169.
93. Max Nordau, *Entartung*, vol. 1 (Berlin: C. Duncker, 1892), esp. 3–71; Roelcke, *Krankheit*, 141–79.
94. Auguste Forel, *Die Vereinigten Staaten der Erde: Ein Kulturprogramm* (Berne and Lausanne: Otto Volkart and E. Peytrequin, 1914).
95. Robert Sommer, 'Eine psychiatrische Abteilung des Reichsgesundheitsamts', *Psychiatrisch-Neurologische Wochenschrift* 12, no. 12 (1910): 295–98.
96. Alois Alzheimer, 'Ist die Einrichtung einer psychiatrischen Abteilung im Reichsgesundheitsamt erstrebenswert?', *Zeitschrift für die gesamte Neurologie und Psychiatrie* 6 (1911): 242–46.
97. Matthias M. Weber, 'Psychiatric Research and Science Policy in Germany: The History of the Deutsche Forschungsanstalt Für Psychiatrie (German Institute for Psychiatric Research) in Munich from 1917 to 1945', *History of Psychiatry* 11, no. 43 (2000): 235–58; Eric J. Engstrom, Wolfgang Burgmair, and Matthias M. Weber, 'Psychiatric Governance, Völkisch Corporatism, and the German Research Institute of Psychiatry in Munich (1912–26): Part 1', *History of Psychiatry* 27 (2016): 38–50; Eric J. Engstrom, Wolfgang Burgmair, and Matthias M. Weber, 'Psychiatric Governance, Völkisch Corporatism, and the German Research Institute of Psychiatry in Munich (1912–26), Part 2', *History of Psychiatry* 27 (2016): 137–52.
98. Emil Kraepelin, 'Ein Forschungsinstitut für Psychiatrie', *Zeitschrift für die gesamte Neurologie und Psychiatrie* 32 (1916): 25.
99. Weber, 'Psychiatric Research', 236–37; Roelcke, 'Entwicklung', 119.
100. Kraepelin, 'Forschungsinstitut', 28.
101. Friedrich Wilhelm Hamdorf, 'Loeb, James', in *Neue Deutsche Biographie*, vol. 15, 1987, 18–19.
102. Weber, 'Psychiatric Research', 239.
103. Ibid., 241.

104. Emil Kraepelin, 'Die Verfassung der Deutschen Forschungsanstalt für Psychiatrie in München', *Zeitschrift für die gesamte Neurologie und Psychiatrie* 55 (1920): 316; Weber, 'Psychiatric Research', 241–42.
105. Roelcke, 'Entwicklung', 119.
106. Emil Kraepelin, 'Die Deutsche Forschungsanstalt für Psychiatrie', *Die Naturwissenschaften* 6, no. 23 (1918): 333 original emphasis; Emil Kraepelin, 'Ziele und Wege der psychiatrischen Forschung', *Zeitschrift für die gesamte Neurologie und Psychiatrie* 42 (1918): 201–5.
107. Kraepelin, 'Forschungsinstitut', 21.
108. Engstrom, 'Psychiatry and Public Affairs', 123–26.
109. Ibid., 127.
110. Emil Kraepelin, 'Hundert Jahre Psychiatrie', *Zeitschrift für die gesamte Neurologie und Psychiatrie* 38 (1918): 270–71.
111. Kraepelin, 'Forschungsanstalt', 333.
112. Ibid., 2.
113. Emil Kraepelin, *Psychiatrie: Ein Lehrbuch für Studierende und Ärzte*, 7th ed., vol. 2 (Leipzig: J. A. Barth, 1904), 815–41; Richard F. Wetzell, *Inventing the Criminal: A History of German Criminology, 1880–1945* (Chapel Hill and London: University of North Carolina Press, 2000), 146–47.
114. Emil Kraepelin, 'Das Verbrechen als soziale Krankheit', *Monatsschrift für Kriminalpsychologie und Strafrechtsreform* 3, no. 1 (1906): 257–79.
115. Eugen Kahn, 'Psychopathen als revolutionäre Führer', *Zeitschrift für die gesamte Neurologie und Psychiatrie* 52, no. 1 (1919): 90–106; Eugen Kahn, 'Psychopathie und Revolution', *Münchener medizinische Wochenschrift* 66, no. 34 (1919): 968–69; Martin H. Geyer, *Verkehrte Welt: Revolution, Inflation und Moderne: München 1914–1924* (Göttingen: Vandenhoeck & Ruprecht, 1998), 98–103.
116. Emil Kraepelin, 'Psychiatrische Randbemerkungen zur Zeitgeschichte', *Süddeutsche Monatshefte* 16 (1919): 171–83.
117. Robert Gaupp, 'Der nervöse Zusammenbruch und die Revolution', *Blätter für Volksgesundheitspflege* 19, nos. 5/6 (1919): 43–46.
118. Kraepelin, 'Randbemerkungen', 181.
119. Kraepelin, 'Hundert Jahre Psychiatrie', 270–71.
120. 'Zweiter Bericht über die Deutsche Forschungsanstalt für Psychiatrie in München zur Stiftungsratssitzung am 30. April 1921', *Zeitschrift für die gesamte Neurologie und Psychiatrie* 70, no. 1 (1921): 349; quoted after Engstrom, 'Psychiatry and Public Affairs', 127.
121. Emil Kraepelin, 'Über Entwurzelung', *Zeitschrift für die gesamte Neurologie und Psychiatrie* 63 (1921): 1–8; Eric J. Engstrom and Matthias M. Weber, '"On Uprootedness" by Emil Kraepelin (1921)', *History of Psychiatry* 21, no. 3 (2010): 340–50.
122. Kraepelin, 'Entwurzelung', 1.
123. Ibid., 5.

124. Ibid., 6.
125. Ibid., 7–8.
126. Ibid., 8.
127. Catherine Fussinger, '"Therapeutic Community," Psychiatry's Reformers and Antipsychiatrists: Reconsidering Changes in the Field of Psychiatry after World War II', *History of Psychiatry* 22, no. 2 (2011): 146–63; Michael Neve, 'A Commentary on the History of Social Psychiatry and Psychotherapy in Twentieth-Century Germany, Holland and Great Britain', *Medical History* 48, no. 4 (2004): 407–12.
128. Hans Roemer, 'Psychische Hygiene', in *Handwörterbuch der psychischen Hygiene und der psychiatrischen Fürsorge*, ed. Oswald Bumke et al. (Berlin and Leipzig: Walter de Gruyter, 1931), 296.
129. Michael Meyer zum Wischen, *'Der Seele Tiefen zu ergründen...' Robert Sommer (1864–1937) und das Konzept einer ganzheitlichen, erweiterten Psychiatrie* (Gießen: Wilhelm Schmitz, 1988); Wilhelm Weygandt, 'Das Leben und Wirken von Robert Sommer', *Zeitschrift für psychische Hygiene* 10, no. 3 (1937): 65–82.
130. Ulrike Enke, 'Die ersten Jahre der psychiatrischen Universitätsklinik Gießen unter ihrem Direktor Robert Sommer', in *Psychiatrie in Gießen: Facetten ihrer Geschichte zwischen Fürsorge und Ausgrenzung, Forschung und Heilung*, ed. Uta George et al. (Gießen: Psychosozial-Verlag, 2003), 59–92.
131. Ernst Rüdin and Hans Roemer, 'Robert Sommer †', *Zeitschrift für psychische Hygiene* 10, no. 1 (1937): 1–2.
132. Robert Sommer, *Bericht über den II. Kurs mit Kongress für Familienforschung, Vererbungs- und Regenerationslehre in Gießen vom 9. bis 13. April 1912* (Halle: Carl Marhold, 1912), 2–6.
133. Meyer zum Wischen, *Robert Sommer*, IX.
134. Weygandt, 'Leben und Wirken', 78–79.
135. UAG, Robert Sommer papers, vol. 36–37.
136. UAG, Robert Sommer papers, vol. 14, 32–33.
137. Roemer, 'Psychische Hygiene', 296; Kauders, 'Geschichte', 14.
138. Radkau, *Das Zeitalter der Nervosität*; Roelcke, *Krankheit*; Killen, *Berlin Electropolis*.
139. Robert Sommer, 'Die Einrichtung von öffentlichen Schlaf- und Ruhehallen', *Die Krankenpflege* 2 (1902): 528.
140. Ibid., 529.
141. Ibid.
142. Robert Sommer, 'Die öffentlichen Schlaf- und Ruhehallen bei der Internationalen Hygiene-Ausstellung in Dresden', *Psychiatrisch-Neurologische Wochenschrift* 13 (1911): 202–5; Robert Sommer, 'Die weitere Entwicklung der öffentlichen Ruhehallen', *Klinik für psychische und nervöse Krankheiten* 6 (1911): 371; Volker Roelcke, 'Prävention in Hygiene

und Psychiatrie zu Beginn des 20. Jahrhunderts: Krankheit, Gesellschaft, Vererbung und Eugenik bei Robert Sommer und Emil Gotschlich', in *Die Medizinische Fakultät der Universität Gießen: Institutionen, Akteure und Ereignisse von der Gründung 1607 bis ins 20. Jahrhundert*, ed. Ulrike Enke (Stuttgart: Franz Steiner, 2007), 398; Johann Susmann Galant, 'Robert Sommers Idee der öffentlichen Ruhehallen und ihre Verwirklichung in Sowjet-Rußland', *Zeitschrift für psychische Hygiene* 1, no. 3 (1928): 91.
143. Sommer, 'Entwicklung', 377.
144. Robert Sommer, 'Die psychische Hygiene der Arbeit und Erholung', in *Bericht über die Erste Deutsche Tagung für psychische Hygiene in Hamburg am 20. Dezember 1928*, ed. Hans Roemer (Berlin and Leipzig: Walter de Gruyter, 1929), 94.
145. Hermann Simon to Gustav Kolb, 21 January 1931, Hermann Simon papers, 926/141.
146. 'Die Halle 51 der Dresdner Hygieneausstellung', *Zentralblatt für Psychotherapie* 3, no. 10 (1930): 629.
147. L. Gaupp, 'Rückblick auf Führungen in der Abteilung des Deutschen Verbandes für psychische Hygiene auf der Internationalen Hygiene-Ausstellung Dresden 1930 und 1931', *Zeitschrift für psychische Hygiene* 5, no. 6 (1932): 164.
148. Galant, 'Robert Sommers Idee der öffentlichen Ruhehallen'; Grégory Dufaud, 'Politiser la médecine: La psychiatrie extrahospitalière en Russie soviétique (années 1920 et début des années 1930)', *Revue d'histoire moderne & contemporaine* 61, no. 3 (2014): 125–48.
149. UAG, Robert Sommer papers, vol. 25, 127.
150. Robert Sommer, 'The Meaning of Recreation and Avocation in Mental Hygiene', in *Proceedings of the First International Congress on Mental Hygiene, Held at Washington D.C., U.S.A. May 5th to 10th, 1930*, ed. Frankwood E. Williams, vol. 2 (New York: The International Committee for Mental Hygiene, 1932), 555.
151. Frank Uekötter, *Umweltgeschichte im 19. und 20. Jahrhundert* (Munich: Oldenbourg, 2007), 20–21.
152. Robert Sommer, 'Die psychische Hygiene des Lärms', *Allgemeine ärztliche Zeitschrift für Psychotherapie und psychische Hygiene* 2, no. 1 (1929): 33–34.
153. Robert Sommer, 'Die nationale und internationale Organisation der psychischen Hygiene', *Deutsches Ärzteblatt* 59, no. 11 (1930): 130–31.
154. Robert Sommer, *Diagnostik der Geisteskrankheiten für praktische Ärzte und Studierende* (Berlin and Vienna: Urban & Schwarzenberg, 1901), 67–68.
155. Ibid., 74–75.
156. Ibid., 75.
157. Sommer, 'Organisation', 130.
158. Sommer, 'Einrichtung', 528.

159. Robert Sommer, *Familienforschung und Vererbungslehre*, 1st ed. (Leipzig: Johann Ambrosius Barth, 1907), V–VI.
160. Ibid., 27–32.
161. Ibid., 2.
162. Ibid., 218–19.
163. Ibid., 220.
164. Robert Sommer, *Familienforschung und Vererbungslehre*, 2nd ed. (Leipzig: Johann Ambrosius Barth, 1922), 192; Robert Sommer, *Familienforschung, Vererbungs- und Rassenlehre*, 3rd ed. (Leipzig: Johann Ambrosius Barth, 1927), 83–84.
165. Sommer, *Familienforschung*, 221.
166. Ibid., 218–25.
167. UAG, Robert Sommer papers, vol. 13, no. 19. Robert Sommer, 'Psychiatrische Erblichkeitsforschung und psychische Hygiene', in *Bericht über die Erste Deutsche Tagung für psychische Hygiene in Hamburg am 20. Dezember 1928*, ed. Hans Roemer (Berlin and Leipzig: Walter de Gruyter, 1929), 96–100.
168. Rüdin and Roemer, 'Robert Sommer', 1.
169. Axel C. Hüntelmann, *Hygiene im Namen des Staates: Das Reichsgesundheitsamt 1876–1933* (Göttingen: Wallstein, 2008).
170. Justus Karl Edmund Boedeker and Wilhelm Falkenberg, *IV. Internationaler Kongress zur Fürsorge für Geisteskranke, Berlin, Oktober 1910: Offizieller Bericht* (Halle: Carl Marhold, 1911).
171. Sommer, 'Abteilung', 295.
172. Ibid., 295–96.
173. Mitchell G. Ash, 'Wissenschaft und Politik als Ressourcen für einander', in *Wissenschaften und Wissenschaftspolitik: Bestandsaufnahmen zu Formationen, Brüchen und Kontinuitäten im Deutschland des 20. Jahrhunderts*, ed. Rüdiger vom Bruch and Brigitte Kaderas (Stuttgart: Franz Steiner, 2002), 32–51.
174. Engstrom, 'Psychiatric Research', 49.
175. Simon D. Shorvon, Giselle Weiss, and Howard P. Goodkin, 'Notes on the Origins of Epilepsia and the International League Against Epilepsy', *Epilepsia* 50, no. 3 (2009): 368–76; R. Percy Smith, 'The International Committee for the Study of the Causes and Prophylaxis of Mental Disease', *British Journal of Psychiatry* 56, no. 234 (1910): 389–405.
176. Sommer, 'Abteilung', 296.
177. Ibid.
178. Robert Sommer, 'Zur Frage einer psychiatrischen Abteilung des Reichsgesundheitsamts', *Psychiatrisch-Neurologische Wochenschrift* 13 (1911): 31.
179. Alzheimer, 'Einrichtung'.
180. Robert Sommer, 'Organisation und Aufgaben eines Reichsinstituts für Familienforschung und Vererbungslehre', *Deutsche Medizinische Wochenschrift*, no. 14 (1914): 708–11.

181. Stefan Zweig, *Die Welt von Gestern: Erinnerungen eines Europäers* (Stockholm: Bermann-Fischer, 1941).
182. Cay-Rüdiger Prüll, 'The Exhausted Nation—Psychiatry and Medicine on the Home Front (1914–1918): The Case of Robert Sommer and the City of Giessen', in *War, Trauma and Medicine in Germany and Central Europe (1914–1939)*, ed. Hans-Georg Hofer, Cay-Rüdiger Prüll, and Wolfgang U. Eckart (Freiburg: Centaurus, 2011), 30–48.
183. UAG, Robert Sommer papers, vol. 28. A line from the same poem concluded Weygandt's obituary for Sommer in 1937, Weygandt, 'Leben und Wirken'.
184. Robert Sommer, 'Die körperliche Erziehung der deutschen Studentenschaft', *Zeitschrift für Schulgesundheitspflege* 29, no. 9 (1916): 395.
185. Prüll, 'Exhausted Nation', 38–43.
186. Robert Sommer, *Krieg und Seelenleben* (Leipzig: Otto Nemnich, 1916).
187. Robert Sommer, 'Krieg und Seelenleben', *Wiener Medizinische Wochenschrift* 65, no. 39 (1915): 1448.
188. Sommer, 'Erziehung'.
189. Ibid., 409.
190. Ibid., 389–409.
191. Robert Sommer, 'Die psychische Hygiene und die Leibesübungen', in *Bericht über die Erste Deutsche Tagung für psychische Hygiene in Hamburg am 20. Dezember 1928*, ed. Hans Roemer (Berlin and Leipzig: Walter de Gruyter, 1929), 95.
192. Prüll, 'Exhausted Nation', 37.
193. Robert Sommer, 'Beseitigung funktioneller Taubheit, besonders bei Soldaten, durch eine experimental-psychologische Methode', *Archiv für Psychiatrie und Nervenkrankheiten* 57 (1917): 574–75; Paul Lerner, *Hysterical Men: War, Psychiatry, and the Politics of Trauma in Germany, 1890–1930* (Ithaca: Cornell University Press, 2003), 116–17.
194. Robert Sommer, *Aerztlicher Notruf zum Ende des Jahres 1918* (n.p.: self-published, 1918).
195. Robert Sommer, *Die Goldmacher: Eine Komödie* (Giessen: von Münchow'sche Univ.-Druckerei, 1921).
196. Ulrike Enke, 'Ein Liebig-Museum in Gießen: Der Psychiater Robert Sommer, die chemische Hexenküche und das Gießener Liebig-Museum', *Mitteilungen des oberhessischen Geschichtsvereins* 89 (2004): 63–86.
197. Sommer, *Goldmacher*, 11.
198. Ibid., 20.
199. Robert Sommer, *Die Werk-Währung* (Giessen: Druck der Oberhessischen Volkszeitung, 1931); Meyer zum Wischen, *Robert Sommer*, 37–38.
200. Sommer, *Werk-Währung*, 12.
201. Karl Marx, *Das Kapital: Kritik Der Politischen Ökonomie*, vol. 1, MEW 23 (Berlin: Dietz, 1962).

202. Sommer, *Werk-Währung*, 15.
203. UAG, Robert Sommer papers, vol. 14, 32–33.
204. Karl Birnbaum to Robert Sommer, 19 December 1927, UAG, Robert Sommer papers, Vol. 66, no. 997.
205. Robert Sommer, 'Clifford Wittingham Beers, A Mind That Found Itself (Eine Seele, die sich fand)', *Zeitschrift für psychische Hygiene* 1, no. 1 (1928): 5–9.

CHAPTER 6

The Rise and Fall of Mental Hygiene

At the beginning of the twentieth century, few people would have had any idea what the term 'mental hygiene' meant. More than a century later, the situation is again similar. In the decade before the Second World War, however, mental hygiene was on the way to becoming an established psychiatric subdiscipline and a part of public health. All over the world, associations for mental hygiene were founded, papers, books, and journals were published, and large-scale national and international conferences gathered hundreds and even thousands of reform-minded psychiatrists. Convinced to be advocates of an idea whose time had come, the protagonists of the mental hygiene movement confidently mapped strategies for how psychiatry could finally escape the constraints of the asylum. Instead of trying to cure or detain the mentally ill, mental hygiene promised scientific methods for the preservation of mental health, proactively preventing mental illness before it could even become an individual problem or a social menace.[1]

As the previous chapter has shown, visions of psychiatric prophylaxis had a long tradition in German-speaking Europe. The idea that mental illness could be prevented before it developed into full-blown pathologies had started with holistic body–mind philosophies and mental dietetics in the first half of the nineteenth century. At the beginning of the twentieth century, the increasing importance of clinical psychiatry, new theories about the social and hereditary causation of mental illness, the influence of the degeneration paradigm and changes in psychiatrists' professional

D. Freis, *Psycho-Politics between the World Wars*,
Mental Health in Historical Perspective,
https://doi.org/10.1007/978-3-030-32702-6_6

self-understanding led to a shift from individual prevention to large-scale socio-medical prophylaxis. The First World War and the upheaval that followed it further fuelled these ideas among German-speaking psychiatrists, and the subsequent expansion of the welfare state promised their realisation. Around the same time, other trends in psychiatry also gathered pace. Against the backdrop of the dismal conditions in psychiatric institutions during and after the war, their resident physicians again began to press for the comprehensive reform of the asylum, introducing new kinds of intra- and extramural treatment. Psychotherapy gained in importance and began a rapid process of professionalisation partly triggered by the psychiatric experiences in the suggestive treatment of 'war neuroses'.

In the mid-1920s, these disparate approaches to the prevention of mental illness and related psychiatric reform efforts came together in the common conceptual and organisational framework of 'mental hygiene'. The idea quickly gained momentum. In 1925, the German Association for Mental Hygiene (*Deutscher Verband für psychische Hygiene*) was founded. The first German conference for mental hygiene was held in Hamburg in September 1928,[2] in the same year as the first volume of the association's journal, a comprehensive handbook followed in 1931.[3] Parallel developments took place elsewhere. The year 1927 saw the creation of mental hygiene subcommittee of the Austrian Society for Public Health (*Österreichische Gesellschaft für Volksgesundheit*) and the Swiss National Committee for Mental Hygiene (NCMH).[4] Mental hygiene became a psychiatric reform movement unparalleled in size, scope, and international range; its history is connected to both the crimes of Nazi psychiatry and to the emergence of 'mental health' as one of the most influential psychiatric paradigms in the post-war period of the Second World War. However, its history in German-speaking Europe has, up to now, not yet been written. This chapter intends to fill this gap.

Before turning to the mental hygiene associations in the German-speaking countries, this chapter takes a short transatlantic detour to the United States in the first decade of the twentieth century, where mental hygiene as an organised movement originated in 1908. Returning the focus to Europe, I focus mainly on the history of the German Association for Mental Hygiene, which was by far the most active and successful in Central Europe. The history of the association was inextricably linked to the social and political history of the inter-war period, situated between the reform ideas of Weimar psychiatry, the rise of eugenics, and the eventual triumph of the racial hygiene paradigm in Nazi psychiatry. Like few other examples, its history encapsulates the tragedy of the inter-war period, where high-flying, utopian ideas of international understanding and humanitarian progress and unparalleled atrocities grew from the same roots. In the United States, mental hygiene became the most important trend in psychiatry in the first half of the twentieth century. Almost immediately after the publication of Clifford W. Beers's (1876–1943) best-selling autobiography *A Mind That Found Itself* in 1908, which recounted his experiences as a psychiatric patient and pilloried the dismal conditions in US asylums, his reform agenda was picked up by laypeople and reform-oriented psychiatrists. In May 1908, a first local organisation, the Connecticut Society for Mental Hygiene, was founded. Less than a year later, in February 1909, the establishment of the NCMH in New York took the programme to a national level. Until it was swallowed by the National Institutes for Mental Health in 1950, the NCMH was an integral part of psychiatry in the United States, propagating institutional reform, psychotherapy, and the prophylaxis of mental illness, playing an important role in the expansion of psychiatry's activities beyond the asylum walls.[5]

A Mind that Found Itself: Mental Hygiene as an International Movement

When telling the history of their cause, European protagonists of mental hygiene usually claimed that their prophylactic ideas stemmed from local traditions in their respective countries. Nevertheless, they also acknowledged that, as an organised movement, mental hygiene had been imported from the United States. More specifically, the movement's own historiography tells us, it was founded in 1908 by Clifford W. Beers, when the former mental patient wrote a best-selling book on what he had experienced and suffered during his confinement in a number of mental institutions.[6] This origin story was bolstered by the fact that the first mental hygiene association, the Connecticut Society for Mental Hygiene was founded just after the publication of Beers's *A Mind That Found Itself* in March 1908.[7] Although a German translation appeared only in 1941 and only in Switzerland, the German-speaking propagandists of the movement would not tire to praise the book as the founding document of mental hygiene and Beers as its founder and spiritual leader.[8]

A Mind That Found Itself offered a compelling narrative for the movement's propaganda. Beers's book told the story of how he fell into a grave mental illness in 1900 and, after attempting suicide, was confined to a series of mental institutions. He denounced the dismal conditions he encountered in these facilities, but also told of his recovery and his pledge to devote his regained sanity to create a movement for the improvement of the conditions of the insane. Mental hygienists later claimed that Beers had not simply recovered, but had 'transformed the destructive powers of psychosis into practical philanthropic energy'.[9] There was a powerful messianic motif in this story of the fall into mental illness and the wilful resurrection as leader of a reform movement. Influenced by Jungian ideas, Heinrich Meng and André Repond—two leaders of the Swiss branch of the movement—later celebrated Beers's experiences as a tale of catharsis, rebirth, and the triumph over egoism and isolation: 'The life of Beers seems to us a symbol: He shaped, from chaos, illness, and madness, childhood and second childhood, a strong ego that became fruitful for the community'.[10]

In the United States, the book was an instant success and reprinted in several editions. It won Beers a national audience and made him the face of the emerging mental hygiene movement. For the following decades, Beers—driven by a profound sense of mission and gifted with considerable energy and a remarkable ability to create networks, mobilise allies, and raise funds—was the main propagandist of mental hygiene in the United States and abroad. However, the story of Beers's solitary invention of mental hygiene was not the whole truth. In reality, *A Mind That Found Itself* was less the founding document of mental hygiene than a part of a larger strategy, 'a propaganda piece for a movement that had already been organized behind the scenes when the book appeared'.[11]

As a Yale graduate, Clifford Beers could tap a large network of influential academics. Even before publishing his autobiography, he had already successfully enlisted some of the leading American physicians and psychiatrists as supporters. Among them were Adolf Meyer (1866–1950), the foremost American psychiatrist of the time, the psychiatrist and eugenicist Stewart Paton (1865–1942), William H. Welch (1850–1934), one of the founders of Johns Hopkins Medical School and thought leader of public health in the United States, and the eminent psychologist William James (1842–1910). From the beginning, these prominent allies shaped the movement for mental hygiene. Before publishing *A Mind That Found Itself*, Beers had invited them to edit his manuscript and gladly accepted most of the changes they proposed. Notably, even the term 'mental hygiene' had been proposed by Adolf Meyer.

Beers's cooperation with leading psychiatrists created a win-win situation. Beers required the psychiatrists' support for his movement and their authentication of his autobiographical account. The psychiatrists, for their part, used his ideas to advance their own reform agenda for the notoriously underfunded and overcrowded asylums, to elevate the public status of their discipline by presenting themselves as reform-minded and progressive, and to draw the attention of philanthropists. Adolf Meyer in particular used the nascent movement for mental hygiene to advertise his 'psychobiology' and to extend the institutional reforms that he had already implemented locally to a national scale.[12] At the same time, however, the psychiatric co-optation of Beers also mitigated his denunciation of institutional abuses. Psychiatrists took control of the nascent movement before it could be picked up by laypeople and turned against their own professional authority. Some of the changes to the manuscript were directly aimed at defusing Beers's criticism of psychiatry, transforming 'the psychiatrists from those being accused and proven guilty of maintaining institutions of poor quality to the central actors in a movement in which the promotion of their profession coincided with the improvement of conditions in mental hospitals'.[13] Nevertheless, the relation between the psychiatrists and Beers as the 'persona of mental hygiene' remained fraught. Beers's history of mental illness interfered with US mental hygienists' masculine and autonomous personality ideal, and the story of his miracle cure cast a poor light on psychiatry's real inability to heal its patients.[14]

After the publication of Beers's autopathography and the founding of the Connecticut Society for Mental Hygiene, the movement slowly but surely gathered momentum. In 1909, the founding of the NCMH took mental hygiene to the national level. It would take another three years until the committee came to life. Only then, a donation by philanthropist Henry Phipps (1839–1930) supplied the financial means necessary to begin operations. Thomas W. Salmon (1876–1927), a physician employed by the US Public Health Service who later became the chief consultant in psychiatry in the American Expeditionary Force, became the first medical director of the committee.[15]

The NCMH was concerned with mental health in the United States, but the movement quickly spread to other parts of the world. As early as 1914, mental hygiene organisations emerged in Canada, South Africa, Australia and Mexico, and in the decade after the First World War the movement again gathered pace. A Canadian National Committee, modelled after the NCMH, was founded in 1918, other national organisations followed in rapid succession: France 1920, Belgium 1921, England 1922, Italy 1924, Germany 1925, and Austria and Switzerland in 1927.[16]

Mental hygiene as an international movement reached its apogee with the 1930 International Congress when 3042 participants gathered for five days in Washington, DC. Although the United States and Canada clearly dominated the congress, it indisputably was an international event. Overall, representatives from twenty-two different national committees took part, most of them from North America, Western and Eastern Europe, but also from the Soviet Union, India, Japan, Siam, Venezuela, and the Union of South Africa. In total, the NCMH assisted in paying the travel expenses for participants from forty-one countries.[17] The programmes and self-understandings of these national groups were anything but uniform and national antagonisms were far from irrelevant; nevertheless, but they all saw themselves as parts of an international movement initiated and led by the Americans.

The establishment of mental hygiene organisations in other countries and the emergence of an international network was a direct outcome of US mental hygienists' propagandistic efforts. In February 1919, Beers proposed an international framework for mental hygiene to complement the NCMH's propaganda by taking it to an international level and foster the founding of similar organisations abroad. The American mental hygiene movement's shift towards internationalisation was part of a broader development in US philanthropism after the First World War—'a continuation of Wilsonianism in the philanthropic and scientific spheres', despite growing political isolationism.[18] However, the international expansion of mental hygiene also reflected the growing tensions between Clifford Beers and the physicians in the NCMH. Unsatisfied with his scope for action in the US mental hygiene movement and irked by Frankwood E. Williams's appointment as the new medical director of the NCMH in 1922, Beers could immerse himself in a new field of work abroad.[19] In 1923, he toured around Europe to advertise his ideas. He was received enthusiastically in Brussels, Paris, and London, where he met political leaders and physicians interested in psychiatric prophylaxis. Among them was the psychiatrist Robert Sommer, who had independently coined the notion of mental hygiene after the turn of the century. Sommer returned to Germany with a mission: to create a German Association for Mental Hygiene and to return Germany psychiatry to the international stage. Beers had not come to Europe with empty hands, but with the offer to fund local mental hygiene initiatives and the promise of organising and funding a large international congress.[20]

It would take more than a decade until the International Committee for Mental Hygiene (ICMH) was finally set up and operating. However, the organising committee reflected mental hygiene's international expansion during the 1920s. In 1919, delegates from only two countries—the United States and Canada—took part in the first meeting; for the second meeting, held in 1922, Auguste Ley from Belgium had joined the committee as its first European member. The third meeting, held in Paris in May 1923, was attended by delegates from eight European countries; at the following meeting in 1927, thirteen European countries were present. At the founding meeting of the international committee during the First International Congress in 1930—on the twenty-second anniversary of the founding of the first mental hygiene society in Connecticut on 6 May 1908—the delegates came from fifty countries.[21]

Mental Hygiene Arrives in Europe

There was a long way to go before the German-speaking countries could join the international movement. Even as mental hygiene flourished in the United States, for a long time, the situation in Germany, Austria, and Switzerland could not have been more different. Until after the First World War, mental hygiene was still unheard-of by medical and lay audiences. Individual parts of what would later be called 'mental hygiene'—such as 'open care', welfare for dismissed patients, or eugenic marriage counselling—were already intensively discussed inside the psychiatric community. Even the term itself was occasionally used, as for example by Erwin Stransky in his manifesto for 'applied psychiatry' in 1918, or by Robert Sommer in a 1902 proposal for the establishment of 'public resting rooms' for the prevention of nervous disorders.[22]

Before the 1920s however, no concrete programme was attached to the term. This only changed when Sommer began to lobby for a German branch of the mental hygiene movement after 1923. Two years later, the German Association for Mental Hygiene (*Deutscher Verband für psychische Hygiene*) was founded. From then on, the movement slowly but surely gathered pace. Austria and Switzerland followed in 1927. The first German conference for mental hygiene was held in Hamburg in September 1928,[23] the first volume of the association's journal was published in 1929, a comprehensive 400-page compendium followed in 1931.[24]

On first sight, the impressive success of mental hygiene in the United States and Clifford Beers's role in the founding and funding of associations abroad support the interpretation that mental hygiene was first and foremost an idea invented in the United States and exported from there to the rest of the world. From this perspective, it would be easy view the American mental hygienists' propaganda through the lens of 'cultural imperialism' and to dismiss the considerably smaller and less effectual mental hygiene organisations in Germany, Austria, and Switzerland as mere subsidiaries of the vastly more influential movement in the United States. However, as a closer look reveals, this was not the case. European mental hygienists saw themselves as parts of a successful international movement. Nevertheless, they were rooted in local traditions and reacted to specific local social and political conditions—as did the NCMH in the United States.[25] The American organisation had something to offer to mental hygiene activists abroad. The concept of 'mental hygiene' was able to bring together existing approaches to prophylaxis, extramural psychiatry, and institutional reform under a common umbrella and provided a catchy brand name to advertise this agenda to psychiatric, medical, political, and lay audiences. At the same time, American mental hygienists offered expertise on organisation and lobbying derived from their own experiences and had some possibilities to give Europeans access to funding by US philanthropic organisations such as the Rockefeller Foundation and the Commonwealth Fund.[26] Nevertheless, there are reasons not to exaggerate the influence of the US movement for the development of mental hygiene in Europe.

Even if their associations and committees were only established in the 1920s following Beers's initiative, local mental hygienists could look back on their own history of psychiatric prophylaxis. In Germany, Austria, and Switzerland, local traditions antedating the ideas of Beers and the NCMH were an integral part of mental hygienists' self-understanding and identity. The genealogy of mental hygiene was, however, just as vague as the term itself. In Germany, Robert Sommer's idea of public resting rooms was widely acknowledged as a direct precursor; the DVPH's chair Wilhelm Weygandt also considered Emil Kraepelin a pioneer of mental hygiene.[27] In Austria, much longer lines of tradition were discussed. As Otto Kauders (1893–1949) argued, the genealogy of mental hygiene—when understood as the effort to 'improve the psychic state of groups of people'—reached back as far as Socrates, Thomas Aquinas, Jean-Jacques Rousseau, and Johann Wolfgang Goethe,[28] and to the Viennese aristocrat, poet, and physician Ernst von Feuchtersleben (1806–1849) in particular.

Moreover, although mental hygiene was clearly dominated by psychiatrists, it was also part of much broader efforts for the preservation of collective health. Often, mental hygienists built their ideas upon pre-existing approaches in public health and social hygiene. The emergence of mental hygiene in the inter-war period was closely related to contemporary developments in public health and to the increasing professionalisation and extension of both state and non-state activities in this field.[29] The larger role of the state in public health and the increasing professionalisation were two reasons why laypeople played a considerably smaller role in the European mental hygiene associations than in the United States, where public health relied strongly on philanthropy.[30]

The connection between mental hygiene and public health was particularly close in Austria, where no independent mental hygiene association existed during the inter-war period. Instead, Austrian mental hygienists founded a working committee under the leadership of Josef Berze (1866–1957), which in October 1928 became a subcommittee of the Austrian Society for Public Health,[31] an independent Austrian Society for Mental Hygiene was established only after the Second World War.[32] The activities of the subcommittee were focused on Vienna with its dense network of public health institutions and organisations. As the Adlerian mental hygienist Rudolf Dreikurs (1897–1972) argued in 1929, many of these private and public initiatives touched on questions of mental hygiene: counselling offices for suicidal individuals, adolescents, psychopaths, alcoholics, open care and counselling for the mentally ill, child guidance offices, welfare for juvenile delinquents, eugenic propaganda, marriage counselling, popular scientific lectures, psychoanalytic sexual counselling, psycho-technic vocational counselling, and the short-lived mental hygiene counselling office at the university clinic. As Dreikurs saw it, the subcommittee's task was not only to 'connect all these institutions and to establish contacts between the neighbouring disciplines, but also to use conferences, radio lectures, publications, etc., so that our movement may penetrate the population more profoundly'.[33]

The situation in Germany was similar. When mental hygiene entered the stage in the mid-1920s, other approaches to public health were already well-established. Mental hygiene's closest older relative was social hygiene, which had crystallised into a discipline after the turn of the century. Like mental hygiene, social hygiene was anything but monolithic. It was an umbrella term that covered a broad range of different approaches and ideas for the 'sanitation of the social environment'.[34] As Paul Weindling writes, 'there were virtually as many theories as theoreticians'.[35] Nevertheless, common trends were discernible. Social hygienists had initially stressed the influence of the social and economic environment on individual and collective health, but then increasingly shifted towards biologically determined theories as eugenics and population policy came to the fore.[36] The Weimar welfare state created an environment in which social hygiene could thrive as the increase in state activity in the field of public health led to the professionalisation of social hygiene as a discipline, which was now taught both at universities and in specialised academies, and became part of the medical curriculum. Simultaneously, public health legislation created additional possibilities for the implementation of new and the extension of existing social hygiene programmes, such as specialised health care for school children, infant welfare, health-care services for patients suffering from tuberculosis and venereal diseases, and—a direct result of the human cost of the war—the welfare the physically disabled.[37]

For mental hygienists in the German-speaking countries, social hygiene was an important model. In some regards, mental hygiene could be considered as an offshoot of the larger social hygiene movement. Before the emergence of a self-professed movement for mental hygiene in the 1920s, many aspects of its agenda had already been part of the debates on social hygiene, and a number of reform-oriented psychiatrists had published and pursued their ideas in this broader context.[38] There was considerable overlap between their proposals and what later became the central demands of mental hygiene: a comprehensive reform of the asylum system, the creation of counselling offices for borderline cases, the prevention of mental illness through the prevention of syphilis and alcoholism, and eugenics. When Robert Sommer introduced the term 'mental hygiene' shortly after the turn of the century, he did not yet have in mind an independent movement, but used the notion as shorthand for the psychiatric aspects of social hygiene—as did Auguste Forel with his 'hygiene of the nerves'.[39] Many ideas of mental hygiene were direct results of the appropriation of social hygiene by psychiatrists and its application to the field of psychiatry.

Even after the founding of specialised associations, mental hygienists in the German-speaking countries usually acknowledged mental hygiene's origins in general and social hygiene. In a programmatic article published in 1928, Hans Roemer, the executive director of the DVPH, described its agenda as form of 'mental social hygiene'.[40] Likewise, his Austrian colleague Erwin Stransky emphasised that mental hygiene and general, somatic hygiene were inextricably connected, so that 'mental hygiene without somatic hygiene is merely a torso'.[41] As Stransky saw it, this connection was a direct expression of the connection between mind and body, and no psychiatric prophylaxis could be successful without taking into account the relation between psychic and somatic factors. For Stransky, any notion of hygiene necessarily comprised racial hygiene; and when he had first used the term 'mental hygiene' in 1918, he had was not referring to the international movement that would spread to Austria some years later, but to the psychiatric aspects of racial hygiene.[42] Stransky's insistence on the somatic foundation of mental hygiene positioned him against the psychoanalysts and Adlerians in Vienna, whose theories focused on intra-psychic processes, and who, different from Germany, were involved in the emerging mental hygiene movement in Austria.

Yet, despite their close connections with social hygiene, mental hygiene clearly saw itself as an independent movement led by psychiatrists, and not as subsidiary of social hygiene. References to older traditions such as von Feuchtersleben's 'dietetics of the soul' stressed German-speaking mental hygienists' independence from the international movement, but also vis-à-vis social hygiene.[43] The emergence and success of a mental hygiene movement in the United States provided reform-oriented psychiatrists with a possibility to unite existing and new ideas for the reform and extension of psychiatry in an internationally connected and independent movement under their own leadership.

When Clifford Beers arrived in Europe in 1923, many aspects of mental hygiene were already there. Most of the ideas propagated by American mental hygiene were already discussed among German-speaking psychiatrists. Prophylactic ideas and eugenics were gaining influence in academic psychiatry, but this was also true for the topic that had been first on Beers's list after his recovery and release—the reform of psychiatric institutions. Like in the United States, mental hygiene in Europe became an umbrella under which academic psychiatrists with their prophylactic approaches came together with reform-minded asylum psychiatrists. Two of the most important proponents of the reform of institutional care came to occupy key positions in the German Association for Mental Hygiene: Gustav Kolb (1870–1938), who introduced 'open care', and Hermann Simon (1867–1947), a pioneer of occupational therapy. While the ideas of academic psychiatrists like Auguste Forel, Emil Kraepelin, and Robert Sommer have been discussed in some detail in the previous chapter, here I give a brief overview over the most important developments in institutional reform in inter-war Germany, focusing on the role for psychiatry's shift towards extramural care and prevention for the emergence of mental hygiene in Germany.

After the First World War, psychiatric institutions in Germany were in crisis. During the war, the conditions in asylums had been catastrophic as tens of thousands of psychiatric inmates had perished due to starvation and illness.[44] After 1918, the situation hardly improved and German institutional psychiatry, once an international model, was in a dismal condition. As Adolf Groß, a resident physician from Konstanz, observed in 1923, the war had abruptly and violently interrupted an era of gradual progress in institutional care.[45] Building expensive modern asylums like before the war was inconceivable now, and even the upkeep of existing institutions and the maintenance of basic humane conditions had become a challenge. Necessities such as coal, potatoes, soap, and bed sheets had become unaffordable, and even more so the medical instruments, drugs, journals, and books for a treatment of patients in keeping with modern medical standards. At the same time, psychiatric institutions were coming under pressure from different sides. The new democratic order threatened the quasi-feudal hierarchies of the asylums from inside, as nurses began to organise in work councils and demand the amelioration of their working conditions and the introduction of an eight-hour day. Externally, psychiatry stood in the centre of a fierce public debate about the brutal treatment of 'hysterical' soldiers during the war and psychiatrists were publicly accused of mistreating and wrongfully confining their patients.[46]

Against the backdrop of this immediate crisis, resident physicians from different asylums drafted extensive programmes for a reform of institutional care. Gustav Kolb, director of the asylum at Erlangen, quickly became the most resolute proponent of institutional reform; as his 1919 reform proposal shaped the subsequent debate and directly led to the introduction of 'open care' in the 1920s.[47] Kolb's ideas were a direct reaction to external, political pressures on institutional care, and he rightly predicted that the upcoming elections would result in a victory of the Social Democrats, which he believed would strengthen the critics of psychiatry. But Kolb's programme was about more than defending the status quo antebellum. He tried to shift the focus of institutional psychiatry from confinement to treatment. This reorientation of psychiatry was not just a reaction to external political and economic pressures, but also an attempt to extend psychiatry's area of authority and to redefine the role of the resident physician.[48]

Kolb's proposal encompassed a range of aspects. He called for the establishment of 'protective courts' (*Schutzgerichte*) to prevent wrongful confinement and abuses. He demanded better funding for public institutions and the gradual closing of private clinics that were only affordable for privileged patients. He agreed to include nurses and non-medical staff in administrative matters pertaining to them, but vehemently rejected their demands for an eight-hour workday. Public prejudices against psychiatry would be countered by educating about the aims and methods of institutional care. The most important and influential part of his proposal was, however, the introduction of 'open care'.

Psychiatric institutions, Kolb argued, were widely seen as 'a cross between prison and hospital'. In the future, this would have to change. To become as 'humane and free as possible', the asylum would have to be transformed from a secluded place of confinement into a modern treatment facility well-integrated into society as hub of a staged system of welfare services.[49] Concretely, Kolb proposed the creation of 'care offices' (*Fürsorgestellen*) attached to existing psychiatric institutions, which would advise, support, supervise, and, if necessary treat mental patients living outside the institution. On the one hand, 'open care' would allow to dismiss patients earlier, thereby reducing the occupancy rate of the asylum and improving psychiatry's efficacy. On the other hand, this form of extramural psychiatry would also be able to reach potential patients before they had to be admitted to an asylum, including 'psychopaths', alcoholics, neurotics, mentally deficient adolescents, released convicts and all other borderline cases. Thus, 'open care' could become a tool of psychiatric prophylaxis.[50]

The second approach to the reform of institutional psychiatry that gained traction in Weimar Germany was Hermann Simon's 'more active therapy' (*aktivere Krankenbehandlung*).[51] This form of treatment, first introduced by Simon during his tenure as director of the asylum of Warstein as early as 1905, was based on the use of occupational therapy for almost every patient. 'More active therapy' was intended as a way to overcome the deficits of the usual treatment methods used in pre-war psychiatry, which mainly tried to keep patients tranquil by keeping them in bed for most of the time, or with long-duration bathing, a method known as hydrotherapy. These methods, Simon believed, were detrimental to the mental state of the patients as they further alienated them from the outside world and made release even more unlikely and challenging. As Simon argued at the first conference of the German Association for Mental Hygiene in 1928, the asylum itself could be pathogenic and cause a mental form of hospitalism:

> We know from old reports that in hospitals and maternity homes the air was ripe with infectious germs, and how hospital gangrene and puerperal fever caused havoc among the wards as a consequence of wound infection which they did catch where they were looking for cure. [...] Likewise, the mental atmosphere of the asylum is impregnated with numerous infectious germs that threaten the sore mental life of the sick looking to be cured: there's the bacilli of unrest and excitation, of constant discontent and incitement, perpetual quarrel and strife, of nasty manners and habits, of hundreds of kinds of fallacy and foolishness.[52]

'More active therapy' promised a pedagogical alternative that combined occupational therapy with the redelegation of responsibility to the patients.[53] Its aim was to enforce order and discipline in the asylum, but also to foster the remaining self-reliance of the patients and to keep them connected to the realities of life outside the institution.[54]

Although Simon had already employed 'more active therapy' before the war, its broader reception only began in 1924, after a presentation at the yearly conference of the German Psychiatric Society at Innsbruck. After the initial reservations of the professional community were overcome, the method was met with great interest, nationally and internationally, and quickly became one of the cornerstones of institutional reform.[55] There were at least three reasons for this success. First, 'more active therapy' promised to transform the asylum from a space of confinement into a facility for effective treatment, and if not to cure, at least to render patients more capable of functioning in society. Second, Simon's 'more active therapy' could complement Gustav Kolb's 'open care' by preparing patients for early release.[56]

Third, the success of 'more active therapy' should also be seen in the context of broader socio-political and socio-economic developments after the First World War. In a rapidly developing and differentiating industrial society, the individual ability to work and perform became increasingly important.[57] Article 163 of the Weimar constitution expressly defined the use of one's 'intellectual and physical abilities for the common good' as a 'moral obligation' of 'every German'. Seen in this light, the intended outcome of different psychiatric therapeutics reflected the characteristics of the ideal citizen in a given historical period and socio-political regime—whereas Wilhelmine psychiatry wanted calm, submissive, and passive patients, Weimar psychiatry tried to use 'more active treatment' to make its patients productive, self-disciplined, and active. Hermann Simon himself was explicit about the work ethics that defined the therapeutic aims of this method: 'Work and performance are the source of all living creature's abilities', he wrote in 1928, and consequently the aim of psychiatric treatment had to be an 'education to performance, self-reliance, and self-responsibility, to preserve our patients from an idiotic existence as parasites, which will rob them of their remaining human dignity and self-esteem'.[58] However, as the future of 'more active therapy' shows, Simon's ideas were not only compatible with the needs of the Weimar welfare state, but also with right-wing social Darwinism. Against the backdrop of the global economic crisis of the late 1920s, Simon eagerly embraced such views and advocated both 'more active therapy' and mental hygiene as ways to counteract the excess of welfare that he found to threaten the health and fitness of the nation.

Auspicious Beginnings

As a self-declared movement, mental hygiene made its first public appearance in Germany in September 1928, when the German Association for Mental Hygiene (*Deutscher Verband für psychische Hygiene*, DVPH) held its first conference in Hamburg-Lichtenberg. In international comparison, Germany was a latecomer. The first association in the United States dated back to 1908; Canada, South Africa, Australia, and Mexico had founded theirs before the First World War. In Europe, mental hygiene arrived only after the war—in France, an association was founded in 1920, followed by Belgium in 1921, England in 1922, and Italy in 1924. The German-speaking countries joined only in the second half of the 1920s, with associations founded in both Austria and Switzerland in 1927.

Given that German psychiatry was leading in terms of academic research and institutional care, the tardy emergence of mental hygiene requires an explanation. As I have shown, many of the individual aspects of mental hygienists' agenda were already discussed long before the American concept of mental hygiene arrived in Europe. Even the term 'mental hygiene' was not unheard of. As early as 1902, Robert Sommer had used the term *psychische Hygiene* to describe his vision of psychiatry prophylaxis.[59] Independently, the Viennese psychiatrist Erwin Stransky had used the same term in his 1918 manifesto for 'applied psychiatry' to refer to the psychiatric aspects of racial hygiene.[60]

One reason for the late emergence of a mental hygiene association in Germany simply was that it took relatively long to organise.[61] As early as

1923, Clifford Beers had encouraged Robert Sommer to lobby for the creation of a German branch of the international movement.[62] It took Sommer two years to drum up sufficient support, so that the German Association for Mental Hygiene was founded in 1925. The association was founded at the annual meeting of the German Psychiatric Society (*Deutscher Verein für Psychiatrie*, DVP) in Kassel, when the assembly unanimously decided that the existing approaches to prophylaxis and reform were to be united in a common association that would represent them on the international stage. Wilhelm Weygandt became the first vice-president and the representative of the larger DVP in the newly founded association.[63] Over the following year, Hans Roemer, Gustav Kolb, and Hermann Simon also became board members.[64] The composition of the board reflected the association's self-understanding: it rallied both reform-minded university scholars and institutional psychiatrists around the flag of mental hygiene, while at the same time retaining its close connection to the established organisations.[65]

On 28 November 1927, the members of the board of the DVPH met for the first time at the hotel *Russischer Hof* in Berlin,[66] were they discussed the upcoming international congress in Washington, DC, plans for a German conference on mental hygiene, and the publication of a new journal. The plans for the journal raised an issue that remained a recurring topic and one of the fault lines of the association—mental hygiene's difficult relationship with the simultaneously professionalising field of psychotherapy. Robert Sommer strongly supported the idea that mental hygiene and psychotherapy were closely related and that both emerging disciplines ought to cooperate: 'Both are parts of an extended psychiatry, which has developed beyond the asylum and in the direction of the treatment and prevention not only of the mental illnesses in the narrow sense, but also of nervous mental states'.[67] Consequently, Sommer proposed a common journal for both psychotherapy and mental hygiene, in which the association would publish its announcements. Roemer, Weygandt, and Kolb disagreed. As they saw it, psychotherapy was still far too controversial, and too close cooperation was a risk to mental hygiene's reputation among psychiatrists. Roemer instead suggested a journal for mental hygiene as a supplement to the well-established *Allgemeine Zeitschrift für Psychiatrie* (AZP). Eventually, two journals with 'mental hygiene' in their title appeared in Germany after 1928—the *Allgemeine ärztliche Zeitschrift für Psychotherapie und psychische Hygiene* (AÄZP), initially edited by Robert Sommer, and the *Zeitschrift für psychische Hygiene*, which was edited by the board of the association and distributed as a supplement to the AZP.

The fledgling association quickly found recognition among political actors in the field of public health. Three state representatives took part in the afternoon session of the Berlin meeting, two from the Ministry of the Interior, and one from the *Reich* Health Office.[68] As undersecretary Max Taute (1878–1934) told the assembled psychiatrists, an organisation tackling the question of prophylaxis and hygiene from a psychiatric perspective had been lacking until now; its founding was expressly welcomed by the Ministry of the Interior. Taute also announced the ministry's financial support for the association's future activities.[69]

This was not an empty promise. In 1927, the association had already received three thousand marks from the Ministry of the Interior; another four thousand would follow in 1928/1929. In the same year, one thousand marks were granted by the Foreign Office for the preparation of the German participation at the International Congress.[70] Unlike the National Council for Mental Hygiene in Britain, the German association did not benefit much from funding by American philanthropic organisations.[71] In 1925, Sommer had received some start-up funding from Clifford Beers, but the sum of three hundred marks covered only the smallest part of the initial expenses.[72] In the case of Austria and Switzerland, there is no evidence of any direct US funding for local mental hygiene activities.

The expertise of the newly founded DVPH was recognised by political actors early on. In 1927, a subsection of the socialist Free Trade Unions (*Freie Gewerkschaften*) had published a memorandum attacking the use of occupational therapy in German asylums, demanding clear limitations to protect psychiatric patients from compulsory labour and economic exploitation. The debate suddenly gained momentum when the trade unions' foray unexpectedly was backed by a Reichstag majority on 26 March 1928. In this situation, the *Reich* Minister of the Interior commissioned a report about occupational therapy from the DVPH. The sixteen-page expert testimony, which was mainly authored by Hermann Simon, defended occupational therapy as an important advance in the treatment of the insane and warned against any legislative obstructions.[73] The DVPH's statement received considerable publicity and successfully changed the direction of the debate.[74]

The first German conference for mental hygiene, held in Hamburg in September 1928, provided the fledgling association with an early success. About two hundred people attended the conference, among them many representatives of the federal government, the German countries, the

Prussian provinces, and municipalities; as well as representatives of medical organisations, the German Hygiene Museum in Dresden, the hygiene institutes of German universities, social hygiene associations, and welfare offices.[75] Wilhelm Weygandt could rightly claim in his opening address that the conference was something new; never before had so many different medical and non-medical actors in the field of mental health care gathered for a meeting.[76] The considerable interest in the DVPH's initial conference clearly showed the acceptance that the young organisation had earned early on, but it also reflected the high expectations that mental hygiene would have to answer to.

At the same time, the conference also documented the association's integration into the international networks of mental hygiene. Representatives of mental hygiene associations from Austria, Hungary, France, the Netherlands, Denmark, and Norway had travelled to Hamburg, and salutatory notes were sent from Italy and Russia. Vice versa, the German mental hygienists affirmed their part in the international movement by sending a greeting telegram to Clifford Beers in New York.[77]

Apart from introducing mental hygiene to Germany, one objective of the conference was to stake out what the field actually contained. The statutes of the DVPH, which were passed at the member meeting held after the conference, defined both mental hygiene and the association's goals ambitiously and in broad terms:

> The term 'mental hygiene' contains, for one thing, efforts for a modern organisation of the open and closed care for the insane and psychopaths according to the principles of mental hygiene (occupational therapy, family and open care, sanatoriums, support societies, etc.), furthermore, mental hygiene and prophylaxis in a narrow sense, and finally, the dissemination of mental hygiene knowledge into all strata of society, and to those groups of people who are professionally concerned with mental hygiene in particular; the practical application of mental hygiene should be promoted not only in psychiatry, but in all fields of social life.[78]

During the conference, papers were held about all topics that could be considered part of the DVPH's responsibilities. However, mental hygiene in 1928 Germany was dominated by institutional reform. Introduced by Gustav Kolb and Hermann Simon, the first of the three sections dealt with the reform of institutional care, and how psychiatric institutions might extend their welfare and counselling activities to non-institutionalised patient populations. Only the second session addressed psychiatric prophylaxis in a broader, socio-medical sense. Notably, the participants almost exclusively discussed the prevention of what Robert Sommer had called the 'exogenous' causes of mental disorder, such as the mental strains of urban life, alcohol, and syphilis, which were to be counteracted mostly through health education.

Eugenics, by contrast, were still marginal in 1928. A single paper about the question of heredity and mental hygiene had been announced by Ernst Rüdin. When Rüdin could not attend the conference; Robert Sommer gave an overview of his own theory of heredity instead. Repeating his prewar views, he argued for voluntary eugenics based on the ideal of 'natural aristocracy', which would have to become the 'principal motif of mental hygiene'.[79] In the following years, however, the association's focus rapidly shifted from institutional reform and education to eugenics. In the wake of the world economic crisis, institutional reform efforts came under economic pressure and concerns for the collective biological health of the body politic moved the fore again. The association's next conference, held in Bonn in 1932, would be devoted entirely to the 'eugenic tasks of mental hygiene'.[80]

The German Association for Mental Hygiene left the 1928 conference well-positioned. It had successfully advertised its agenda to a large professional audience and secured the support of political actors from all levels of the administration and of various organisations in the field of public health and welfare. Moreover, the DVPH had clearly established itself as a branch of the larger international movement for mental hygiene. The association's early success was mirrored by its membership. By 1930, the DVPH already had seventy-five individual members both in Germany and abroad, and thirty-eight corporate members, among them several psychiatric institutions, provincial societies for the support of the mentally ill, and other welfare institutions. Growth continued over the next years; in 1932, the number of individual members had reached 102, including many directors of major psychiatric institutions and many of the most renowned academics in the field.[81] Simultaneously, public interest in mental hygiene also grew. From 1928 on, Robert Sommer received many inquiries about mental hygiene and its aims from German medical, scientific, and popular scientific periodicals.[82]

International Reintegration

From the mid of the 1920s, one event mesmerised the adherents of psychiatric prophylaxis and institutional reform all over the world: the planned international congress for mental hygiene, to be held in Washington, DC. It would finally bring together everyone working in the field, unite the many national branches of the movement, and see the founding of the ICMH, turning mental hygiene into a truly international movement. First announced to take place in 1925, financial and organisational issues repeatedly led the congress to be postponed, so that it eventually only took place in 1930. Nevertheless, the congress became a major success for the international movement. More than three thousand representatives from many countries and continents gathered for six days in an atmosphere of great optimism. However, while the congress marked the moment in which mental hygiene came closest to becoming a truly global movement, the fault lines that would lead to its dissolution were already visible.

Even years before mental hygienists from all over the world flocked to Washington, DC in 1930, the international congress already loomed large over the Atlantic. In fact, Clifford Beers's promise during his trip to Europe in 1923 to host and fund a large international meeting was directly connected to the subsequent founding of mental hygiene associations in Germany, Austria, and Switzerland. Among the European psychiatrists who met Beers in 1923 and joined the Organising Committee was Robert Sommer, who went on to become the first to drum up support for the creation of the German and Austrian branches of the international movement.[83] Initially, he mainly pointed to his own pre-war advocacy of mental hygiene, arguing that this development had been interrupted by the war in Germany, but had continued and gained momentum in the United States and France, where it was now experiencing a breakthrough. To not be left behind in the international competition, German and Austrian psychiatry had to revisit their own prophylactic ideas.[84]

At the 1925 conference of the German Psychiatric Association in Kassel, Sommer repeated his argument in a more compelling way. The international movement for mental hygiene, he claimed, offered a way to reintegrate German science into the international scientific community. Alluding to the common trope of the war as a large-scale experiment, Sommer said: 'In the history of the sciences the great war that lies behind us has been – political, military, and economic aspects apart – a very peculiar experiment, consisting in the almost total separation of the German people from all international intellectual relations'.[85] In many regards, Sommer argued, German science had stood the test and had developed and flourished autonomously. In some fields, however, the 'hitherto hostile foreign countries' now threatened to surpass Germany. In the United States, France, and Russia, mental hygiene had emerged as an 'intellectual and social movement', while Germany stood apart and was left behind.[86] What had to be done now was to unite the existing approaches to psychiatric prophylaxis nationwide, and to bring them back into the international 'politics of comparison'.[87] This was not only a call for German psychiatry's international reintegration, but also meant Sommer's own return to the international stage where he had already been active prior to the war.

In Germany, Austria, and Switzerland, Clifford Beers became the figurehead of the mental hygiene movement. By praising Beers as their charismatic founder and leader, representatives of European associations presented themselves as members of a dynamic international movement led by the successful NCMH in the United States. On the one hand, this was an affirmation of the movement's internationalist aspirations; on the other hand, it also was an advertising strategy designed to bolster reputation and legitimacy in different national environments. Unsurprisingly, Beers's most ardent supporter in Germany was Robert Sommer. In the first issue of the *Zeitschrift für psychische Hygiene*, he introduced an audience of German psychiatrists to Beers's achievements with an adulatory review of *A Mind That Found Itself*. He depicted Beers's autobiography not only as the founding document of mental hygiene as a movement, but also as an extraordinary piece of literature 'with a great wealth of characteristic words' reminding the amateur playwright Sommer of William Shakespeare. The exceptional quality of Beers's prose, Sommer claimed, was one reason the book had not yet been translated into German.[88]

However, Sommer's enthusiasm for Beers and his dedicated internationalist stance was not the consensus among German mental hygienists. His fellow board member Hermann Simon, for example, was fairly sceptical about Sommer's scientific internationalism and the use of Clifford Beers for the association's propaganda. As he saw it, Beers was of little value to mental hygiene in Germany and his ideas might even be detrimental to psychiatry's interests. In a 1931 letter to fellow board member Hans Roemer, he wrote:

> Time and again, I must urge to leave Beers out of it when possible. In the long run, he can be no mentor to us. When reading his book carefully, one

> has to say: his approach may perhaps be useful and economically successful for the American mentality (sensation!); for he has financed mental hygiene with his book (non olet!). That is not for our mentality! [...] Why do we still refer to Beers in all of our programmatic announcements (lately again Sommer in the short paper that he sent us)? Would it not be a pathetic display of our whole aspirations if these announcements were not to count for themselves but were only deemed valuable because the American Beers has initiated them in a book written for America, which has totally different aims. All this, we must not utter publicly, but we can show some restraint towards Mr. B[eers].[89]

Despite some common anti-American stereotypes, Simon's opposition to Beers was more than just an expression of his staunch German nationalism. His difference of opinion with Sommer, as well as his reservations against international networks in general reflected an inherent tension inside the DVPH. Robert Sommer was a professor of psychiatry at the University of Giessen, for whom international connections were an important source of reputation in the scientific community and an inherent part of his self-understanding. For the asylum director Hermann Simon, however, scientific reputation mattered far less than the support of local and national authorities and networks. Against the backdrop of the world economic crisis, Simon had to follow another rationale, focusing on state funding for psychiatric institutions instead of cultivating international scientific networks with their costly conferences and congresses. Moreover, as an asylum director Simon was sensitive to the potential dangers that Beers's denunciation of the mistreatment of psychiatric inmates meant for the interests and public reputation of the profession.

Prior to 1930, Robert Sommer's internationalist position prevailed. Many of the DVPH's activities were aimed at the planned international congress in Washington, DC. As far as Sommer was concerned, even the 1928 conference in Hamburg was merely a 'rehearsal' for the international event to come, and in fact, some of the papers presented there reappeared two years later in Washington, DC, clumsily translated.[90] Moreover, the participation of a German delegation at the international congress was also supported by state authorities. In 1928/1929, the DVPH had already received 1000 marks for travel expenses from the Foreign Ministry; additionally, the Ministry of the Interior apparently ramped up its funding before the event.[91] Apart from the financial support, the Ministry of the Interior also backed the delegation by designating Robert Sommer, Wilhelm Weygandt, and Hans Roemer as official German delegates.[92]

In the association's announcement of the congress shortly before the delegates' departure, gleeful anticipation was palpable.[93] Emphatically lauding a meeting that, for the first time in history, would 'bring together representatives [of mental hygiene] from all nations for an exchange of their experiences and for an agreement about the aims and methods of their work', the board members celebrated an event that would bring international rapprochement and social progress. Echoing the NCMH's propaganda and its focus on social adaptation, they envisioned mental hygiene as overcoming its purely 'defensive' prophylactic tasks and turn into a 'productive' force for the well-being of society at large. Anticipating a rhetoric of positive 'mental health' that would only gain wider influence after the Second World War, the aim of mental hygiene was seen in 'the preservation and promotion of the mental health and welfare of the individual and the community through the most rational integration of the individual into the whole of society'.[94] The approaches existing in Germany—from occupational therapy, open care, psychotherapy, social pedagogy, psychotechnical vocational counselling to eugenics—would have to be developed in this direction. Like the utopian ardour, the internationalist idealism in the German mental hygiene movement was never as pronounced as on the eve of the first international congress. Robert Sommer lauded the mental hygiene movement for creating 'humane relations between the peoples of all continents' and the board of the DVPH joined in[95]:

> There is no nation that has nothing to contribute to the common progress, and no nation that has nothing to gain from this common progress! May the united efforts of the nations succeed in the fight against the public prejudice against the mentally ill, and everything that has to do with them, in victoriously ending the fight that no nation has ended yet, and to create a new global opinion based on modern knowledge. May the standing International Committee for Mental Hygiene, which will be the visible outcome of the congress, succeed in making the concern for mental health and general human welfare the common goal of the whole civilised world.[96]

The First International Congress on Mental Hygiene indeed became a seminal event for the movement and marked its heyday before the Second World War.[97] With 3042 participants from fifty-two countries, it was the largest and most international meeting of mental health professionals held by that time. From 5 to 10 May 1930, forty-four papers covered almost all of the topics that comprised mental hygiene's encompassing agenda.

The congress clearly documented that the movement had come a long way since the founding of the Connecticut Society for Mental Hygiene in 1908, on the day twenty-two years before the formal inauguration in Washington, DC by NCMH president William A. White. Since, mental hygiene had grown into a movement that could mobilise thousands of professionals from psychiatry, related fields, and public health. Three professional organisations held their annual meetings parallel to the larger mental hygiene congress: the American Psychiatric Association, the American Society for the Study of the Feebleminded, and the American Psychoanalytic Association. This kind of interdisciplinary cooperation among the psy-ences would have been unthinkable in inter-war Germany. Mental hygiene also had become an international movement spanning over five continents, with representatives from twenty-two different national committees attending the conference. Moreover, the congress was supported by several US federal agencies and Herbert Hoover (1874–1964), then the thirty-first President of the United States, accepted the honorary presidency. In the United States at least, mental hygienists had successfully positioned themselves in the first line of politically recognised public health experts.[98]

The meeting was clearly international, but the American hosts dominated the congress. In terms of total participants, the United States outnumbered all other countries combined; less than ten per cent came from abroad. One reason was that transatlantic travel in the 1930s was still expensive and time-consuming. In the programme, the Americans' dominance was less pronounced; twenty-eight of the forty-four papers were given by Americans. Despite the tardy emergence of mental hygiene associations in the German-speaking countries, they were well represented. Eighteen Germans attended, which made them the second-largest group of foreigners after the Canadians. Six participants came from Switzerland, four from Austria.[99] The number of lectures is also revealing: With five papers, the Germans were second only to the Americans. Using mental hygiene to improve German psychiatry's standing on the international stage was beginning to pay off.[100]

Of course, content mattered more than mere numbers. The programme of the First International Congress on Mental Hygiene showed a movement that was mainly concerned with the reform of psychiatric institutions, the establishment of community care, and the education and adjustment of specific populations, such as 'feebleminded', borderline cases, neurotics, 'psychopaths', problem children and adolescents, as well as criminals. The two-volume documentation of the congress ran up to more than 1500 pages, and it will be neither possible nor necessary to give a comprehensive overview. Instead, I will briefly highlight two of the German contributions to the congress: Hans Roemer's reflections about mental hygiene and public opinion, and Ernst Rüdin's lecture on eugenics. Both papers clearly illustrate the limitations of internationalism and show how German mental hygienists tried to use the international congress as a stage for specifically German debates.

Hans Roemer's talk in Washington, DC reflected the self-understanding of progressive German psychiatrists and their self-ascribed role in enlightening the public. One of the major challenges faced by psychiatrists, Roemer argued, was the public bias against them and their patients. Outdated prejudice against the mentally ill lived on in the public opinion, 'like dark shadows, coming from a gloomy, painfully conquered past'. Psychiatric institutions were still seen in the light of conditions long overcome—'prison-like insane asylums, dark dungeons, gloomy rows of cells, cruel corporal and spiritual coercive measures'. Roemer blamed patients' families who 'projected onto the asylum and the physicians' their frustration about their sick relatives, as well as former patients, 'psychopaths' in particular, who tried 'for more or less morbid reasons to stir up public opinion' against psychiatry. The press was also to blame. Driven by sensationalism, journalists unjustly attacked psychiatry: 'They do not spare their reproaches when an insane person causes disaster; on the other hand, they like to take the part of those who complain at being confined'. All these prejudices directly impaired psychiatrists' ability to treat their patients. They prevented people suffering from mental disorders from being recognised as sick and in need of treatment and being brought to appropriate facilities, they helped outdated legislation to remain in effect, and the notion that psychiatric institutions were merely places of confinement effectively hindered psychiatrists' attempt to secure the necessary public funding for modern occupational therapies and open care.[101]

Roemer's complaints were not entirely new. For a long time, psychiatrists had painted themselves as the ones who had to enforce a modern, scientific understanding of mental illness against outdated metaphysical, moral, and superstitious beliefs.[102] And in the late nineteenth century already, psychiatry had found itself in the focus of public attention when a bourgeois 'anti-psychiatric' movement had begun to voice concerns about abuses of power in the asylum and the courtroom in a plethora of pamphlets and brochures, and newspapers regularly revealed dismal conditions in psychiatric institutions and other psychiatric scandals. As the topic entered parliamentary debates and psychiatry's opponents became more organised in the first decade of the twentieth century, psychiatrists discussed how they could defend their professional reputation.[103] Robert Sommer's plans for a psychiatric department of the *Reich* health office, for example, would also have had a forensic section tasked with countering misleading press reports about the abuse of psychiatric expertise in the courtroom.[104] In the aftermath of the First World War, the debate reignited and became politicised as anti-psychiatry mixed with revolutionary rhetoric, celebrating the end of psychiatry's 'reign of terror' in the service of the *ancien régime*.[105] And psychiatrists not only felt threatened by attacks from political activists, but also by their depiction in literature and movies. In particular, Heinrich Mann's (1871–1950) 1917 novel *Die Armen* ('The poor') struck a nerve and led to an extensive debate in a major psychiatric journal.[106]

And yet, Roemer's outlook for the future was optimistic. Recent years had brought a reorientation in 'the general thought of Germany' and a climate more suitable for the reform of psychiatry. Through the teachings of Sigmund Freud, Alfred Adler, Carl Jung, and Ernst Kretschmer, psychological knowledge had penetrated wider circles of the public and prepared a fertile ground for the expansion of psychiatric social services, psychotherapy, and 'a pedagogy of cure aiming at a thoughtful self-government'.[107] Moreover, Roemer claimed, the post-war crisis had also increased the need for a 'systematic economy of human beings' that was already beginning to reshape welfare, health care, and penal legislation. This, still ongoing, shift in public opinion would eventually allow for psychiatry to become an integrated part of public health and social services, transforming the psychiatrist from the alienist of old into a public health and welfare expert with a strong influence on state legislation.[108]

Ernst Rüdin's (1874–1952) lecture revealed the growing discrepancies between mental hygiene in the United States and Germany. The only paper about eugenics at a congress otherwise dominated by ideas of community care, adjustment, and institutional reform, it showed where the German mental hygiene association, and German psychiatry in general, were headed in the next years. At the time of the Washington, DC congress, the Swiss-born Rüdin was the most eminent psychiatric geneticist and arguably the most influential propagandist of eugenics in Germany. As he would continue to play a crucial role in German mental hygiene, a brief sketch of his biography is useful. From the onset of his scientific career, Rüdin had tried to combine academic research and public activism. In 1905, together with his brother-in-law Alfred Ploetz (1860–1940), he founded the Society for Racial Hygiene (*Gesellschaft für Rassenhygiene*). Over the following years, he joined his teacher Emil Kraepelin in diagnosing an impending 'degeneration' of the German people and advocated systematic, state-led eugenics, including the sterilisation of alcoholics and the mentally ill. In 1917/1918, he was appointed director of the genealogic-demographical department of Kraepelin's newly founded German Research Institute for Psychiatry (DFA) in Munich, the first research facility for psychiatric genetics worldwide. After a short stint as chair of psychiatry at the University of Basel after 1925, he returned to Munich in 1928, after his demands for a triplication of the budget of the genealogic-demographical department had been met. In 1931, he became director of the DFA. The transfer of power to the Nazis in 1933 intensified Rüdin's alliance with the state; in 1933, he became chair of the DVPH, now renamed German Association for Mental Hygiene and Racial Hygiene, in 1935 the *Reich* leader of the neurological and psychiatric professions. Rüdin was one of the central figures of Nazi psychiatry and contributed to the creation of the scientific and institutional framework for the forced sterilisation and, after 1941, the mass murder of mental patients.[109]

Rüdin's 1930 lecture in Washington, DC was an attempt to incorporate the nascent movement for mental hygiene into psychiatric eugenics and racial hygiene—a move that would eventually be successful in Germany. Rüdin incorrectly claimed that mental hygiene had focused almost exclusively on the well-being and health of 'those already born'. Caring for the mentally ill and preventing the development of full-blown mental disorder was important but, in Rüdin's view, it also meant that preventive measures had come too late: 'It would be better, however, if such persons were not born at all, and that calls for eugenics'.[110] By preventing hereditary mental illness through eugenics, mental hygiene would be able to more efficiently focus its efforts and resources on those for whom preventive measures aimed at environmental factors could actually have an effect. In 1930 however, Rüdin did not yet go as far as to advocate coercive sterilisation of mental patients but argued that marriage counselling and voluntary sterilisation would be the best way to achieve his eugenic goals.[111] Yet, his ambiguous and conspicuously tactical statement—'At this time, I personally should not care to consider any coercive measures'—was far apart from Robert Sommer's categorical and moral rejection of coercive eugenics.[112] When the political opportunity for a more radical approach presented itself in 1933, Rüdin was ready to act without hesitation.[113] In an equally elusive manner, Rüdin affirmed the global reach of eugenics without subscribing to internationalism in science and public health:

> I am of the opinion that mental hygiene and eugenics should be of equal interest for all social classes, races, peoples and countries. May every people, every race, every country work independently in these matters in order to attain to the high aims set by mental hygiene and, within it, by eugenics.[114]

To an American audience, Rüdin's paper brought little new. Even before the First World War, eugenics were well-established in the United States and a broad range of different organisations advocated the sterilisation of the 'unfit'. When Rüdin crossed the Atlantic to propagate eugenics, twenty-four states had already passed sterilisation laws, which often also allowed for coercive measures.[115] In the context of the mental hygiene movement, however, the situation was more complicated. Mental hygiene in the United States had initially been part of a larger eugenic alliance but was shifted from nature to nurture after the First World War. By 1930, the NCMH's activities focused on education and adjustment for specific groups of mental patients and borderline cases, on community care, and on mental health education and counselling for the general population. Rüdin's attempt to unite mental hygiene and eugenics came at a time when in the United States, both movements were already drifting apart. Rejecting social Darwinism and the therapeutic pessimism on which eugenics were based, the American Foundation for Mental Hygiene celebrated their belief in scientific progress instead:

> Science takes exception to the law that only those whom nature deems the fittest shall survive. [...] The knowledge so gained forms a sacred trust of civilization for the maintenance of the strong, for the refitting of the weak and sick to their health and opportunity, and for their deliverance to a useful life in the community and that pursuit of happiness which is the proper promise of creation.[116]

Hence, Rüdin's attempt to unify mental hygiene and eugenics received mixed reactions at the congress. Charles B. Davenport, one of the most eminent US eugenicists, unsurprisingly came out in support of Rüdin. Abraham Myerson, professor of neurology at Tufts College and director of research at the Boston State Hospital, vehemently criticised Rüdin's disregard for environmental factors. He also attacked the core of Rüdin's reasoning when he questioned the underlying Kraepelinian nosology, arguing that diseases like dementia praecox and schizophrenia were no stable units from which laws of heredity could be derived, but 'loosely defined and ill-understood entities' in a 'classification that is changing year by year'.[117]

The conflict between eugenics and adaptation was the main unresolved issue in the international movement for mental hygiene. While individuals like Robert Sommer were able to bridge the gap between nature and nurture for themselves, the movement as a whole could not. In the following years, this inherent fault line became one of the reasons for the gradual dissolution of the international movement before the Second World War. In 1930 however, optimism still prevailed. Among the participants of the First International Congress, the consensus was mental hygiene's global rise was only beginning. Clifford Beers was enthusiastic about the success of the congress and saw his role as the charismatic leader of an international movement confirmed. His next trip, he wrote in a circular letter to representatives of the various national associations, would lead him to New Zealand and Australia aboard the S.S. Aorangi—'a 22,000 ton liner capable of floating the founder of the mental hygiene movement!'—to propagate his ideas there. In Beers's optimistic outlook, the humanitarian progress of mental hygiene proceeded alongside the advances of technology:

> When travel by airplane becomes absolutely safe, we shall expect a large number of members of the International Committee to come to annual celebrations of our National Committee, and I hope to live long enough to see air traveling so safe that I can fly to different parts of the world to attend meetings of the various mental hygiene organizations which are part of our international work.[118]

Consequently, one of the major items on the agenda of the congress had been the founding of an ICMH tasked with spreading mental hygiene globally.[119] Planning for the International Committee had been going on for more than a decade, before the Washington, DC congress finally offered the possibility to gather the world's leading mental hygienists for a founding meeting. Its professed goal was to create a common framework for the many existing national mental hygiene associations, to support the creation of new ones, and thereby to help transform mental hygiene into a truly international and global movement. It was to

> encourage and promote in every country the establishment of a duly authorized voluntary national society for mental hygiene, for the conservation of mental health, the reduction and prevention of nervous and mental disorders and mental defect, the scientific and humane care and treatment of those suffering from any of these disorders.[120]

The internationalism of the ICMH was, however, not without limitations. Like the 1930 congress, the committee was conspicuously dominated by mental hygienists from the United States. Its president, chairs, treasurer, and general secretary were all Americans, and so were most of the members of the governing board and council. The committee's founding document explicitly stated that its permanent secretariat was to be set up in the United States.[121] Moreover, the entire approach of the ICMH clearly reflected a form of philanthropism specific to the United States, relying strongly on lay participation and private donations. The ICMH's organisational structure and objectives closely were modelled after the NCMH, which had been at the centre of the American movement's meteoric rise in the previous decades.[122]

However, despite the American dominance, it is unjust to claim that the ICMH was a tool for 'cultural imperialism', as Mathew Thomson has done.[123] The notion of 'cultural imperialism' poses more questions than it actually answers, as it implies that the committee's activities were part of a coherent and intentional state-led agenda, illegitimately trying to supersede indigenous approaches to psychiatric prophylaxis and institutional reform abroad. This was clearly not the case. While the committee was led by American mental hygienists whose vision of philanthropism was based on their experiences in the United States, it was not part of any formal state policy. Moreover, unlike, for example, the German Association for Mental Hygiene, the ICMH did not receive state funding but solely relied on private donations. Moreover, even if led by Americans, the committee nevertheless was as a truly international affair. Apart from the key functionaries mentioned above, the numerous vice presidencies, honorary presidencies, boards and councils members were mental hygienists from many countries and continents, so that the committee could rightly claim to represent mental hygiene as an international, and even as a global movement. Most of the leaders of the various national organisations were part of the committee in one way or another. As for the German-speaking countries, Robert Sommer became one of the committee's six vice-presidents and a member of the governing board and the executive committee, while Josef Berze, Hans

Roemer, and André Repond represented the Austrian, German, and Swiss mental hygiene organisations, respectively, as honorary vice-presidents of the ICMH.

The committee's internationalist commitment was underlined by the decision to hold the next international congress on mental hygiene in Paris, France. However, the international movement would not able to replicate the success of the first congress. Initially set to take place in 1933, the Paris congress had to be postponed several times for organisational and financial reasons, and eventually only happened in 1937.[124] By then, the global political landscape had changed. Against the backdrop of rising political tensions and the ongoing Spanish Civil War, the number of participants hardly exceeded even one-tenth of those of the Washington, DC congress. The German branch was drifting further apart from the US-led international movement. Unlike in 1930, in 1937 the optimistic rhetoric of mutual progress could not hide the centrifugal forces that had existed in the movement from the beginning anymore.

Crisis, Radicalisation, and Demise

'The outlook is bright and the possibilities are great in the whole field of mental hygiene', John Robert Lord (1874–1931) of the British delegation emphatically declared on occasion of the 1930 congress.[125] This view was shared by the vast majority of delegates from all over the world. Mental hygiene seemed to be on the rise and solving the problem of mental illness only a question of time. Wilhelm Weygandt, of the German delegation, issued a very long-term prognosis: 'If mental hygiene shows the same great gains in the next four thousand years as in the last, in the year 5930 there will be no more cases of insanity [...]'.[126]

Weygandt's long-term vision may have been too bold for some, and too cautious for others, but the experience of mental hygiene as a booming international movement clearly stimulated the local branches in Europe, as did the prospect of holding a similar congress in the near future. Shortly after the return of the German delegation from Washington, DC, board member Hermann Simon penned a detailed itinerary of the next steps.[127] Apart from disseminating the results of the international congress through various channels, Simon was concerned with strengthening the association's connections with other actors in the field of mental and public health care, with different organisations in psychiatry and neurology, in other areas of hygiene, as well as with state and municipal authorities. The

German Association for Mental Hygiene would also have to intensify its public outreach to both professional and lay audiences. Moreover, Simon noted, mental hygienists would have to identify and formulate their vision more positively, with regard to education, sexual reproduction, vocational choices, recreation and sports, but also 'culture, civilization, and art' as well as their 'world view'.

A consensus about what 'mental hygiene' actually was did not emerge in the German-speaking countries during the inter-war period. Nevertheless, in the early 1930s, several attempts were made to unify and systematise the outlook of mental hygiene. In Austria, Erwin Stransky published a 'guide to mental hygiene' (*Leitfaden der psychischen Hygiene*) in 1931, in which various authors, most of them Viennese, discussed different aspects of mental hygiene, its relation to psychiatry, psychotherapy, and other areas of hygiene, as well as its intended impact on education, sexual reproduction, eugenics, criminology, and 'contemporary civilisation' in general.[128]

In the same year, the German psychiatrists Oswald Bumke, Gustav Kolb, and Hans Roemer, together with Eugen Kahn, who in 1929 had left Germany for a position as professor of psychiatry and mental Hygiene at Yale, published another, even more comprehensive 'dictionary of mental hygiene and psychiatric care' (*Handwörterbuch der psychischen Hygiene und psychiatrischen Fürsorge*).[129] In seventy-two entries and on more than four hundred pages, psychiatrists and hygienists from Germany and Switzerland discussed a very broad range of topics. The reform of the mental health-care system and eugenics took up the most space, but numerous other articles about less prominent aspects of mental hygiene—from food, clothing, and the prevention of noise to the psychiatric aspects of the relation between community and society, of love and the joy in life—document as just how encompassing its protagonists envisioned their socio-medical project. However, the dictionary also shows that there hardly was a common definition of 'mental hygiene' on which all authors could have agreed. And the publication of the dictionary itself was a sign of rifts in the German movement for mental hygiene. One member of the association's board, Gustav Kolb, was among the editors, and two other board members, Hermann Simon and Hans Roemer, had contributed articles. But the dictionary had bypassed Robert Sommer's plans for an 'international guide to psychiatric prophylaxis and mental hygiene' that was soon to be printed. Sommer's three-hundred-page manuscript eventually went unpublished.[130]

Together with national and international conferences and congresses and the publication of a special journal, the almost simultaneous publication of two handbooks reinforced the impression that mental hygiene entered the 1930s in good shape. The last decade had seen the emergence and professionalisation of a previously unseen number of actors in the wider area of mental health care and psychiatric prophylaxis, which was not limited to psychiatrists but also included pedagogues, care workers, and public health officials. Mental hygiene promised to unify and foster these activities, while at the same time securing psychiatrists' leadership of the movement.[131] There was, however, a conspicuous gap between aspirations and realities. In sharp contrast to many high-flying plans, the realities on the ground were sobering. The economic situation was one important reason. The world economic crisis had hit the Weimar Republic hard, and with soaring unemployment and dwindling state revenues, the welfare system came under intense pressure. Mental health care was struck by the onset of the depression as massive budget cuts threatened to unravel the results of reforms that had only really begun in the second half of the 1920s.

The international movement for mental hygiene was directly affected. Globally, the economic crisis made transatlantic travel and large-scale international conferences unaffordable, and the internationalist seeds planted in 1930 never came to fruition. In Germany, the crisis triggered a momentous change in priorities, shifting mental hygienists' focus from institutional reform to eugenics. Many German psychiatrists, including some of the future leaders of the emerging movement, had already advocated eugenics as the best kind of psychiatric prophylaxis from the turn of the century on. The German Association for Mental Hygiene, however, was initially a mouthpiece of reform ideas such as open care and occupational therapy championed by its board members Gustav Kolb and Hermann Simon. At the first German conference on mental hygiene in 1928, speakers had advocated institutional reform, the extension of psychiatry's welfare activities and had stressed the importance of counselling and education. The second conference in 1932, by contrast, was devoted entirely to eugenics as a means of psychiatric prophylaxis. Even before the Nazis made compulsory sterilisations on eugenic indications state policy in 1933, German psychiatrists and mental hygienists were already in line. At the turn from the 1920s to the 1930s, mental hygiene experienced a paradigm shift, but eugenics were not simply a break away from earlier reform ideas. Institutional reform, new therapeutics, and eugenics were in fact intricately connected.

With increasing poverty and a seeming dissolution of social norms, expensive attempts to improve the treatment of the mentally ill seemed less relevant and affordable in the late 1920s and early 1930s than even some years before. The therapeutic optimism of the recent years notwithstanding, state officials again saw the main function of psychiatric institutions in confinement and social control. These priorities were apparent in the 1931 police administration law (*Polizeiverwaltunggesetz*), which—to the great displeasure of the psychiatric profession—confirmed that the responsibility for the decision to confine mentally disordered individuals lay exclusively with the police and which ignored medical indications in favour of public safety. The decline of German psychiatry and the shift back to confinement directly affected the patient numbers and the average duration of their stay: In 1929, the asylums had reached their highest capacity yet, treating more than 300,000 patients a year while reducing the average length of stay to six months. By 1932, the total number of patients had dropped by 50,000, but with 218 days the average length of stay had increased by almost a month, climbing back to pre-1914 levels.[132]

In this desperate situation, eugenics promised a way out of the impasse. For several decades, proponents of eugenics and racial hygiene had sedulously asserted that the most efficient way to deal with mental illness was not to treat individual patients, but to target the population. Instead of the expensive confinement and therapy of individual mental patients, eugenicists promised to prevent mental illness before it could become a burden and a menace to society. This argument had been the core of eugenicists' propaganda since the end of the nineteenth century; in times of economic and political crisis, both medical colleagues and political decision makers became far more likely to lend an ear. In the natal crisis of the Weimar Republic in 1918/1919, many psychiatric articles and pamphlets had propagated eugenics for national reconstruction after the lost war. Eugenics never completely vanished from the debate during the 1920s, but in the republic's final crisis, it moved to the fore again, now as a way to cut psychiatry's costs and to subject the care for the mentally ill to an imperative of rationality and efficiency.[133]

The same was also true for the most radical form of racial hygiene, which did not only want to prevent future generations of mental patients from being born, but also to get rid of the living. In 1920, jurist Karl Binding and psychiatrist Alfred Hoche had contemplated the 'destruction of life unworthy of life' (*Vernichtung lebensunwerten Lebens*) in their now notorious treatise.[134] After triggering a heated debate, Binding and Hoche's foray faded as German post-war economy and society consolidated and more optimistic perspectives regarding the treatment of the mentally ill began dominated psychiatric discourse in the 1920s. Against the backdrop of economic crisis, however, the idea of relieving the nation of the burden of the mentally deficient regained momentum.[135] In 1932, Berthold Kihn (1895–1964), professor of psychiatry in Erlangen argued that a 'more radical approach against the inferior' was needed. The current economic crisis did not allow for any waste of resources, and 'among the needless expenses we have to count the sustainment of surplus existences (*Ballastexistenzen*) (Hoche) by public means'.[136]

One year later, the Nazis' rise to power offered radical eugenicists the possibility for a political alliance that enabled them to realise long-held aspirations. On 14 July 1933, the Law for the Prevention of Hereditarily Diseased Offspring (*Gesetz zur Verhütung erbkranken Nachwuchses*), which allowed compulsory sterilisations for a variety of purportedly hereditary diseases, was published; it came into effect on 1 January 1934.[137] The killing of the mentally ill, although overtly propagated by numerous psychiatrists and racial hygienists for decades, was a moral transgression on another scale. The mass murder of psychiatric patients and disabled individuals as part of different 'euthanasia' programmes only began in 1939 and in relative secrecy.[138]

Juxtaposing the crimes of Nazi psychiatry to the reform programmes of Weimar psychiatry may be tempting. However, to describe psychiatry's radicalisation and the triumph of the eugenics paradigm in the 1930s as a break away from earlier, more humane reform ideas would be overly simplistic. Eugenics and Nazi 'euthanasia' were ideologically related, but not identical, and many eugenicists—like the DVPH board member Hans Roemer—supported eugenics, but categorically rejected the idea of killing the mentally ill in the name of racial hygiene.[139] Historians have compellingly shown the considerable intellectual and personal continuities between Weimar and Nazi psychiatry and eugenics. Moreover, as the history of the mental hygiene movement in the German-speaking countries illustrates with exceptional clarity, institutional reform, new therapeutic approaches, and eugenics were by no means mutually exclusive. Robert Sommer, for example, understood mental hygiene as a two-pronged strategy, which necessarily had to include the prevention of both 'endogenous' and 'exogenous' mental disorders; the former through research in heredity and eugenics, the latter through changes in individual and collective lifestyles.[140] Leading eugenicists like Ernst Rüdin and his colleague Hans Luxenburger used very similar arguments when speaking to psychiatric audiences.[141]

The view that eugenics and new therapeutics were two sides of the same coin was common among German psychiatrists in the late 1920s and early 1930s. The introduction of new therapeutic methods and the promise to treat and cure at least some groups of mental patients by implication redrew and reinforced the distinction between 'curable' and 'incurable' patients. At the same time, psychiatry's therapeutic advances also triggered a new kind of 'therapeutic actionism' which aroused hopes that the problem of mental illness could be solved for good. Consequently, the suitability of individual patients for occupational therapy became the most important criterion in the selection of psychiatric inmates for annihilation in the 'T4' programme.[142] More recent research has also taken into account the role of the new somatic cures, like electroconvulsive therapy (ECT) and insulin coma therapy (ICT), which entered psychiatrists' armoury in the 1930s, and has largely confirmed this interpretation.[143]

Hermann Simon, who in 1929 began to systematically reflect on the broader implications of his approach to the reform of institutional care, provides a particularly clear-cut example for the connection between mental hygiene, institutional reform, and psychiatry's eugenic radicalisation.[144] In the early 1920s, his concept of 'more active therapy' had made him one of the most prominent advocates of institutional reform; a reputation that led Robert Sommer to invite Simon to join the board of the German Association for Mental Hygiene in 1927.[145] Simon's 'more active therapy' was based on the consistent use of occupational therapy, but from the beginning on, the underlying concept of work was double-edged. On the one side, occupational therapy likely was a real improvement for parts of the asylum population in comparison with previous attempts to immobilise and sedate them. Simon's approach fitted the needs of mid-1920s Weimar psychiatry on various levels. It promised to reduce length of stay in the asylum, had patients contribute to the operations of the institution, and prepared them to be reintegrated into working life and society, all of which could help ease the economic burden of the mentally ill for both the health-care system and society at large. On the other side, however, Simon's approach also widened the gap between those patients who were able to work and those who were not. 'More active therapy' was connected to a highly ideological concept of labour as citizen's duty. Simon's work ethics linked the value of a human being to his or her ability and willingness to work, and the notion that some patients could be cured prepared the dehumanisation of others. In a 1929 treatise about the philosophical implications of 'more active therapy', Simon argued that the reform of institutional care might have unwelcome side effects. Keeping the patients active kept them in a better shape, extending the lifespan of the sick and elderly, and thus contributed to the overcrowding of the asylums. As he insinuated, passive euthanasia by denying some patients the benefits of the new treatment methods was a legitimate choice:

> If we were to keep all these highly senile and the other 'weak ones' in bed, there is no doubt that within a year most of them [...] would have their bronchopneumonia or cardiac insufficiency and perish. What if this were my conviction, and I would nonetheless keep them lying in bed, how does this relate to § 211 of the penal code [sanctioning abandonment]? I am not joking; and even less do I think of accusing colleagues who think and act different than I do of a criminal offence.[146]

Simon's approval of neglecting patients and leaving them for dead at first seems incompatible with the therapeutic optimism of one of the most eminent psychiatric reformers of his time. Although he campaigned for the reform of institutional care, Simon was in fact, and somewhat paradoxically, wary of contemporary advances in mental health care, and medical care in general. In 1929, he introduced 'more active treatment' to a world view equally based on a social-Darwinist notion of the survival of the fittest, a dichotomist juxtaposition of health and sickness, and a utilitarian approach to of medicine, in which the nation and the healthy individual took precedence over the sick.

Reacting both to the political and economic crisis and his frustration about the practical limits of 'more active therapy', Simon proposed a voluntaristic notion of sickness, which morally blamed sick and weak patients for their inability and alleged unwillingness to participate in occupational therapy. With this notion of mental illness as a moral failure, occupational therapy became a pedagogical intervention. The prevalent approach in the treatment of mental illness, Simon argued, was to keep patients calm and passive, thereby allowing them to continue to be weak and sick, and to develop an egoistic sense of entitlement. 'More active therapy', by contrast, was supposed to foster the healthy parts of a patient's personality, teaching self-sufficiency and demonstrating that one could still contribute to society instead of relying on it. While 'more active therapy' had emerged in the context and as part of the Weimar welfare state, Simon saw it as a way to counteract an excess of welfare that reallocated scarce resources from the healthy to the sick and created incentives for sickness. A healthier society, he believed, would not be achieved through more medicine, but only with less. In a 1931 letter to fellow DVPH board member Hans Roemer, he asked:

> A private question: Could it be that we physicians exaggerate the fight against death, and its forward post, sickness?? Do we fight this battle with means which, even when the best possible result is achieved, are out of proportion? [...] I gradually come to realise that a good part of mental hygiene, if it really is supposed to benefit a nation, should consist in renouncing the exaggerations of modern medicine. But what a hornets' nest we would get into![147]

Mental hygiene, as Hermann Simon came to envision it in the late 1920s, did not only target mental patients, but the health of the nation. Translating his experiences from the asylum into a social-Darwinist view of society at large, he vehemently argued against the corrupting effects of modern life, culture, and civilisation. Spoiling and pampering mental patients, Simon claimed, would not cure them, but only create more and worse symptoms instead; the same being true for civilised life in general, which weakened individuals' and the nation's fitness in the constant 'struggle for survival'. The alliance of modern medicine and the welfare state acted against nature, undermining the health of those still healthy, and burdening them with the care for the sick, until the sick would finally overcome the healthy. In this apocalyptic scenario, Simon believed that mental hygiene had to stem the tide, advocating the laws of nature and defending the healthy against the sick: 'Our efforts have again to come to the relief of *health*, which today is almost helpless against the burden of everything weak and inferior'.[148]

Simon's social-Darwinist vision of mental hygiene, which became the dominant theme in his correspondence with other board members in the late 1920s, was rooted in a profound sense of national crisis. The nation, and not the sick individual, moved to the centre of his concept of mental hygiene. In a 1929 letter to Robert Sommer, he wrote: 'Mental hygiene must work towards an education of a tough and vigorous people, which is able to stand up to the hard times that await us'.[149] 'Nation, toughen up!' (*Volk, werde hart!*) became Simon's mantra in the early 1930s, reflecting worries about the economic and social hardships and the crisis of the asylum in the wake of the economic crisis, as well as widespread fears of degeneration, and popular Nietzschean tropes. However, despite his wordy evocation of the health and strength of the nation, the details of his programme of national reconstruction remained in the vague. Economic considerations about the cost of medical care were one important aspect, but other statements show that Simon could also imagine the national 'struggle for survival' as military conflict:

> 'Nation, toughen up!' To fight, I need a sword made from solid metal: Steel, not gold nor lead. In our bitter struggle for survival, our whole nation – due to wealth and security – is too much attuned to the rear and the home front, and too little to the trenches and their rough conditions of life.[150]

For the future of the German Association for Mental Hygiene, Simon's views on the national 'struggle for survival' had two immediate consequences—the separation of German mental hygiene from the international movement as part of which it had emerged, and a shift towards the advocacy of state-led eugenics. In 1930, Simon had been a member of the official German delegation at the First International Congress on Mental Hygiene in Washington, DC. However, unlike others in the delegation, he had not been overly enthused about his trip to the United States. On his return, he left the writing of success stories about the German delegation's success on the international stage to Robert Sommer and Hans Roemer and complained that the number of lectures and the mixture of languages had made it impossible for him to follow anyway.[151] Against the backdrop of the economic downturn, he became even more wary of large-scale international conferences. Participating in the upcoming meeting of European mental hygienists in Paris in 1932 would mostly be a waste of scarce resources:

> As I see it, the work in our own house is much more important than the international fuss that is prepared in Paris. Let the rich foreign countries seek heaven in their own fashion and let us use the scarce means that are available to us for our own benefit. We will not be able to make a great impression in Paris anyway. For I do not know who should finance this delegation. And that we are a nation that is being sucked out, nobody knows that better than the enemy powers assembled in Paris.[152]

Other German mental hygienists, like Robert Sommer, were nationalists of one sort or another, but their nationalism was one in which nations peacefully competed for prestige on the international stage. Simon, by contrast, came to advocate a more bellicose nationalism, in which nations and their scientists encountered each other as opponents in a zero-sum game. The reduction in scope of scientific and medical activities to the own nation was one side of an interpretation of mental hygiene narrowed to maintaining the health of the body politic in a time of existential crisis. The other side was a growing belief that forceful eugenic measures were the only workable approach to psychiatric prophylaxis. The concentration of mental hygiene on eugenics, persistently pushed by Simon in his correspondence with other members of the DVPH in the early 1930s, was the direct result of a world view based on economic concerns, the belief that the German nation was beleaguered from all sides, as well as an adulation of health and strength, and the concomitant rejection of welfare and medical care for the weak and sick: 'For the relief of the nations from the nightmarish burden of the inferior and weak has to happen, if the unfit and inferior is [!] not to devour the fit'.[153]

In the mid-1920s, Hermann Simon as a reform-oriented asylum physicians had connected the emerging movement for mental hygiene to practical efforts for institutional reform to improve the situation of mental patients; by the end of the decade, he had become the main advocate of a shift away from the asylum and individual patients, and towards public and state-led interventions for the collective health of the nation. By 1933, Simon had severed the tie between institutional reform and mental hygiene; in preparation for the next international congress in Paris, then planned to take place in 1935, he argued that topics pertaining to the asylum system should not be discussed at a conference about hygiene.[154]

Although Simon's radicalisation during the economic crisis was representative of a broader shift in both psychiatry and society in the early 1930s, his socio-medical views were not shared by all protagonists of the German movement for mental hygiene. As I have shown in the previous chapter, Robert Sommer, despite his support of eugenics, vehemently and consistently rejected all coercive measures and unequivocally defended the right to live of the mentally ill. Hans Roemer's position was more ambiguous. He supported eugenics, and after 1933, defended the Nazi's policy of forced sterilisation, but he nevertheless recognised what dangers the eugenic mindset held. In a direct reply to Simon's latest reflections on the future of mental hygiene in 1932, Roemer argued that 'eugenic aspects are undoubtedly indispensable for mental hygiene, but there is the danger of one-sided exaggeration, which can then lead to the misunderstanding and the mistake that by this means one can breed the super-human (*Übermensch*)'.[155] Moreover, Roemer also defended psychiatry's medical commitment to the sick and the importance of public welfare against the 'spirit of ruthlessness, egoism, and brutal force coming from the realm of naturalism and the ruthless struggle for survival'. If the community's responsibility for individual lives were to be reduced to an economic consideration about a person's value for society, Roemer clear-sightedly argued, the 'destruction of life unworthy of life' was a logical consequence—'be it directly or through the denial of the means of subsistence, and then there is no distinction anymore between the incurable ill, the feebleminded, the criminal, the disabled, and finally, he who is thought to be a political enemy of the nation'. Simon dismissed Roemer's criticism and replied by emphatically recapitulating his views. In particular, he rejected Roemer's warning against eugenic excess: 'Eugenics have never sought to breed the super-human. As far as I have followed the literature, they have only pursued the more obvious goal, to prevent the breeding of the *sub-human*. In the end, it is the *sub-human* who kill their own nations'.[156]

While Roemer and Sommer warned against the consequences of overly radical interpretations, there was no general opposition to eugenics as such in the German Association for Mental Hygiene. Quite the contrary, psychiatric eugenics became the sole topic of the second conference on mental hygiene, which took place in Bonn in May 1932, almost four years after the initial conference in Hamburg.[157] Economic difficulties were one reason for the delay, another was that the preparations for the international congress in Washington, DC had tied up the resources of the association in the previous years.[158] To reduce the travel expenses for its two hundred participants, the conference took place immediately after the yearly general assembly of the German Psychiatric Society. Despite the global economic crisis, and despite Hermann Simon's calls for a severing of international networks, German mental hygiene was still well-integrated in the European movement, with representatives from Switzerland, the Netherlands, Finland, Norway, and France attending the conference. Austria, however, was absent.

Robert Sommer opened the 1932 conference by talking about the 'eugenic tasks of mental hygiene', putting on display his profound uneasiness about this topic. Arguing in two directions at the same time, Sommer tried to defend the thematic choice against both the proponents and the opponents of eugenics. On the one side, he stressed that mental hygiene's interest in eugenics was not an opportunistic reaction to the topic's boom during the depression. Eugenics had been an integral part of mental hygiene's agenda from the beginning on, and a direct consequence of its two-pronged approach targeting both endogenous and exogenous forms of mental disorder. Insinuations that mental hygiene had only recently turned towards eugenics were 'totally mistaken', and Sommer defended mental hygienists' expertise in an increasingly crowded field.[159] On the other side, however, Sommer also defended the thematical choice against reproaches that mental hygiene had abandoned its more holistic approach:

> While the association has chosen to place psychiatric eugenics at the centre of the II. German conference, it has to be stressed that it does not intend a dogmatic limitation to endogenous causes and genetics, but will also continue to examine and combat exogenous causes with the same rigor. Only for technical reasons was it necessary to focus on the prevention of pathogenic genetic constitutions (*pathogene Keimbeschaffenheiten*), which today is at the fore of public interest.[160]

Even as Sommer insisted that nothing had changed, the 1932 conference in Bonn showed how and where mental hygiene had shifted in the previous years. Unlike in 1928, where a broad range of different approaches had been discussed, the second conference was totally dominated by eugenics as the singular topic. As the economic downturn caused severe cutbacks in the funding of psychiatric institutions, the collective health of the nation had effectively supplanted any notion of improving the living conditions of mentally disordered individuals. Ernst Rüdin and his colleague Hans Luxenburger made few references to any form of psychiatric care beyond the sterilisation of the potential parents of future mental patients.[161] Rüdin repeated an argument that he had already used in Washington, DC in 1930 when he claimed that individual mental hygiene could only be effective and efficient when 'its attempts to educate and cure can be made with hereditarily flawless human material'.[162] Whereas for Rüdin eugenics prepared the ground for individual treatment and prophylaxis, for Luxenburger, this relation was reversed. The more effectively psychiatrists would prevent mental illness from developing and cure the mentally ill, the more important eugenics became, as symptom-free carriers of hereditary disease could spread it more easily to the next generation than those who were visibly sick.

However, there was little at stake for Rüdin and Luxenburger in 1932. As the other papers and the discussion at the conference demonstrated, they were already preaching to the choir. The odd exception was Robert Sommer, who took the focus on eugenics as an opportunity to revisit his own theory of 'natural nobility'.[163] Unlike Rüdin and Luxenburger, who represented the mainstream of German eugenics, Sommer again argued that a healthier society could not be achieved through coercive measures like the sterilisation of the unfit, but only through a social and intellectual mass movement in which all parts of society voluntarily participated. At the centre of the tacit conflict between the founder of the German mental hygiene movement and more aggressive eugenicists like Rüdin, Luxenburger, and Simon was not just a different understanding of the ethical boundaries of social medicine, but also a different conception of mental hygiene's relation to the state. Although they largely agreed on both the importance of hereditary factors in the development of mental illness and on the necessity of some form of socio-medical intervention, the old-fashioned liberal Sommer did not see the state, but society as the solution to the problem. Sommer imagined the eugenic regeneration of the nation as a result of a kind of grass-roots movement that would spread the idea of hereditary health through rational insight and an idealist belief in the common good. Most of his colleagues, by contrast, found top-down, state-led interventions to be the more viable way to improve and maintain the health of the nation. Consequently, the fact sheet on the prevention of hereditary mental illness, in which the German Association for Mental Hygiene tried to summarise and popularise its position, remained vague, and referred both to the importance of individual choices and the necessity of a legal framework for voluntary sterilisation.[164] The notion of 'natural nobility' that Sommer had included in his draft did not make it into the published version.[165]

The immediate future of course belonged to the forceful state-led approach advocated by Rüdin and Luxenburger. Little more than a year after the 1932 conference, in July 1933, the Nazi authorities passed the Law for the Prevention of Hereditarily Diseased Offspring (*Gesetz zur Verhütung erbkranken Nachwuchses*), which allowed the forced sterilisation of the carriers of supposedly hereditary defects. Most of the diseases indicated by the law were neurological or psychiatric, namely congenital mental deficiency, schizophrenia, manic-depressive insanity, hereditary epilepsy and Huntington's chorea, although the law also mentioned hereditary muteness and deafness, all kinds of hereditary bodily malformations, and severe alcoholism.[166] Mental hygiene, however, had already been on this path before.

From Mental Hygiene to Racial Hygiene

The German mental hygiene movement's shift towards racial hygiene was a gradual process that had begun long before 1933. In the last years of the Weimar Republic, the German Association for Mental Hygiene (DVPH) had increasingly come to see itself as the avant-garde of psychiatric eugenics and the health policies of the 'Third Reich' did not impose a new paradigm. And yet, the year 1933 was a caesura. As the Nazi authorities made eugenics state policy, some of mental hygienists' main demands were implemented, and even quicker than the most zealous proponents of eugenics had thought possible. This was, however, not a triumph of mental hygiene, but created an ambiguous situation that held risks and chances. Overtaken by events, the association found itself in danger of being superseded by other organisations, or just bypassed by the new powers-that-be. Simultaneously, the introduction of a far-reaching eugenic sterilisation legislation created attractive opportunities for medical experts. From May 1933 onwards, the association's leaders rushed to establish ties with Nazi officials to specify their position in the new system and secure their standing as eugenic experts.[167]

In the end, these efforts were at least partly successful. Under the leadership of Ernst Rüdin, the association retained its relative independence for two more years, before being turned into a subcommittee of the newly created Association of German Psychiatrists and Neurologists. With Rüdin as their new chair, mental hygienists moved considerably closer to the political and scientific centre of psychiatry in the 'Third Reich'. As Matthias Heinrich Göring and Carl Gustav Jung—whose General Medical Association for Psychotherapy (*Allgemeine Ärztliche Gesellschaft für Psychotherapie*) also struggled to secure its position under the changed political circumstances—wrote on the occasion of Robert Sommer's seventieth birthday in 1934, that while before the caesura of 1933 it had been 'a relatively small association, today it is of utmost importance'.[168] But this success came at a cost. Two of the most important characteristics of mental hygiene in the inter-war period—its multifaceted approach and its integration into an international network of related associations—were gradually lost as mental hygiene was reduced to a synonym for racial hygiene and became a foreign policy tool of the Nazi regime.

As the internal correspondence of the association shows, after January 1933, the board members plunged into hectic activity to establish contacts with the new authorities and secure and specify their position. As early as

14 March 1933, Hermann Simon had argued that, given the new situation, leading eugenicists like Ernst Rüdin or Hans Luxenburger would have to be added to the association's board.[169] By the end of May, the situation was already becoming clearer. In a circular letter to the members of the board, Robert Sommer urged that the DVPH immediately get in touch with the new government, or risk to be left out in the ongoing forcible coordination (*Gleichschaltung*) of racial hygiene.[170]

Hermann Simon took the lead. As he wrote in an extensive reply to Sommer, the DVPH had to 'get in with the new times', and had to act quickly, 'for the events are precipitating, and he who does not get on board in time, will remain standing on the platform after the express train has passed!' Mental hygienists had to intensify their propaganda efforts to remain visible for the political authorities. The remaining fact sheets on the prevention of hereditary mental illness, which had been printed in 1932, had to be distributed quickly, so that a new version, 'formulated in a more trenchant way, according to the new situation', could be published soon. And any reference to the voluntariness of eugenic sterilisation would have to be blackened out—a redaction that Simon had already and eagerly made in his own copies. Controversial as it was among mental hygienists in the late Weimar Republic, this question had now been answered by politics: 'Coercion or no coercion is a matter of the political state, not the physician's advice!'[171]

Furthermore, Simon argued, the association would have to connect with the new state institutions for public health education and racial hygiene and offer its services—something that he proactively did in a private letter to the Education Office for Population Policy and Racial Hygiene (*Aufklärungsamt für Bevölkerungspolitik und Rassenpflege*) on the very next day.[172] While these measures might help securing the association's position in the short run, in the long run, its forcible coordination into the system of Nazi organisations would be inevitable, and without being part of this system, formal contacts with government authorities and the allocation of state funding would become impossible. Again, Simon quickly tried to take matters in his own hand and had already requested to join the NSDAP in April 1933. As his request was still pending by June, he repeated his earlier proposal, 'to include a younger person, who is already long and firmly connected with the state of today', that is, Ernst Rüdin. Another way to combine the association's propaganda with attempt to link itself to the new powers-that-be, would be offering classes on mental hygiene in strategic locations: 'At this time, Munich would be the most opportune, because this is where the centre of the NSDAP is, and where it is easier to get in touch with its acting and influential bodies'. The flipside of these efforts was the reallocation of the association's resources from the international stage to national politics; a shift that Simon had already called for in the late 1920s, and again in 1933: 'Today, our *international relations* are less important than the national ones. I strictly warn against still using any significant amounts for their cultivation'.[173] As Simon wrote to Sommer, this also meant that a planned German publication of the proceedings of the Washington, DC congress could be shelved: 'Let's leave the Washington congress dead and buried. No one in Germany cares about it, now that we have to think and worry about other, more important things'.[174]

But while Hermann Simon in Gütersloh was trying to bring German mental hygiene in line with the new political situation, the future of the association was being decided in Berlin and Munich. As Hans Roemer notified the other board members on 25 June 1933, he had received a phone call from Ernst Rüdin, who had been appointed as a commissioner for the *Reich*'s racial hygiene activities.[175] Rüdin had requested to meet with executive director Roemer to discuss how the association could be integrated in the 'forthcoming racial hygiene activities'. Simon emphatically urged Roemer to meet with Rüdin as soon as possible: 'Now we have to hurry! And all personal emotions and sensitivities have to be put aside in favour of the goal ahead of us. The opportunity is offering itself to us, and we have to grasp it, for the sake of our higher duties'.[176]

A few days later, Robert Sommer, who had been the association's chair since 1925, resigned. Given Sommer's long-standing and public misgivings about the coercive eugenics favoured by the new authorities, a political reason for this decision seems likely; however, neither the internal correspondence of the association nor Sommer's own papers offer much to confirm or refute this interpretation.[177] In any case, the resignation was also a tactical move with an eye to the upcoming negotiations with Rüdin as representative of the Nazi state. As Simon pointed out, the vacancy of the chair could become a tactical gift to Rüdin: 'In fact, in the present situation, our association needs a strong liaison with Rüdin and his institute; and we can only win Rüdin over by offering him the *leading* position in the association'.[178] When Roemer met Rüdin in Munich on 3 July 1933, the latter was willing to accept the position—in addition to the chair of the German Society for Racial Hygiene, which he had recently been appointed to by the Ministry of the Interior. Although Rüdin confidentially assured Roemer that he was willing to maintain the independence of the German

Association for Mental Hygiene, at this point, mental hygiene had already inched closer towards racial hygiene.[179]

On 16 July 1933, the board members of the DVPH—Wilhelm Weygandt, Hans Roemer, Hermann Simon, Paul Nitsche, and the present and future chairs, Robert Sommer and Ernst Rüdin, respectively—met in Kassel to discuss the future of mental hygiene in the 'Third Reich'.[180] Rüdin arrived well-prepared—a few days earlier, Simon had already briefed him about the views of the other board members in a personal letter, in which he also distanced himself from the 'sensitivities' of some of his colleagues.[181] Moreover, Rüdin had not come with empty hands. As commissioner of the Ministry of the Interior, designated chair of the German Society for Racial Hygiene, and chair of the second working committee on racial hygiene of the scientific advisory council of the Ministry of the Interior, he was in a position to promise state resources for the activities of the German Association for Mental Hygiene, provided that they were used for eugenic propaganda. Rüdin's nomination was accepted unanimously, while Robert Sommer received a newly created, largely symbolic position of honorary chair.

Under their new leadership, mental hygienists could secure their connection to the state and improve their position in the psychiatric profession, as Rüdin personified the connected interests of the state and his profession like few others.[182] Rüdin added another item to his growing list of political and professional functions, but also gained a political asset. The association was supposed to serve as springboard for eugenic propaganda inside the psychiatric profession (as opposed to the German Society for Racial Hygiene and other bodies tasked with public propaganda). One of its next activities would be to conduct a seminar on racial hygiene for 'psychiatrists interested in questions of racial biology', planned to take place in October 1933 on the premises of Rüdin's German Research Institute for Psychiatry in Munich. The meeting in Kassel resulted in what Hermann Simon had persistently argued for in the last years.

Mental hygiene had left the individual patient behind and became indistinguishable from racial hygiene, while at the same time moving closer to the state than it had ever been before. However, different from what Hermann Simon had envisioned, this reorientation did not yet bring the separation of German mental hygiene from the international movement. Instead, the association was to continue its international activities, namely the preparations for the second international congress in Paris, then planned for 1935, as a foreign policy tool of the 'Third Reich' and as a means to legitimise German racial hygiene policies abroad. As the members of the board agreed, 'the international relations should continue to be maintained in the interest of the state, and in the interest of Germany, and should also be used to inform foreign countries about the development [of psychiatric eugenics] in Germany'.[183]

That this would not be an easy task was something that Hans Roemer found out two months later, when representatives of the European mental hygiene associations met in Rome in September 1933.[184] Roemer received a tepid reception:

> At the beginning of the meeting, [...] a certain reticence was clearly noticeable from the representatives of the other European organisations, most of which we already knew from Washington. My Hitler-badge [the NSDAP membership badge] received much attention.[185]

Roemer's paper on the role of the family in mental hygiene was well received, but the issue of Germany's eugenic policies led to controversy. Notably, it was one of the leading psychiatrists from fascist Italy, Sante de Sanctis (1862–1935), who most forcefully objected to the sterilisation of mental patients, while the Belgian Auguste Ley (1873–1956) and the Swiss André Repond came out in support.[186] As a publication of de Sanctis's statement was planned in the high-circulation *Corriere della Sera*, Roemer informed the German embassy about the course of the meeting. In the eyes of the German diplomats, de Sanctis's opposition was a tactical move in line with the Mussolini government's position, which rejected eugenics as not to antagonise the Apostolic See. The release of de Sanctis's statement to the press was to demonstrate publicly that Italian psychiatry would not follow the German lead. Eugenics were, however, not the only point of contention. The persecution of Jewish physicians had not gone unnoticed by mental hygienists in Europe and was the main reason Roemer's attempts to bring the next European meeting to Germany failed for now:

> For my incessant efforts to voice our invitation, doubts were repeatedly raised about the possibility to speak freely in Germany. [The Dutch psychiatrist K. H.] Boumann openly said that the treatment of Jewish colleagues ran contrary to the fulfilment of our wish. [Eugenio] Medea, who like Bond is Jewish, would personally have liked to come, especially as he, like some other participants of the conference, gratefully remembers his training in Germany. After the meeting of the European commission, [Auguste] Ley told me that

one should give some time to a meeting in Germany, as the treatment of the emigrants had upset many.[187]

In fact, it only took another five years for the European mental hygienists to overcome their reservations against Nazi Germany as a venue for their meetings, on which later more. Back in Germany in 1933, the main challenge was to define mental hygiene's role and position in the changed political situation. The outcome of the Kassel meeting was made public in the next issue of the *Zeitschrift für psychische Hygiene*.[188] To reflect its new orientation, the association renamed itself 'German Association for Mental Hygiene and Racial Hygiene', and a closer cooperation with the German Psychiatric Association was envisioned. Mental hygiene's new course found its clearest expression in a programmatic article appositely entitled 'The psychiatrist and the new time' in the following issue.[189] It was authored by Hermann Fritz Hoffmann (1891–1944), a psychiatric geneticist who previously had shown little interest in politics and who had just succeeded the recently retired Robert Sommer as chair of psychiatry in Giessen.[190] As Hoffmann argued, psychiatry had always been torn between two incompatible goals—on the one hand, psychiatrists had to care for their patients and treat them; on the other hand, their task was also to secure the welfare of the collective, which often meant to protect society from their own patients. The Nazi government, Hoffmann claimed, had solved this conflict:

> Of these conflicting approaches, in past times, the care for the individual welfare of the sick person had priority, and was often determinative; in the national-socialist state, the psychiatrist has not only the right, but also an obligation to primarily follow the interests of the community, and to integrate, if not to subordinate, the individual interest of the sick person to these. His helping hand should be guided by the ideals, which the new state embodies in our national community (*Volksgemeinschaft*), and to which every healthy member of our nation (*Volksgenosse*) has to bow. It is an insight and a principle of National Socialism that the individual is only rated by what his worth, his significance, and his achievements are for the whole of the nation.[191]

As the previous chapters have shown, psychiatrists concerned with the prophylactic possibilities of their discipline had contemplated this shift away from the sick individual for a long time, in particular in times of social and political crisis, as after the First World War and during the global economic crisis at the end of the 1920s. The sterilisation law that the Nazi state passed in July 1933 was a milestone in this shift. Hoffmann extensively commented on and legitimised the sterilisation law and discussed the diagnostic and practical details of its implementation—a recurring topic in psychiatric professional journals from 1933 onwards. As for many others, for Hoffmann the law was only a beginning: 'It is not only to serve practical measures, but it also wants to pursue an ideational goal, bringing the thought and the reflection of racial hygiene to our people'.[192] As he saw it, the next step would be to complete negative with positive eugenics: 'Who in the perspective of racial hygiene has the right to have children, in the national-socialist state has also the duty to have children'.

Over the following years, the association was, however, less concerned with Hoffmann's phantasies of national rebirth and eugenic breeding of racial elites, and more with providing the practical expertise for the racial hygiene policies of the 'Third Reich'. In 1934, the association organised a seminar on racial hygiene and hereditary biology. Conducted with the express authorisation and funding by the Ministry of the Interior and chaired by Ernst Rüdin, during the nine-day seminar in Munich, more than a hundred physicians from university clinics and asylums were briefed about the scientific basis and practical application of the sterilisation law.[193] The seminar lectures were quickly published in a volume of almost four hundred pages, the most comprehensive overview of Nazi Germany's racial hygiene policies by then.[194] While racial hygiene triumphed, the term 'mental hygiene' was side-tracked. Hans Roemer's opening address contained the only explicit mention of mental hygiene during the seminar.[195]

In 1933 already, the participants of the board meeting in Kassel had agreed that the continued existence of a German Association for Mental Hygiene and Racial Hygiene would only be temporary. In line with the forcible coordination (*Gleichschaltung*) of all parts of German society by the Nazi regime, the mental hygiene association was to be united with the German Psychiatric Association, as well as with the General Medical Association for Psychotherapy (*Allgemeine Ärztliche Gesellschaft für Psychotherapie*).[196] From the mental hygienists' perspective, the planned merger was neither a necessity-driven political decision, nor pre-emptive obedience, but promised the possibility of embedding their agenda more firmly in the psychiatric mainstream. Nonetheless, a resolution passed at the Kassel meeting stipulated that, even after the merger, mental hygienists would retain a certain degree of autonomy and some prerogatives, including the right to accept non-psychiatrists as members, to collects and administer their own member fees, to continue publishing their own journal, and to remain part of the international and European networks for mental hygiene.[197]

The merger eventually happened in early September 1935.[198] Different from what had been planned two years earlier, the mental hygienists did, however, not join the German Psychiatric Association. Instead, the association became a committee in the newly created Society of German Neurologists and Psychiatrists (*Gesellschaft deutscher Neurologen und Psychiater*, GDNP), which in turn was the result of the unification of the German Psychiatric Association and the Society of German Neurologists (*Gesellschaft deutscher Nervenärzte*) under the leadership of Ernst Rüdin.[199] Rüdin had been among the signatories of the 1933 resolution, and as head of the GDPN, he also had the political leverage with the state and the psychiatric profession to allow the committee for mental hygiene to retain some parts of its former independence inside the new association. Appointed by Rüdin, Hans Roemer would continue to manage the committee, which kept its own finances, its non-psychiatric members, as well as its journal. As Rüdin and Roemer wrote in the public announcement of the merger, the new set-up strongly increased their clout as mental hygienists would now speak 'on behalf of the representatives of German psychiatry and neurology'.[200]

In some regards at least, in 1935, mental hygiene's prospects in Germany seemed good. As part of the neurological and psychiatric professional organisation, it was closer to becoming integrated into the research and practice of both disciplines than it had before. Mental hygiene also had the long-standing support of the leading man in German psychiatry, Ernst Rüdin, who had been a member of the association since the late 1920s and its chair from 1933 to 1935, and who had already used the international movement for mental hygiene as a stage for his own eugenic agenda in Washington, DC in 1930. Rüdin was listed as a co-editor of the *Zeitschrift für psychische Hygiene* until its seventeenth and final volume in 1944 and continued to participate in the meetings of the international movement until 1939. At the same time, the prophylactic approach that was at the core of mental hygiene gained importance in German psychiatry. On the occasion of the unification of the psychiatric and neurological associations, Rüdin issued guideline for the role of both disciplines in the 'Third Reich': The principle that 'prevention is better than care' was to be applied to 'the whole body of our nation'.[201]

The direct consequences of German psychiatry's increasing occupation with the collective health of the nation are well known. Between 1934 and 1945, more than 400,000 people were forcibly sterilised on the grounds of the Law for the Prevention of Hereditarily Diseased Offspring; several thousand of them, mostly women, died due to complications during the procedure. With the beginning of the Second World War, Nazi racial hygiene entered a new phase, shifting its attention from future generations to the present. Between September 1939 and August 1941, more than 70,000 disabled people and mental patients were murdered in the 'euthanasia' programme later known as 'Aktion T4'. After the programme was discontinued, mainly due to protests by churchmen, decentralised killings continued, leading to an estimate of more than 200,000 additional deaths.[202] Although the improvement of the conditions for the mentally ill had been one the expressed goals of the mental hygiene movement in Germany in the second half of the 1920s, its propaganda for psychiatric eugenics and its participation in the scientific legitimisation of racial hygiene had helped to prepare the ground for 'euthanasia'. Some of its protagonists were directly connected to the mass killings.

Ernst Rüdin, as *Reichsleiter* of the German psychiatrists and neurologists and as the 'Third Reich's' most eminent eugenicist was a particularly prominent example for the manifold connections between mental hygiene and racial hygiene.[203] But other members of the association were even more directly involved. Paul Nitsche (1876–1948) had been a member of the extended board of the German Association for Mental Hygiene since the end of the 1920s and joined its five-member board after the resignation of Gustav Kolb in 1932. Nitsche actively participated in the development of killing methods; in February 1940, he became an expert for the 'T4' programme and medical director of the central office at the eponymous Tiergartenstraße 4 in Berlin. After the cancellation of 'T4', he participated in the '14f13' or 'prisoner euthanasia' programme.[204] Another 'T4' expert was Kurt Pohlisch (1893–1955), who joined the committee for mental hygiene and the editorial board of the *Zeitschrift für psychische Hygiene* in 1938.[205] The names of other psychiatrists involved in Nazi medical crimes appear in the periphery of the mental hygiene association, as participants at the conferences and as authors in the journal. This corresponds with the perpetrator profile identified by historians. Since its emergence, mental hygiene rallied not only zealous eugenicists, but also reform-minded psychiatrists who wanted to overcome psychiatry's notorious therapeutic nihilism with new treatment methods. Although the debates in the movement shifted back and forth between these two positions, they were not mutually exclusive, but inherently connected. The hope that some groups of patients could be successfully treated fuelled the view that caring for chronic and untreatable patients was a waste of resources at the expense of those that could be healed. Hence, for many perpetrators of Nazi 'euthanasia' the killings were not only a eugenic intervention for the health of the present and future body politic, but also part of an ambitious reform of psychiatry, clearing the overcrowded institutions from hopeless cases and freeing resources for a better and more efficient treatment of the remaining patients.[206]

Despite its close alignment with Nazi health policy, as an organised movement, mental hygiene played only a marginal role in German psychiatry after 1935. Instead of increasing the importance of mental hygiene, the rise of racial hygiene pushed other prophylactic approaches aside and reduced mental hygiene to another synonym for psychiatric eugenics—a process that already started at the beginning of the 1930s. This narrowing of mental hygiene was reflected in the contents of the *Zeitschrift für psychische Hygiene*, which continued to appear until 1944 on a steadily decreasing number of pages. Apart from an intensive debate about alcoholism and drug abuse at the end of the 1930s, psychiatric eugenics clearly dominated. The only area in which mental hygiene retained independent relevance was the representation of German psychiatry in the framework of the international movement, continuing until the beginning of the Second World War. And while Nazi Germany armed for war, its most prominent psychiatrists engaged in propaganda that played on international hopes for peace.

Peace for Our Time

From 19 to 25 July 1937, mental hygienists from forty-two countries gathered in Paris for the Second International Congress on Mental Hygiene.[207] The event, which had been in preparation since then, was supposed to continue what had started seven years earlier in Washington, DC. But the movement was not able to repeat this success. Due to rising political tensions in Europe, the ongoing Spanish Civil War, and dire economic conditions, the congress, which was initially planned for 1933, was postponed several times. Despite the *Exposition Internationale des Arts et Techniques dans la Vie Moderne* taking place in Paris at the same time, and several parallel medical congresses, no more than three to four hundred participated, most of them Europeans. This was only about one-tenth of the participants of the 1930 congress, and ten countries which had been present in

Washington, DC had not even sent delegations to Paris, the Soviet Union among them.[208]

The 1930 congress had stood under the sign of international cooperation, and the fault lines of the movement had been coated under a rhetoric of mutual progress. In 1937, long-standing political and scientific divides came to the fore. While many other topics such as institutional reform, education, and the creation of international standards in terminology were also discussed, the question of heredity and the German eugenics legislation clearly dominated the meeting. A heated debate following the lecture by Ernst Rüdin, head of the German delegation, about the role of eugenics in psychiatric prophylaxis dispelled the illusion of mental hygiene as a unified movement. Unsurprisingly, what Rüdin presented were the official positions of the 'Third Reich'; based on a detailed overview of the latest results of the genetic research by German psychiatrists, he argued that heredity played a key role in the development of mental illness, and, due to its dramatic impact on public health, compulsory measures were both necessary and legitimate.[209] At least two papers directly contradicted Rüdin. The Polish-French psychiatrist Françoise Minkowska (1882–1950) pointed out that the mechanisms and the role of heredity were still far too little understood as to allow for such drastic and irreversible measures.[210] The American Howard W. Taylor used the experience after almost three decades of compulsory sterilisation legislation in California to show that the actual effects of such measures on the prevalence of mental illnesses were much smaller than commonly assumed. Even if all feebleminded were to be sterilised, Taylor claimed, 'it would require 8,000 years to eliminate these defects'.[211]

German and American perceptions of the congress differed strongly. In the German mental hygienists' journal, Hans Aloys Schmitz (1899–1973), a child psychiatrist and colleague of Kurt Pohlisch in Bonn,[212] proudly reported that the audience had largely joined in with Rüdin's call for 'active eugenic measures' and that misunderstandings about the German legislation had quickly been cleared up. The American *Psychiatric Quarterly* by contrast stressed the 'unanimity of opinion in opposition to compulsory sterilization' and quoted extensively from Taylor's statement, which was almost completely absent from the German account.[213] Despite the growing rift in the movement, Rüdin still appealed to its internationalist and progressive ethos to serve the 'Third Reich's' international propaganda. With Nazi Germany preparing for war, its leading psychiatrist called for peace in the name of racial hygiene:

> Not loudly and solemnly enough, not too often, can eugenics raise its warning voice against the genocidal (*völkermörderisch*) scourge of war. Today, this is probably its most important role in the prophylaxis of mental disorders; because for victors and vanquished alike, war only leaves the mentally inferior to reproduce, while the carriers of mental balance and mental health are carried off by the thousands, even by the millions. [...] The coming age must serve the peaceful development and competition of racial hygiene among the cultured nations, and psychiatric eugenics in particular.[214]

This was not only Rüdin's voice speaking, but also that of the official propaganda of the 'Third Reich' targeted at an international audience. One way in which German science and politics served as 'resources for each other' after 1933 was that scientists contributed to the foreign policy of the Nazi state by internationally projecting the image of Germany as a scientific world power. Moreover, scientists in medicine and genetics lent their expertise to provide the legitimacy for the regime's racial hygiene policies—not only in Germany, but also abroad.[215] Consequently, the participation of German scientists at international conferences was closely monitored by the Nazi authorities. In 1934, a German Congress Centre (*Deutsche Kongress-Zentrale*) was established as a division of Josef Goebbels's Ministry for Propaganda and Public Education (*Ministerium für Propaganda und Volksaufklärung*); from 1936, the participation of German scientists at conferences abroad had to be authorised by the centre. Critical scientists were barred from travelling abroad, and those who were allowed to travel were required to organise in delegations with a delegation leader, meet with German officials at their destination, and had to submit reports of their activities. By 1938, the German Congress Centre issued a set of rules that scientific delegations had to follow when representing Germany on the international stage. In particular, members of the delegation were not to contradict each other on matters pertaining to Nazi ideology and had to present a unified front against every criticism of the official German position.[216] Against this backdrop, Rüdin's appeal to the pacifist ethos of the international movement for mental hygiene became its tragic epigraph.[217] Three years later, German troops invaded the venue of the Second International Congress on Mental Hygiene, and a third congress, planned for 1940 'somewhere in South America' never happened.[218]

However, before the war eventually severed the networks of the international movement for mental hygiene, two more large meetings took place in Europe; one in Munich in August 1938, and another Lugano in Switzerland in June 1939. Both were part of the European Assembly on Mental Hygiene (*Europäische Vereinigung für psychische Hygiene*), with previous meetings having been held in Rome (1933), Brussels (1935), and London (1936). In Munich as well as in Lugano, mental hygiene's role in fostering international understanding and the prevention of a looming war was solemnly and verbosely conjured—cynically in the first case, desperately in the second.

When representatives of the European mental hygiene associations gathered for their fifth meeting in Munich from 22 to 25 August 1938, the political situation had drastically deteriorated since the congress in Paris. Earlier in the same year, Nazi Germany had annexed Austria, and during the summer, German demands over the Sudetenland and threats against Czechoslovakia had become increasingly aggressive. By August, Europe was on the brink of war. Troops were being mobilised, and diplomatic efforts to mitigate the crisis remained without result. Less than three weeks before the infamous Munich Agreement, Ernst Rüdin opened the V. European Assembly on Mental Hygiene in the same city and welcomed delegates from abroad, representatives of the state, the city of Munich, the Wehrmacht and the party with his own version of 'peace for our time'.[219] This kind of international congress, he claimed, would foster both professional and private exchange, and thus contribute to the mutual understanding of nations: 'May the Munich Conference on Mental Hygiene not only lead to a productive scientific discussion of current problems, but also to a personal rapprochement of its participants and to a peaceful understanding of the nations to which we belong!'[220] That this statement was in line with Germany's propaganda was also corroborated by a declaration of loyalty (*Ergebenheitstelegramm*) cabled to Adolf Hitler on the same day:

> The participants of the V. European delegate conference on mental hygiene assembled in Munich and the representatives of 11 European nations present their respectful compliments to the Führer and Reich Chancellor. The conference not only wants to serve current and scientific discussions, but also the peaceful political and personal understanding among the nations of Europe. Rüdin.[221]

More than a hundred participants had come to the conference, which took place in the lecture hall of the psychiatric and neurological clinic of the

University of Munich. Although the political situation was fraught, twenty-eight foreigners were among them—not counting the Austrians, who now were listed as representatives from the German *Ostmark*. Most of the participants were mental health-care professionals, but the state authorities also showed considerable interest. Both the Ministry of the Interior and the *Reich* health office had sent their delegates, and so had the health administrations of several federal states, the Wehrmacht, and the Nazi party.[222] This was a reflection of the penetration of most aspects of science and society by the Nazi state, but it also showed the relevance that the 'Third Reich' attributed both to the eugenic brand of mental hygiene represented by Rüdin and to the international representation of German science. Herbert Linden (1899–1945), delegate of the Ministry of the Interior, stated on behalf of Minister Wilhelm Frick (1877–1946): 'The German government gives utmost attention to the efforts of mental hygiene. In these nerve-racking times, the mental health of the population must be particularly cared for'.[223] As Linden, who soon would become one of the managers of the 'euthanasia' programme, believed, mental hygiene fit in seamlessly with Nazi public health policy, which—from 'strength through joy' to racial hygiene—was aimed at 'maintaining the health of the productive'.[224]

The Munich conference dealt with three topics, eugenics, drug abuse, and occupational therapy. Unsurprisingly, eugenics were the primary focus, with the Swiss psychiatrist and psychotherapist Walter Morgenthaler and Ernst Rüdin discussing 'marriage prophylaxis and mental hygiene'.[225] Morgenthaler advocated the introduction of a variety of measures to promote marriages that would produce healthy offspring, including marriage counselling and health certificates. Notably, he was especially concerned about how eugenics policies might unintendedly affect gender relations on an evolutionary scale. By increasing the competition on the matrimonial market, eugenic policies would create a situation in which determined and energetic women would have an advantage. Morgenthaler pondered: 'If this kind of selection, which directly breeds a type of strong and reckless woman, is for the good of the whole nation is questionable'.[226]

While Morgenthaler's lecture was mostly theoretical, Rüdin directly referred to existing German eugenic legislation, namely the Law for the Protection of the Hereditary Health of the German People (*Gesetz zum Schutze der Erbgesundheit des deutschen Volkes*, 18 October 1935) barring individuals with a number of purportedly hereditary diseases from marriage. Rüdin repeated one of the main ideologemes of Nazism—'the common interest precedes the self-interest'—and maintained that decisions about marriage and procreation had to be subordinated to the collective health of the nation. However, as specific guidelines were concerned, the 'Third Reich's' eminent geneticist took a probing stance. With clear scientific indications not yet available, eugenic counselling for couples was still to be left to the discretion of individual physicians. Rüdin's moderation was not just an attempt to tone down his views in front of an international audience. From a eugenic perspective, the 1933 Law for the Prevention of Hereditarily Diseased Offspring had already created the possibility to remove carriers of hereditary illnesses from the nation's genetic pool; and while this law targeted individuals with diseases that were relatively easy to recognise, the complementary marriage law was only relevant in cases that fell below a certain diagnostic threshold or in which the hereditary defect was latent in the present generation.

But even as eugenics dominated mental hygiene in Germany, other issues continued to occupy mental hygienists internationally. The second panel of the meeting was devoted to a topic that was gaining in relevance.[227] As L. Stanojewitsch from Belgrade pointed out, alcoholism had become less prevalent than it had been before the First World War, but a new challenge to public health was emerging in the form of various drugs and intoxicants. While physicians already had recognised the problem, there was no coherent policy and legislation yet. This new phenomenon was a side effect of the rise and diversification of a chemical industry in the first third of the twentieth century; but medicine itself was also part of the equation. Unlike alcoholism, against which psychiatrists had campaigned for decades by then, new forms of drug abuse used substances introduced as pharmaceuticals, which were often provided by physicians and pharmacists. Statements from delegates of various countries showed that many European states faced similar problems, but in Nazi Germany the topic could not be separated from racial ideology. The German delegates who lectured about the prevention of drug abuse, the aforementioned Kurt Pohlisch and his protégé Friedrich Panse (1899–1973) both were zealous adherents of racial hygiene and would become experts in the 'T4' programme two years later.[228] For Pohlisch, the drug problem was rooted in biology, as those who became addicted were usually hereditarily defective 'psychopaths'. Moreover, he claimed, the use of different drugs by different nations corroborated the idea of racial differences; in particular believed, the fact that in European countries Jews were far more likely to be morphine addicts than alcoholics was proof of their distinct racial biology.[229]

The third panel of the Munich meeting revisited an older topic—occupational therapy. In mental hygiene discourse since the late 1920s, occupational therapy had lost some of its momentum as a form of reform psychiatry and had been almost entirely side-tracked by eugenics. In everyday asylum life, it was still a common form of treatment, although the relative number of patients who were occupied dropped as cuts in the funding of the asylum system reduced the available resources and the ratio of nurses per patients. At the same time, however, the economic crisis also produced incentives to exploit the workforce of the patient population in agriculture and for the maintenance of the institution. Research in the history of occupational therapy is still fragmentary and has in many cases focused only on individual institutions. Nevertheless, recent studies indicate that for occupational therapy, the year 1933 was no clear-cut caesura and that there was no sudden shift from a 'good', therapeutic to a 'bad', exploitative use of work in the asylum.[230] As I have discussed in more detail earlier in this chapter, with its specific concept of work, occupational therapy could transition seamlessly from the Weimar welfare state to the Nazi's utilitarian understanding of health care. In his writings and his correspondence, Hermann Simon had already carried out this transition long before 1933. The increasing separation of patients according to their ability or perceived willingness to work and the retraction of resources from untreatable patients had already been an integral part of the theory and practice of occupational therapy before 1933. The economic crisis and Nazi health policy amplified these tendencies, but it was only with 'euthanasia' that this rationale reached a deadly conclusion.[231]

There were two reasons why occupational therapy, after a period of absence from mental hygiene discourse in Germany, reappeared in 1938. First, it was a matter of national prestige and part of the propagandist function of the conference. Since the mid-1920s, occupational therapy had received considerable international attention, and Hermann Simon's Gütersloh clinic had become somewhat of a pilgrimage site for reform-minded asylum psychiatrists from abroad. Although it was widely adopted in many countries, it was still perceived as a genuinely German invention, and therefore, a discussion about the advances and accomplishments of occupational therapy was a possibility to showcase German psychiatry's therapeutic achievements.

Second, the Munich conference also coincided with a generational change in the history of occupational therapy, marking the end of Hermann Simon's career, and the rise of Carl Schneider (1891–1946) as main theorist of psychiatric therapy.[232] Both men were present at the conference and participated in the discussion about occupational therapy. Simon, seventy-one years old at this time, had already retired in 1934. While his relation with the Nazi authorities was uneasy, he did not depart from his markedly social-Darwinist views about occupational therapy and the importance of work for society.[233] In 1938, Simon briefly returned for a number of professional meetings to draw a resume of his activities in the previous decades.[234] At the same time, his younger colleague Schneider was preparing his seminal textbook on the 'treatment and prevention of mental disorders' (*Behandlung und Verhütung der Geisteskrankheiten*) that would be published in the following year.[235] While previous psychiatric textbooks had focused on diagnosis, Schneider shifted the focus towards therapy; his book was the first comprehensive and systematic summary of the range of new therapeutic methods available to psychiatrists on the eve of the Second World War.[236] Largely based on Schneider's own experiences at the university clinic of Heidelberg, it was a characteristic expression of therapeutic optimism at the end of the 1930s, relying equally on eugenics, a range of different shock treatments, and the use of occupational therapy. Although the title promised a textbook on 'treatment and prevention', the focus clearly was on treatment. Schneider occasionally used the term 'mental hygiene' but his concept of preventive psychiatric was largely limited to eugenics, and to some specialised care for hereditarily defect borderline cases.[237] Other aspects of mental hygiene, Schneider claimed, had been realised as part of the 'national socialist regeneration of Germany', which had improved the physical and mental health of the people and marked a new phase in the fight against alcohol, syphilis, and morphine addiction:

> The importance for mental hygiene of the many truly socialist institutions of the Third Reich, of the N.S. organisation Strength through Joy, of physical exercise, of education in various formations, of health guidance in the Hitler Youth and of the public health guidance in general with its care for all working Germans, cannot be overstated.[238]

While his concept of occupational therapy was clearly influenced by Simon, Schneider went beyond the model provided by his older colleague in two ways. On the one hand, his vision of psychiatric reform was far more comprehensive and systematic; to Schneider, occupational therapy was the 'foundation' of an integrated system of mental care.[239] On the other hand, he also extended the use of occupational therapy from chronic patients in the asylum, for whom Simon had originally devised his method, to acute cases in the university clinic. But this was not the only way in which Schneider surpassed Simon. The dialectic of 'healing and annihilation' was already spelled out in Simon's writings, but it was Schneider who proceeded to action. Schneider advocated the killing of untreatable patients as a last resort and complementary part of psychiatry's therapeutic reorientation; as an expert in the 'T4' programme, he became directly involved in the murder of psychiatric patients after 1940. As a keen scientist, Schneider used the exceptional situation during the war and the 'euthanasia' programme to conduct research on the brains of dissected victims. On Schneider's behest, numerous mentally disabled children were sent to the Eichberg asylum, where they were murdered so that their brains could be used for his research.[240]

Little more than a year before Nazi Germany began its attacks on Poland and on the lives of the mentally ill, the Munich conference conveyed an illusion of normalcy. Against the backdrop of rising political tensions and German psychiatry's gradual radicalisation, the participants of the V. European Assembly on Mental Hygiene enjoyed a close-packed social programme. On Monday, they dined in the ceremonial hall of the old city hall, and on the following day received a reception by the *Reich* government in a lavish lake house in Munich's English Garden. There, the foreign guests were greeted on behalf of the Minister of the Interior Wilhelm Frick and his head of department Arthur Gütt (1891–1949) by undersecretary (*Ministerialdirigent*) Fritz Cropp (1887–1984).[241] The personal connection between mental hygiene and Nazi Germany's racial hygiene policies was close. Arthur Gütt was the main responsible for the Law for the Prevention of Hereditarily Diseased Offspring, while Fritz Cropp—together with his subordinate Herbert Linden, who had held the welcome address—soon became directly involved in the organisation and administration of 'T4'. On Thursday, 25 August 1938, the participants of the conference visited the mental institution at Eglfing-Haar in the vicinity of Munich. In the following years, about two thousand patients were transferred from there to the killing centres of the 'euthanasia' programme; later, the asylum itself became the site of numerous killings.[242]

At the time of the conference, these atrocities of Nazi psychiatry still lay in a not-so-far future, but state-sanctioned eugenic policies were already in place and the radicalisation of racial hygiene was conspicuous in many statements of the German delegates. Nevertheless, while critics of eugenics, political opponents of the 'Third Reich', and Jewish mental hygienists would have stayed away from the event, the delegates of the European mental hygiene associations played along. In the conference proceedings published in Germany, no public criticism of the Nazi's medical and racial policies was recorded. Instead, Eugenio Medea (1873–1967), delegate from fascist Italy, spoke on behalf of the European associations when he lauded 'German psychiatry, the city of Munich, and the rise of the Third Reich with words of enthusiasm'.[243]

Comprehénsion Mutuelle

The next European assembly, held in Lugano in the south of Switzerland from 4 to 6 June 1939, was the last meeting of the international movement for mental hygiene before the Second World War. It also was an event of a different kind. Whereas the Munich conference in 1938 had been a propaganda event by and for the 'Third Reich', in the following year the Swiss hosts tried to rekindle mental hygiene's cosmopolitan and utopian spirit—with sobering results. For the first time in the history of the European assemblies, a single topic had been set as an overarching theme for the whole conference, and in the context of the summer of 1939 the choice of topic—*comprehénsion mutuelle*, 'mutual understanding'—could hardly have been any more political. The aim of the conference was to create a sort of mutual understanding not only among the mental hygienists from different European countries, but also among their nations. There was something quixotic about this attempt to stop a war that by then already seemed unavoidable with a meeting of psychiatrists. Remembering the conference in Lugano, the Swiss psychiatrist Max Müller (1894–1980) later wrote:

> The mood was particularly sombre at a conference that [André] Repond as president of the Swiss Committee for Mental Hygiene convened in Lugano after the meeting of the SGP [*Schweizer Gesellschaft für Psychiatrie*, Swiss Psychiatric Association] in June 1939. It was supposed be international, and was to deal with a single topic, comprehénsion mutuelle! Did Repond really believe that a meeting and an understanding of psychiatrists from different countries could still change anything about what was unavoidably coming to us? I do not think this can be ruled out. There were true believers in progress like him, [Walter] Morgenthaler, [Oscar] Forel, and others more, who seriously believed that 'mental hygiene' only had to be sufficiently organised and supported internationally in order to change great politics and the world in general.[244]

Switzerland was the right place for such a meeting. A proud tradition of neutrality had kept the country out of the First World War, and in the decades since, it had become the home of many institutions of the League of Nations. By then, the rise of fascism and the escalating political tensions in Europe had revealed the League's structural deficiencies and its inability to secure a peaceful post-war order. Nevertheless, in 1939 the organisers of the mental hygiene assembly could still appeal to a lofty vision of enemy nations meeting on neutral ground to peacefully resolve their differences that seemed more plausible in Switzerland than it would have elsewhere. The other reason the theme of mutual understanding was particularly well-set against the panorama of the Swiss Alps was that, as a multi-language society, the Swiss had long-standing experience with such problems in everyday life. Among the organisers of the conference, there may well have been some hope that this spirit of understanding—together with the Swiss confederates' proverbial sense of liberty, equality, and civic duties—would also rub off on their international visitors. In his Italian welcome address, the socialist state counsellor (*conseiller d'état*) of the canton of Ticino, Gugliemo Canevascini (1886–1965), connected the notion of mutual understanding to the 'immortal and transboundary' principles of the Swiss polity, which would have to become 'the basis of tomorrow's Europe'.[245] Inspired by these principles, mental hygiene would become a utopian idea leading the way through troubled times:

> Certainly, to speak of mutual understanding, of prophylaxis and of cure, while in the world rivalry, discord, and hate prevail, while the nations are concentrating their efforts and squandering their wealth on weapons and preparations for war, might seem anachronistic and perhaps tragically ironic.
>
> But you are men of safe faith, who look at the future. – And you think like I do, that mental hygiene will also take hold with the men leading the nations, that reason will still triumph, and that the nations, after the hardships that have been suffered, will come to understand each other and finally establish the basis for a solid and fruitful collaboration.[246]

This was an emphatic utopianism that had completely vanished from the German debates on mental hygiene after the First International Congress in Washington, DC back in 1930. It had not survived the economic crisis, the rise of the Nazis, and the death of Robert Sommer as its most dedicated voice in 1937. In Switzerland, by contrast, the roots of this kind of psycho-utopianism were older and more resilient. Decades before the emergence of an international movement for mental hygiene, Auguste Forel had blended individual psychiatric prophylaxis, radical eugenics, pacifism, cosmopolitanism, and socialist ideas into a psycho-political ideology of his own.

The group of men that dominated the Swiss Committee for Mental Hygiene in the inter-war period—André Repond, Walter Morgenthaler, Hans W. Maier, and Auguste Forel's son Oscar Forel—did not subscribe to the same socialist agenda, but remained loyal to the central utopian moments of Forel's thought—including, but not limited to, eugenics.[247] Their understanding of psychiatry and mental hygiene was much broader than that of most of their German colleagues. In particular, and as the programme of the Lugano conference shows, Swiss mental hygienists were far more inclined to include psychoanalysts in their meetings, and psychoanalytic ideas into their own writings. This may have been a result of their scientific upbringing. Repond, Morgenthaler, and Maier had been students of Eugen Bleuler at the Burghölzli hospital in Zurich, where they had seen that psychoanalysis and mainstream psychiatry were not mutually exclusive.[248] Notably, their efforts to move beyond the traditional disciplinary boundaries of psychiatry were not limited to mental hygiene and predated the emergence of the movement in the German-speaking countries. Together with Erwin Stransky and Karl Jaspers, Maier and Repond had been among the original members of the editorial board of Morgenthaler's 'Studies in applied psychiatry' (*Arbeiten zur angewandten Psychiatrie*) in the early 1920s, while Oscar Forel later joined the editorial board for the final instalment in 1941.

The idea that mental hygiene could be far more than only the prevention of mental illness on an individual and collective scale was particularly pronounced in the Swiss branch of the movement well before the 1939 conference. For the Swiss committee's president André Repond, mental hygiene went far beyond a mundane programme for the reform of psychiatric institutions. He was convinced that, as a holistic reform project, mental hygiene would not only change mental health care, but could remake society at large. Like many protagonists of the mental hygiene movement in the United States, Repond adhered to an optimistic interpretation of psychoanalysis, believing that the irrational and atavistic impulses in the individual psyche could be kept in check when the underlying dynamics were rationally understood. Moreover, as the same mechanisms were also to be found in collective psychology, mental hygienists' knowledge about the human soul and their expertise in the prevention of mental illness could become a remedy for political ills. This kind of psycho-political intervention, Repond believed, was urgently needed in this time of crisis. Echoing the psychiatric diagnoses of the immediate post-war period of the First World War, he wrote as early as 1931:

> In Europe right now, we are witnessing the violent irruption of archaic, irrational forces into politics. The relations among the nations are ridden by aggressive tendencies. Anxious reticence, the wish for oppression, for the suppression of others, the politics of the great European nations today amount to nothing more than that. Collective hysteria, an anxiety neurosis; that is what the diagnosis of current European politics would have to be.
>
> The question is how psychology, in a way that is elucidating and mitigating, can intervene in this disastrous play of irrational powers. For without doubt, it is about the subsistence or the destruction of civilisation.[249]

Repond's view of politics was based on the psychoanalytic re-reading of Gustave Le Bon's crowd psychology in Sigmund Freud's 1921 *Group Psychology and the Analysis of the Ego*.[250] Like many of his colleagues, he was particularly concerned with the relation of the masses and their charismatic leaders, which he considered an extension of individual psychology. While members of the mass recognised in the leader a father-figure with which they could identify, the leaders themselves were often driven 'by the unhealed wounds of childhood' or by the need to 'finally act out the revolt against their father that they never dared'.[251] Where Repond departed from Freud was that for him, psychology could not only be projected from the individual and the family to society and politics in terms of diagnosis, but also in terms of therapy. For him, mental hygiene's political role was to educate the masses about the psychological dynamics of politics, enabling them to see through the 'empty phrases' of demagogues, and to choose better leaders. The underlying utopian vision was one of rational politics, purged from dangerous irrational, emotional, and atavistic impulses. Psychology was to be used to exorcise emotions from politics—or, as some might say, the political from politics.

Eight years later, the political situation in Europe had not improved. The rise of the Nazis in Germany had given the issue of charismatic leaders in politics a whole new relevance, and the kind of psycho-educative intervention on the part of mental hygiene envisioned by André Repond seemed more urgent now than ever. The choice of *compréhension mutuelle* as the overarching theme of the Lugano conference was a direct expression of this sense of mission, and the Swiss setting added to the symbolism. However, while Gugliemo Canevascini as a socialist state official could explicitly mention the political implications of the theme, this was more problematic for some of the international participants. Throughout the conference, they often avoided straight-forward political implications of mutual understanding, framing in more general terms and different disciplinary contexts. Of course, the inherent broadness and elusiveness of the theme was a necessary condition for the conference to even take place under the given political circumstances. At the same time, this broad and abstract topic also shifted mental hygiene away from intra- and extramural clinical psychiatry, touching on questions of philosophy, sociology, and anthropology instead.

In the case of Ernst Kretschmer's (1888–1964) markedly clinical lecture about 'constitutional retardation and the problem of social contacts', elusiveness became deliberate avoidance. Only at the very end did the political context briefly appear, when Kretschmer identified 'dramatic verve, protests, and defiant rebellion against what is awe-inspiring, lasting, established, and authoritative' in adult life as residues of infantile retardation; but this was a conservative staple rather than Nazi ideology.[252] The second lecture given by a German is more difficult to interpret. The psychotherapist Hans von Hattingberg (1879–1944) spoke about the 'role of the polar psychological types in understanding'; starting from Goethe and Schiller, it was a philosophical and psychological reflection on the characteristics of 'introverted' and 'extroverted' personality types as described by Carl Jung in 1921.[253] Following lengthy and relatively abstract deliberations, the lecture took a surprising turn for the political when Hattingberg used the example of Jacques Rivière's (1886–1925) *Les Allemands* ('The Germans') to illustrate his ideas.[254] In this 1919 book, the French writer Rivière had recounted his experiences as a prisoner of war during the First World War and his insights into the German national character that he gained during this time. In 1939, this obviously was a politically charged topic at an international conference. As Hattingberg saw it, Rivière's description of the Germans confirmed his own view that the long-standing conflict between France and Germany was a conflict between introvert and extrovert national characters. The lecture ended on a somewhat enigmatic note with Hattingberg quoting Rivière's statement that the extrovert Germans had started the First World War to be recognised and understood by the introvert French, and to realise their own identity through action.[255] It remains unclear whether this was a psychological essentialisation of the

Franco-German 'hereditary enmity', a defence of the German position, or if Hattingberg tried to speak from a position of equidistance.

As telling as the content of the lectures is who gave them. Ernst Kretschmer and Hans von Hattingberg did not represent the biologistic paradigm of racial hygiene advocated by Ernst Rüdin and the likes, who had dominated the German branch of the mental hygiene movement for a decade by then. Instead, both had strong connections to the emerging field of psychotherapy; an approach that, despite Robert Sommer's efforts to integrate it in the mid-1920s, never became a part of mental hygiene in Germany. Kretschmer was as a co-founder and, from 1930 to his resignation in 1933, president of the General Medical Society for Psychotherapy.[256] Hattingberg was an eclectic therapist, co-founder of the German General Medical Society for Psychotherapy in 1933, and from 1939 head of the research department of the German Institute for Psychological Research and Psychotherapy, also known as the 'Göring-Institute'.[257]

Kretschmer and Hattingberg's relations with the authorities of the 'Third Reich' were complicated. In both cases, historians have grappled with the details of their biographies and political views and have reached no unequivocal conclusions. As a detailed discussion would go far beyond the scope of this study, some brief remarks will have to suffice. On the one hand, both men were certainly no dissidents—they would not have been allowed to travel to Switzerland in the first place if the authorities would have had any serious doubts about their political loyalties. In fact, Kretschmer and Hattingberg were well-established members of the medical and scientific community of the 'Third Reich', involved in the eugenic policies or in the attempts to create a new, specifically German form of psychotherapy (*Neue Deutsche Seelenheilkunde*), respectively. They used the possibilities offered by the political circumstances to their advantage, and occasionally included elements of the official ideology in their writings. On the other hand, they were no Nazi zealots, and neither of them joined the party. In the case of Hattingberg, a certain reticence and distance towards the regime can be discerned from his private correspondence, but there is no evidence of public opposition.[258] Kretschmer, by contrast, had a public reputation for being critical of the Nazis. In June 1933, he resigned from his position as president of the psychotherapists' association, a move that historians have read as a result of a political decision. In the next years, his relation with Nazi colleagues and authorities remained fraught, but the situation never escalated and Kretschmer retained his scientific position and prestige.[259] What was important in Lugano in 1939, was that both Hattingberg and Kretschmer could pass as German mental hygienists who were not too closely affiliated with the Nazi state and its racial hygiene policies. This is what made them acceptable to other participants of the conference, but from the Nazi regime's point of view, this was also what made them suitable scientific ambassadors of Germany for this specific setting.

But the prominent role of Kretschmer and Hattingberg also hints to another aspect of the Lugano conference. *Compréhension mutuelle* could not only mean the understanding and rapprochement among hostile nations and their psychiatric representatives through mental hygiene, it could also refer to a mutual understanding inside and among the different psy-ences. The mental hygiene movement was not been an exclusively psychiatric movement; from the beginning on, the idea of preventing mental illness and improving mental health care beyond the clinic and the asylum not only appealed to psychiatrists working in these institutions, but also to members of other emerging disciplines—psychotherapists of different schools, psychologists, pedagogues, social workers, and others more. However, while it was generally agreed that these professions had a role to play in mental hygiene, the movement was clearly dominated by the psychiatrists, a tendency reinforced by the rise of eugenics and biologistic approaches.[260] In Germany in particular, psychotherapists had increasingly been pushed to the margins of the movement. For German psychiatrists like Ernst Rüdin or Carl Schneider, eugenic sterilisation was the only effective form of mental hygiene, and all other approaches were merely subsidiary activities that would gradually become irrelevant as eugenics proceeded.[261]

In Switzerland by the end of the 1930s, mental hygiene was seen in much broader terms. The reason was not that the local branch of the movement was in other hands; like elsewhere, its leaders were mostly psychiatrists with a firm belief in eugenics. There was, however, a strong local tradition of a psychiatric involvement with psychotherapeutic and psychoanalytic approaches and ideas that had already begun before the First World War, and still shaped the outlook of prominent Swiss psychiatrists a generation later. At the same time, this openness towards other approaches also went hand in hand with a much broader understanding of the philosophical, sociological, and anthropological implications of mental hygiene. Although he was himself an asylum director, the president of the Swiss national committee André Repond was the most vocal advocate of this holistic concept of mental hygiene. In Washington, DC in 1930 already, Repond had argued that mental hygiene had to overcome the boundaries of clinical psychiatry and even of medicine in general.[262] By integrating psychoanalytic perspectives, mental hygiene could develop into a psycho-social practice for the sick and healthy alike and would no longer be limited to the treatment of mental patients and neurotics. To do so, Repond believed, mental hygiene had to develop a philosophy of its own; and while he remained vague about the details of this philosophy, he was certain that its social and cultural ambit would soon lead to a conflict with the churches and other social authorities with similarly encompassing claims. In a wording strongly reminding of Erwin Stransky's post-war writings about 'applied psychiatry', Repond claimed that as a kind of secular religion, mental hygiene would eventually pave the way for a 'complete regeneration of the human mind', and mental hygienists would become priest-like 'experts of the human mind'.[263]

Repond's vision of mental hygiene went beyond social medicine, it was psycho-utopianism at its best. His ideas, however, emerged at an inherent fault line of mental hygiene that was directly connected to medical questions. As Robert Sommer had recognised almost four decades earlier, the prevention of mental illness was necessarily based on a theory of its causation. Mental hygiene was torn between the two poles between which psychiatry has oscillated throughout its history. The rift between biological and psycho-social explanations of mental illness went through the mental hygiene movement, and while some of its protagonists based their scientific self-understanding on the laboratory, biology, and the sciences, others tended towards psychological interpretation, hermeneutics, and the humanities and social sciences.[264] Far-reaching socio-medical and utopian ideas were not exclusive to either side, but took different shapes with psycho-pedagogical projects on the one side, and eugenic bio-politics on the other.

In the years before the Second World War, Swiss mental hygienists' penchant for psycho-social and pedagogical utopianism was reinforced by the arrival of the German émigré Heinrich Meng (1887–1972). Meng, a psychiatrist and psychoanalyst who had been a co-founder and member of the short-lived Frankfurt Psychoanalytic Institute (*Frankfurter Psychoanalytisches Institut*) in 1929, emigrated from Germany to Basel in 1933 after the Nazis had forcibly closed the institute, demolished its library, and publicly burned the books.[265] Unlike many other German emigrants, he was welcomed with open arms in Switzerland—not least by André Repond, who recognised him as a 'comrade-in-arms' (*Kampfgefährte*).[266] In fact, although Meng's career, with the exception of his training analysis with Paul Federn in Vienna in 1921, had been limited to Germany, he was part of the same school as the Swiss mental hygienists. During his time as a student in Freiburg in the first decade of the century, Meng had made the acquaintance of Auguste Forel and had been profoundly impressed by his demeanour and his ideas. 'Social hygiene, mental hygiene, the education of the people, socialism, and pacifism were the main topics of our conversations', he later remembered in his autobiography, omitting Forel's radical views about eugenics and race.[267] Already as a student, Meng had tried to put the prophylactic ideas adopted from Forel into practice; in Freiburg in 1909, he participated in the creation of a local lodge of Forel's teetotal 'Good Templars'.[268]

Before 1933, Heinrich Meng was not affiliated with the mental hygiene movement, and German mental hygienists had shown little interest in his attempts to put psychoanalysis in the service of public health. Nevertheless, psychiatric prophylaxis had been a crucial part of his work. Together with Paul Federn, he published a popular guide to psychoanalysis in 1926 (*Das psychoanalytische Volksbuch*). Under the heading 'hygiene', the book contained a whole nine chapters about the various uses of psychoanalysis for the prevention of mental disorders in adolescence and adult life.[269] At the time of its publication, it was not only the first attempt to popularise psychoanalysis through an explanation in laypeople's terms, but also the most systematic and ambitious exploration of its potentials in social medicine and public health. Then already, Meng was particularly concerned with the application of psychoanalytic concepts and methods in pedagogy, and this educational approach became the pivotal element of his professional activities in the decades to follow.

It was only after his arrival in Switzerland that Meng joined the movement for mental hygiene. Not licensed to work as a physician, his activities and publications during his first years in Basel were mostly devoted to pedagogical topics, and it was through pedagogy, not through medicine, that he found his way to mental hygiene. In 1936, a group of teachers and educators proposed the introduction of mental hygiene as a subject in teacher training and the creation of a corresponding teaching position for Meng. However, as the medical faculty considered mental hygiene a part of its domain and Meng was trained as a physician, the lectureship was eventually associated with the medical school in 1937 as the first position of its kind at a European university. Despite this disciplinary detour, he explicitly considered himself part of the international movement for mental hygiene, but took his inspirations from the United States rather than from Germany, which had as much to do with German mental hygienists' biologistic approach as with the general political situation.[270] In the following years, Meng became one of the central figures of the movement in Switzerland, and the views that he laid out in his lectures and publications decisively shaped the local understanding of mental hygiene during and after the Second World War.[271]

Although his position as lecturer was attached to the medical faculty, Meng's scope remained much broader. Psychoanalysis, psychotherapy, and pedagogy were the points of departure, but his understanding of mental hygiene drew on 'biology, psychopathology, sociology, anthropology, genetics, law, and philosophy', and his lectures attracted students and auditors from a similar range of disciplines.[272] With this encompassing scope and against the backdrop of what he saw as a 'world in upheaval', Meng's concept of mental hygiene unavoidably reached far into the social and political sphere, but the political aspects often had to be toned down: 'In the first lecture, no names of personalities who in 1937/38 played a destructive role in world-history were named'.[273] With political tensions building in Europe, foreigners in neutral Switzerland were eyed with suspicion, and Meng, who sympathised with socialism, had to answer to accusations of being a Soviet spy operating a secret transmitter, as well as a Nazi in disguise.[274] Explicitly political statements and political activities of foreigners were hardly tolerated, but this did not mean that Meng did not touch on the psycho-politics of mental hygiene. In particular, he taught a seminar on 'utopia from Plato to Freud', arguing that a utopian concept of politics had to go beyond purely rational aspects and had to include the unconscious.[275]

For a German émigré like Meng, the conference in Lugano must have been an emotional event. On the one hand, the overarching idea of mutual understanding clearly was compatible with his own psycho-political understanding of mental hygiene, on the other hand however, the meeting also involved a confrontation with representatives of the Nazi regime that had forced him to emigrate six years earlier. This was not necessarily the case with Kretschmer and Hattingberg, who had kept a certain distance from politics, but the Swiss-German Ernst Rüdin and Hermann Hoffmann, who were also present at the conference, were loyal adherents of the Nazi state. Together with his precarious position as a foreigner in Switzerland, these tensions at the conference may have been one reason why Meng refrained from openly discussing the political aspects of *compréhension mutuelle*. Instead, he asked about the psychological and pedagogical methods to 'prompt someone else to become an understanding human being, who lives in an active social contact with his fellow human beings'.[276] This was far away from the foreign policy aspects of politics, but entailed the very political question of how the very foundation of life in society had to be arranged. As Meng believed, the upbringing of social individuals was based on two preconditions—an education that fostered the development of a stable ego able of adapting to dynamically changing realities, and a society 'structured in a way that allows for a healthy rapport between individuals'. Meng's perspective was distinctly Freudian, and he argued that a successful form of pedagogy had to find ways to productively integrate both 'eros and aggression'.[277] However, he left the societal implications of his theory undeveloped. It was Hans von Hattingberg who picked up Meng's vision of psycho-pedagogy and found the coalescence of love and aggression to be realised in the historical figure of the crusader and the present-day figure of the worker, 'who directs his whole aggression against the resistance of the matter to serve mankind'. This was an unanticipated political twist, as it moved Meng's ideas away from his own moderate left-wing perspective and used them to frame in psychoanalytic terms a heroic cult of sacrifice and work that was a key part of Nazi ideology and propaganda.[278]

The 1939 conference in Lugano was a failure, and not only when measured by its most lofty goals. The war was not prevented and the mutual understanding did not happen. In the end, the European movement for mental hygiene was not even able to improve the mental well-being of its own members. As Max Müller remembered:

> The congress in Lugano became a total fiasco. Many people came from abroad, Germans and French in particular. There was nothing in the sort of mutual conversation, or even a willingness to do so. The Germans – I remember [Ernst] Kretschmer, [Ernst] Rüdin, [Hermann] Hof[f]mann – were very buttoned up, isolated themselves, and mocked our frontier fortifications, which then were in full play, but mostly did not think about getting in touch with others (there were also Swedes and Italians). Some of them surely would have liked to, but did not dare. The French too were behaving with suspicion and reserve. Thus, the lectures became vacuous monologues; Repond tried in vain at least to produce one of the famous 'resolutions', which everybody would have signed. One dispersed even more depressed than one had arrived.[279]

The meeting in Lugano marks the sad and surreal end of the mental hygiene movement in Europe before the Second World War. Less than three months after the conference, the war severed the international networks and almost simultaneously, German medicine, led by a number of physicians closely connected to the local branch of mental hygiene, crossed moral lines as the 'euthanasia' programme began. The mass murder of the disabled and mentally ill was the logical conclusion of a vision of racial hygiene that proponents of mental hygiene had advocated and radicalised in the previous decades. In the eyes of the perpetrators, it was part of the fulfilment of the promise of mental hygiene, to prevent mental illness in present and future generations, to improve mental health care, and to create a society free from the scourge of mental illness.

In Germany, mental hygiene would not recover from its involvement in these crimes. After the war, the term *psychische Hygiene* by and large disappeared from public and professional debates and, discredited by its close connection with racial hygiene, the movement did not re-emerge in its pre-war form. In Austria and Switzerland, the situation was different. The term and the movement survived, although *psychische Hygiene* was increasingly supplanted by the synonymous, but catchier term *Psychohygiene* that had rarely been used in the inter-war period. Another influential terminological change took place in London in 1948, where mental hygienists from all over the world resumed the tradition of the large-scale international congresses that had begun in Washington, DC in 1930 and Paris in 1937, and had been interrupted by the war. The International Congress on Mental Health held in London marked the rebirth as well as the end of the pre-war movement for mental hygiene, now named 'mental health', the term that is still in use to the present day.[280]

In Switzerland, Heinrich Meng and André Repond continued their work after the war,[281] and in 1949, Repond became the second president of the newly founded World Federation of Mental Health—the direct successor organisation to the ICMH.[282] In Austria, the post-war period became a kind of 'golden age' of mental hygiene. What had only been a sub-committee of the Austrian Society for Public Health before 1938, now became the independent Austrian Society for Mental Hygiene (*Österreichische Gesellschaft für Psychische Hygiene*) in 1948.[283] One of the driving forces in the reestablishment of mental hygiene in Austria was Erwin Stransky, who had used the notion of mental hygiene as early as 1918; a revised and updated edition of his 1931 textbook was published in 1955.[284] In the 1950s, Austria became a focal point for the international movement, and in 1953, the sixth international congress on mental hygiene was held in Vienna.[285] Only a few years later, the Viennese psychiatrist Hans Hoff (1897–1969) became president of the World Federation for Mental Health, which together with the World Health Organisation and UNESCO proclaimed 1960 the 'World Year of Mental Health'. The Austrian Society for Mental Hygiene participated with an extensive series of lectures and events.[286]

However, it was not only the international institutions and networks of mental hygiene that reappeared after the Second World War. Facing the global devastation of the recent war and the looming threat of a third, nuclear, world war, the idea of psychiatric prophylaxis again came to embody a utopian promise of progress and world peace. Like the notion of mental hygiene in the inter-war period, mental health reached far beyond the immediate medical aspects of psychiatric prophylaxis and promised to guide the way into a better future:

> The fact that men and women everywhere are looking for guidance in world affairs, as well as in dealing with the problems of their own community, constitutes the greatest challenge ever presented to social scientists and psychiatrists. Two world wars in a single generation, and the possibility of a much more devastating one in the not distant future, have made clear to everyone the urgency of the crisis. More directly and more clearly than ever before, the question must be faced as to whether survival is possible without adapting human institutions so that men can live together as world citizens in, a world community, in which local loyalties are rendered compatible with a wider allegiance to mankind as a whole.[287]

Notes

1. Erwin Stransky, 'Wesen und Programmatik der psychischen Hygiene', in *Leitfaden der psychischen Hygiene*, ed. Erwin Stransky (Vienna: Urban & Schwarzenberg, 1931), 1.
2. Hans Roemer, ed., *Bericht über die Erste Deutsche Tagung für Psychische Hygiene in Hamburg am 20. September 1928* (Berlin and Leipzig: Walter de Gruyter, 1929).
3. Oswald Bumke et al., *Handwörterbuch der psychischen Hygiene und der psychiatrischen Fürsorge* (Berlin and Leipzig: Walter de Gruyter, 1931); Erwin Stransky, ed., *Leitfaden der psychischen Hygiene* (Vienna: Urban & Schwarzenberg, 1931).
4. Helmut Gröger, 'Die Entwicklung der psychischen Hygiene von der Bewegung zur psychiatrischen Disziplin - der österreichische Weg', *Schriftenreihe der Deutschen Gesellschaft für Geschichte der Nervenheilkunde* 18

(2012): 221–31; Hans Jakob Ritter, *Psychiatrie und Eugenik: Zur Ausprägung eugenischer Denk- und Handlungsmuster in der schweizerischen Psychiatrie 1850–1950* (Zurich: Chronos, 2009), 161–63.

5. Hans Pols, 'Managing the Mind: The Culture of American Mental Hygiene, 1910–1950' (PhD thesis, University of Pennsylvania, 1997); Hans Pols, '"Beyond the Clinical Frontiers:" The American Mental Hygiene Movement, 1910–1945', in *International Relations in Psychiatry: Britain, Germany, and the United States to World War II*, ed. Volker Roelcke, Paul Weindling, and Louise Westwood (Rochester: University of Rochester Press, 2010), 111–33.
6. Clifford W. Beers, *A Mind That Found Itself: An Autobiography* (New York: Longmans, Green, and Co., 1908); Otto Kauders, 'Geschichte der psychischen Hygiene', in *Leitfaden der psychischen Hygiene*, ed. Erwin Stransky (Vienna: Urban & Schwarzenberg, 1931), 12; Norman Dain, *Clifford W. Beers: Advocate of the Insane* (Pittsburgh: University of Pittsburgh Press, 1980).
7. Robert Sommer, 'Clifford Whittingham Beers, A Mind That Found Itself (Eine Seele, die sich fand)', *Zeitschrift für psychische Hygiene* 1, no. 1 (1928): 8.
8. Clifford W. Beers, *Eine Seele die sich wiederfand: Autobiographie des Begründers der 'Geistigen Hygiene'*, trans. Otto Reuter (Basel: Benno Schwabe, 1941).
9. Heinrich Meng and André Repond, 'Vorwort', in *Eine Seele die sich wiederfand: Autobiographie des Begründers der 'Geistigen Hygiene'*, ed. Clifford W. Beers (Basel: Benno Schwabe, 1941), 5; see also William A. White, 'The Origin, Growth, and Significance of the Mental-Hygiene Movement', in *Proceedings of the First International Congress on Mental Hygiene, Held at Washington D.C., U.S.A. May 5th to 10th, 1930*, ed. Frankwood E. Williams, vol. 1 (New York: The International Committee for Mental Hygiene, 1932), 523–33.
10. Meng and Repond, 'Vorwort', 12.
11. Pols, 'Managing the Mind', 31.
12. Ibid., 31–33, 40–42; Susan D. Lamb, *Pathologist of the Mind: Adolf Meyer and the Origins of American Psychiatry* (Baltimore: Johns Hopkins University Press, 2014).
13. Pols, 'Managing the Mind', 46–47.
14. Ibid., 62–63.
15. Ibid., 132–33; William L. Russel, 'A Brief Account of the Life and Work of Dr. Salmon', in *Proceedings of the First International Congress on Mental Hygiene, Held at Washington D.C., U.S.A. May 5th to 10th, 1930*, ed. Frankwood E. Williams, vol. 1 (New York: The International Committee for Mental Hygiene, 1932), 515–23.

16. Dain, *Beers*, 209; Kauders, 'Geschichte', 13–14; André Repond, 'Die Bewegung für psychische Hygiene in der Schweiz', *Zeitschrift für psychische Hygiene* 1, no. 6 (1928): 188; Francesco Cassata, *Building the New Man. Eugenics, Racial Science and Genetics in Twentieth Century Italy* (Budapest and New York: Central European University Press, 2011), 118–34.
17. Mathew Thomson, 'Mental Hygiene as an International Movement', in *International Health Organisations and Movements, 1918–1939*, ed. Paul Weindling (Cambridge: Cambridge University Press, 1995), 285.
18. Ibid., 284–85.
19. Dain, *Beers*, 208–9.
20. Ibid., 219–23; Thomson, 'Mental Hygiene', 285.
21. Frankwood E. Williams, ed., 'The Founding of the International Committee for Mental Hygiene', in *Proceedings of the First International Congress on Mental Hygiene, Held at Washington D.C., U.S.A. May 5th to 10th, 1930*, vol. 1 (New York: The International Committee for Mental Hygiene, 1932), 32–49.
22. Erwin Stransky, 'Angewandte Psychiatrie: Motive und Elemente zu einem Programmentwurf', *Allgemeine Zeitschrift für Psychiatrie und psychisch-gerichtliche Medizin* 74, nos. 1–3 (1918): 43; Robert Sommer, 'Die Einrichtung von öffentlichen Schlaf- und Ruhehallen', *Die Krankenpflege* 2 (1902): 529.
23. Roemer, *Bericht*.
24. Bumke et al., *Handwörterbuch*; Stransky, *Leitfaden*.
25. Thomson, 'Mental Hygiene', 298–99.
26. Ibid., 290–96.
27. Frankwood E. Williams, ed., 'World View of Mental Hygiene', in *Proceedings of the First International Congress on Mental Hygiene, Held at Washington D.C., U.S.A. May 5th to 10th, 1930*, vol. 1 (New York: The International Committee for Mental Hygiene, 1932), 101.
28. Kauders, 'Geschichte', 11–12.
29. Gabriele Moser, '"Die Zukunft gehört der prophylaktischen Medizin:" Sozialhygiene, medizinisches Präventionsverständnis und Gesundheitsbegriff Ende der 1920er Jahre', in *Sozialmedizin, Sozialhygiene und Public Health: Konzepte und Visionen zum Verhältnis von Medizin und Gesellschaft in historischer Perspektive*, ed. Udo Schagen and Sabine Schleiermacher (Berlin: Forschungsstelle Zeitgeschichte im Institut für Geschichte der Medizin, 2002), 15–20.
30. Harry Oosterhuis, 'Outpatient Psychiatry and Mental Health Care in the Twentieth Century: International Perspectives', in *Psychiatric Cultures Compared: Psychiatry and Mental Health Care in the Twentieth Century. Comparisons and Approaches*, ed. Marijke Gijswijt-Hofstra et al. (Amsterdam: Amsterdam University Press, 2005), 249.

31. Heinrich Kogerer, 'Psychische Hygiene in Österreich', *Zeitschrift für psychische Hygiene* 2, no. 4 (1929): 114.
32. Gröger, 'Entwicklung', 226.
33. Rudolf Dreikurs, 'Der gegenwärtige Stand der psychischen Hygiene in Wien', *Volksgesundheit: Zeitschrift für soziale Hygiene* 3, no. 10 (1929): 221.
34. Alfons Labisch, *Homo Hygienicus: Gesundheit und Medizin in der Neuzeit* (Frankfurt am Main and New York: Campus, 1992), 146–47.
35. Paul Weindling, 'Public Health in Germany', in *The History of Public Health and the Modern State*, ed. Dorothy Porter (Amsterdam and Atlanta: Editions Rodopi, 1994), 124; Adolf Gottstein, 'Soziale Hygiene und Gesundheitsfürsorge', in *Handwörterbuch der psychischen Hygiene und der psychiatrischen Fürsorge*, ed. Oswald Bumke et al. (Berlin and Leipzig: Walter de Gruyter, 1931), 331–33.
36. Weindling, 'Public Health', 124.
37. Gottstein, 'Soziale Hygiene und Gesundheitsfürsorge', 333–38; Weindling, 'Public Health', 125–26; Wolfgang U. Eckart, *Medizin und Krieg: Deutschland 1914–1924* (Paderborn: Schöningh, 2014), 395–400.
38. Alfred Grotjahn and Ignaz Kaup, *Handwörterbuch der sozialen Hygiene*, 2 vols (Leipzig: F.C.W. Vogel, 1912).
39. Adolf Dannemann, 'Irrenwesen', in *Handwörterbuch der sozialen Hygiene*, ed. Alfred Grotjahn and Ignaz Kaup, vol. 1 (Leipzig: F.C.W. Vogel, 1912), 523.
40. Hans Roemer, 'Was Will Die internationale Bewegung für geistige Hygiene?', *Zeitschrift für psychische Hygiene* 1, no. 2 (1928): 38.
41. Stransky, 'Wesen und Programmatik', 5.
42. Stransky, 'Angewandte Psychiatrie', 43; Stransky, 'Wesen und Programmatik', 3–5.
43. See, for example, Hans Roemer, 'Psychische Hygiene', in *Handwörterbuch der psychischen Hygiene und der psychiatrischen Fürsorge*, ed. Oswald Bumke et al. (Berlin and Leipzig: Walter de Gruyter, 1931), 296–312.
44. Hans Ludwig Siemen, *Menschen blieben auf der Strecke ...: Psychiatrie zwischen Reform und Nationalsozialismus* (Gütersloh: Jakob von Hoddis, 1987), 29–30; A. Richter, 'Über die Ernährungsverhältnisse in der Irrenanstalt Buch während des Krieges 1914/1918 und deren Folgen', *Allgemeine Zeitschrift für Psychiatrie und psychisch-gerichtliche Medizin* 75 (1919): 407–23.
45. Adolf Groß, 'Zeitgemäße Betrachtungen zum wirtschaftlichen Betrieb der Irrenanstalten', *Allgemeine Zeitschrift für die Psychiatrie und psychisch-gerichtliche Medizin* 76, no. 1 (1923): 60–74.
46. Hans Ludwig Siemen, 'Die Reformpsychiatrie der Weimarer Republik: Subjektive Ansprüche und die Macht des Faktischen', in *Nach Hadamar:*

Zum Verhältnis von Psychiatrie und Politik im 20. Jahrhundert, ed. Franz-Werner Kersting, Karl Teppe, and Bernd Walter (Paderborn: Ferdinand Schöningh, 1993), 100; Heinz-Peter Schmiedebach, 'Eine "antipsychiatrische Bewegung" um die Jahrhundertwende', in *Medizinkritische Bewegungen im Deutschen Reich (ca. 1870–ca. 1933)*, ed. Martin Dinges (Stuttgart: Steiner, 1996), 127–60.

47. Gustav Kolb, 'Reform der Irrenfürsorge', *Zeitschrift für die gesamte Neurologie und Psychiatrie* 47 (1919): 137–72; Gustav Kolb, 'Inwieweit sind Änderungen im Betriebe der Anstalten geboten?', *Psychiatrisch-Neurologische Wochenschrift*, nos. 17/18 (1920): 133–39; Astrid Ley, 'Psychiatriekritik durch Psychiater: Sozialreformerische und professionspolitische Ziele des Erlanger Anstaltsdirektors Gustav Kolb (1870–1938)', in *'Moderne' Anstaltspsychiatrie im 19. und 20. Jahrhundert: Legitimation und Kritik*, ed. Heiner Fangerau and Karen Nolte (Stuttgart: Franz Steiner, 2006), 195–220.
48. Ley, 'Psychiatriekritik', 195–96.
49. Kolb, 'Reform der Irrenfürsorge', 141–42.
50. Ley, 'Psychiatriekritik', 202; Kolb, 'Reform der Irrenfürsorge', 156–57.
51. Bernd Walter, 'Hermann Simon: Psychiatriereformer, Sozialdarwinist, Nationalsozialist?', *Der Nervenarzt* 73, no. 11 (2002): 1047–54; Thomas Beddies, '"Aktivere Krankenbehandlung" und "Arbeitstherapie:" Anwendungsformen und Begründungszusammenhänge bei Hermann Simon und Carl Schneider', in '*Heroische Therapien:' Die deutsche Psychiatrie im internationalen Vergleich 1918-1945*, ed. Hans-Walter Schmuhl and Volker Roelcke (Göttingen: Wallstein, 2013), 268–86.
52. Hermann Simon, 'Krankenbehandlung in der Heilanstalt, insbesondere Beschäftigung, in ihren Beziehungen zur psychischen Hygiene', in *Bericht über die Erste Deutsche Tagung für psychische Hygiene in Hamburg am 20. Dezember 1928*, ed. Hans Roemer (Berlin and Leipzig: Walter de Gruyter, 1929), 20.
53. Heinz-Peter Schmiedebach and Stefan Priebe, 'Social Psychiatry in Germany in the Twentieth Century: Ideas and Models', *Medical History* 48, no. 4 (2004): 461.
54. Siemen, 'Reformpsychiatrie', 104.
55. Between 1925 and 1930, more than seven hundred visitors came to see Simon's Gütersloh clinic as a model for institutional reform, seventy from abroad, Walter, 'Hermann Simon', 1049.
56. Simon, 'Krankenbehandlung', 24; Schmiedebach and Priebe, 'Social Psychiatry', 461–62.
57. Monika Ankele, 'Arbeitsrhythmus und Anstaltsalltag: Eine Einführung in den Sammelband', in *Arbeitsrhythmus und Anstaltsalltag: Arbeit in der Psychiatrie vom frühen 19. Jahrhundert bis in die NS-Zeit*, ed. Monika Ankele and Eva Brinkschulte (Stuttgart: Franz Steiner, 2015), 11.

58. Simon, 'Krankenbehandlung', 22, 24.
59. Sommer, 'Einrichtung'; Robert Sommer, 'Eine psychiatrische Abteilung des Reichsgesundheitsamts', *Psychiatrisch-Neurologische Wochenschrift* 12, no. 12 (1910): 295–98.
60. Stransky, 'Angewandte Psychiatrie', 43.
61. On the history of the German Association for Mental Hygiene, see Hans-Walter Schmuhl, *Die Gesellschaft Deutscher Neurologen und Psychiater im Nationalsozialismus* (Berlin: Springer, 2016), 31–35; Siemen, *Menschen blieben auf der Strecke*, 89–94; Bernd Walter, *Psychiatrie und Gesellschaft in der Moderne: Geisteskrankenfürsorge in der Provinz Westfalen zwischen Kaiserreich und NS-Regime* (Paderborn: Ferdinand Schöningh, 1996), 286–96.
62. Robert Sommer, 'Zu dem internationalen Kongress für psychische Hygiene', *Wiener Medizinische Wochenschrift* 75, no. 18 (1925): 1060–61.
63. Minutes of the DVPH board meeting in Berlin, 28 November 1927, Hermann Simon papers, 926/193. Robert Sommer, 'Die nationale und internationale Organisation der psychischen Hygiene', *Allgemeine Zeitschrift für die Psychiatrie und psychisch-gerichtliche Medizin* 83, nos. 5/6 (1926): 391–94.
64. Hermann Simon to Wilhelm Weygandt, 11 October 1926, Hermann Simon papers, 926/193.
65. See also Robert Sommer to Gustav Kolb and Hermann Simon, 8 June 1927, Hermann Simon papers, 926/193.
66. Minutes of the DVPH board meeting in Berlin, 28 November 1927, Hermann Simon papers, 926/193.
67. Robert Sommer, 'Psychotherapie und psychische Hygiene', *Allgemeine ärztliche Zeitschrift für Psychotherapie und psychische Hygiene* 1, no. 1 (1928): 9–10; Robert Sommer, 'Psychotherapie und psychische Hygiene', *Allgemeine ärztliche Zeitschrift für Psychotherapie und psychische Hygiene* 1, no. 2 (1928): 129–34.
68. Axel C. Hüntelmann, *Hygiene im Namen des Staates: Das Reichsgesundheitsamt 1876–1933* (Göttingen: Wallstein, 2008).
69. Minutes of the DVPH board meeting in Berlin, 28 November 1927, Hermann Simon papers, 926/193, 14.
70. Robert Sommer and Hans Roemer, 'Niederschrift über die erste Mitgliederversammlung des Deutschen Verbandes für psychische Hygiene in Hamburg in der Staatskrankenanstalt Friedrichsberg am 19. September 1928', *Zeitschrift für psychische Hygiene* 1, no. 5 (1928): 134–35.
71. Mathew Thomson, 'Mental Hygiene in Britain during the First Half of the Twentieth Century: The Limits of International Influence', in *International Relations in Psychiatry: Britain, Germany, and the United States to World War II*, ed. Volker Roelcke, Paul Weindling, and Louise Westwood (Rochester: University of Rochester Press, 2010), 134–55.

72. Minutes of the DVPH board meeting in Berlin, 28 November 1927, Hermann Simon papers, 926/193, 1.
73. 'Zur Frage der Arbeitstherapie in den Heil- und Pflegeanstalten', *Zeitschrift für psychische Hygiene* 2, no. 2 (1929): 50–61. See also DVPH to the *Reich* Minister of the Interior, 30 July 1928, Hermann Simon papers, 926/139.
74. Walter, *Psychiatrie und Gesellschaft*, 291–95.
75. Roemer, *Bericht*, 151–57; Robert Sommer, 'Die I. Tagung des Deutschen Verbands für Psychische Hygiene in Hamburg-Friedrichsberg vom 19.-21. Sept. 1928', *Allgemeine ärztliche Zeitschrift für Psychotherapie und psychische Hygiene* 1 (1928): 619–22.
76. Wilhelm Weygandt, 'Über die Aufgaben des deutschen Verbandes für psychische Hygiene und die erste deutsche Tagung', in *Bericht über die Erste Deutsche Tagung für psychische Hygiene in Hamburg am 20. Dezember 1928*, ed. Hans Roemer (Berlin and Leipzig: Walter de Gruyter, 1929), 8.
77. Roemer, *Bericht*, 4.
78. 'Satzungen des Deutschen Verbands für psychische Hygiene', *Zeitschrift für psychische Hygiene* 1, no. 5 (1928): 137–40.
79. Robert Sommer, 'Psychiatrische Erblichkeitsforschung und psychische Hygiene', in *Bericht über die Erste Deutsche Tagung für psychische Hygiene in Hamburg am 20. Dezember 1928*, ed. Hans Roemer (Berlin and Leipzig: Walter de Gruyter, 1929), 96–100.
80. Hans Roemer, 'Die Zweite Tagung für psychische Hygiene in Bonn am 21. Mai 1932', *Zeitschrift für psychische Hygiene* 5, nos. 3/4 (1932): 65–80.
81. List of members of the DVPH, 1930, with handwritten additions until 1 May 1932, Hermann Simon papers, 926/139.
82. UAG, Robert Sommer papers, Vol. 67.
83. Minutes of the DVPH board meeting in Berlin, 28 November 1927, Hermann Simon papers, 926/193, 1.
84. Sommer, 'Zum dem internationalen Kongress'.
85. Sommer, 'Die nationale und intrernationale Organisation', 391.
86. Ibid.
87. Martin Kohlrausch and Helmuth Trischler, *Building Europe on Expertise: Innovators, Organizers, Networkers* (Houndmills, Basingstoke: Palgrave Macmillan, 2014), 1.
88. Sommer, 'A Mind That Found Itself'.
89. Hermann Simon to Hans Roemer, 21 May 1931, Hermann Simon papers, 926/141.
90. Robert Sommer, 'Schlusswort', in *Bericht über die Erste Deutsche Tagung für psychische Hygiene in Hamburg am 20. Dezember 1928*, ed. Hans Roemer (Berlin and Leipzig: Walter de Gruyter, 1929), 136.
91. Robert Sommer to Hermann Simon, 20 February 1930, Hermann Simon papers, 926/140, 2.

92. Robert Sommer et al., 'Zum Ersten Internationalen Kongreß für psychische Hygiene', *Zeitschrift für psychische Hygiene* 3, no. 2 (1930): 33.
93. Ibid.
94. Ibid., 34.
95. Robert Sommer, 'Die nationale und internationale Organisation der psychischen Hygiene', *Deutsches Ärzteblatt* 59, no. 11 (1930): 131.
96. Sommer et al., 'Zum Ersten Internationalen Kongreß', 35.
97. Frankwood E. Williams, *Proceedings of the First International Congress on Mental Hygiene, Held at Washington D.C., U.S.A. May 5th to 10th, 1930*, 2 vols (New York: The International Committee for Mental Hygiene, 1932).
98. John R. Shillady, 'The Story of the Congress', in *Proceedings of the First International Congress on Mental Hygiene, Held at Washington D.C., U.S.A. May 5th to 10th, 1930*, ed. Frankwood E. Williams, vol. 1 (New York: The International Committee for Mental Hygiene, 1932), 21–22.
99. Ibid., 23.
100. Hans Roemer, 'Eine humanitäre Bewegung: Der Erste Weltkongreß für psychische Hygiene', *Frankfurter Zeitung*, 20 July 1930.
101. Hans Roemer, 'To What Extent Does Public Opinion Help, and to What Extent Does It Impair the Work of Mental Hygiene?', in *Proceedings of the First International Congress on Mental Hygiene, Held at Washington D.C., U.S.A. May 5th to 10th, 1930*, ed. Frankwood E. Williams, vol. 1 (New York: The International Committee for Mental Hygiene, 1932), 267–71.
102. See, for example, Emil Kraepelin, 'Hundert Jahre Psychiatrie', *Zeitschrift für die gesamte Neurologie und Psychiatrie* 38 (1918): 161–275.
103. Schmiedebach, 'Eine "antipsychiatrische" Bewegung', 145–52.
104. Sommer, 'Abteilung', 296.
105. 'Revolution Im Irrenwesen', *Die Irrenrechts-Reform* 62 (1919): 160.
106. Hermann Haymann, 'Irrenärztliche Bemerkungen zu Heinrich Mann's neuem Buch', *Zeitschrift für die gesamte Neurologie und Psychiatrie* 39 (1918): 225–28, as well as several comments and replies in the same journal.
107. Roemer, 'Public Opinion', 273.
108. Ibid., 279.
109. Volker Roelcke, 'Ernst Rüdin: Renommierter Wissenschaftler, radikaler Rassenhygieniker', *Der Nervenarzt* 83, no. 3 (2012): 303–10; Volker Roelcke, 'Psychiatrische Wissenschaft im Kontext nationalsozialistischer Politik und Euthanasie: Zur Rolle Ernst Rüdins und der Deutschen Forschungsanstalt für Psychiatrie/Kaiser-Wilhelm-Institut', in *Geschichte der Kaiser-Wilhelm-Gesellschaft im Nationalsozialismus: Bestandsaufnahme und Perspektiven der Forschung*, ed. Doris Kaufmann, vol. 1 (Göttingen: Wallstein, 2000), 112–50.
110. Ernst Rüdin, 'The Significance of Eugenics and Genetics for Mental Hygiene', in *Proceedings of the First International Congress on Mental*

Hygiene, Held at Washington D.C., U.S.A. May 5th to 10th, 1930, ed. Frankwood E. Williams, vol. 1 (New York: The International Committee for Mental Hygiene, 1932), 473.

111. See, for example, Ernst Rüdin, 'Erbbiologisch-psychiatrische Streitfragen', *Zeitschrift für die gesamte Neurologie und Psychiatrie* 108 (1927): 296.
112. Rüdin, 'Significance', 483.
113. Roelcke, 'Ernst Rüdin', 306.
114. Rüdin, 'Significance', 483.
115. Ian Robert Dowbiggin, *Keeping America Sane: Psychiatry and Eugenics in the United States and Canada, 1880-1940*, 2nd ed. (Ithaca, NY: Cornell University Press, 2003); Wendy Kline, 'Eugenics in the United States', in *The Oxford Handbook of the History of Eugenics*, ed. Alison Bashford and Philippa Levine (Oxford: Oxford University Press, 2010).
116. Williams, *Proceedings*, i.
117. Rüdin, 'Significance', 490.
118. Clifford W. Beers, 'To Those Interested in the International Work', 18 December 1930, Hermann Simon papers, 926/140, 5.
119. Williams, 'Founding'.
120. Ibid., 43.
121. Ibid.
122. Thomson, 'Mental Hygiene', 283–84.
123. Ibid., 283.
124. Clifford W. Beers, 'To Those Interested in the International Work', 18 December 1930, Hermann Simon papers, 926/140, 7. 'Der II. Internationale Kongreß für psychische Hygiene', *Zeitschrift für psychische Hygiene* 9, no. 4 (1936): 127–28.
125. Williams, 'World View of Mental Hygiene', 103.
126. Ibid., 102.
127. 'Vorschläge für die weitere Arbeit des Verbandes', Hermann Simon papers, 926/141.
128. Stransky, *Leitfaden*.
129. Bumke et al., *Handwörterbuch*. On Eugen Kahn, see Volker Roelcke, 'Psychiatry in Munich and Yale, ca. 1920–1935: Mutual Perceptions and Relations, and the Case of Eugen Kahn (1887–1973)', in *International Relations in Psychiatry: Britain, Germany, and the United States to World War II*, ed. Volker Roelcke, Paul Weindling, and Louise Westwood (Rochester: University of Rochester Press, 2010), 156–78.
130. UAG, Robert Sommer papers, Vol. 25.
131. Franz Sioli, 'Ausbildung der mit psychischer Hygiene befaßten Personenkreise', in *Handwörterbuch der psychischen Hygiene und der psychiatrischen Fürsorge*, ed. Oswald Bumke et al. (Berlin and Leipzig: Walter de Gruyter, 1931), 31–34.

132. Hans Ludwig Siemen, 'Reform und Radikalisierung: Veränderungen der Psychiatrie in der Weltwirtschaftskrise', in *Medizin und Gesundheitspolitik in der NS-Zeit*, ed. Norbert Frei (München: Oldenbourg, 1991), 99–102.
133. Robert Gaupp, 'Die Unfruchtbarmachung geistig und sittlich Minderwertiger: Erweitertes Referat, erstattet auf der Jahresversammlung des Deutschen Vereins für Psychiatrie am 2. September 1925 in Kassel', *Zeitschrift für die gesamte Neurologie und Psychiatrie* 100 (1926): 139–81.
134. Karl Binding and Alfred Hoche, *Die Freigabe der Vernichtung lebensunwerten Lebens: Ihr Maß und ihre Form* (Leipzig: F. Meiner, 1920).
135. Siemen, *Menschen blieben auf der Strecke*, 104–6.
136. Berthold Kihn, 'Die Ausschaltung der Minderwertigen aus der Gesellschaft', *Allgemeine Zeitschrift für Psychiatrie* 98 (1932): 394; Siemen, *Menschen blieben auf der Strecke*, 105.
137. 'Gesetz zur Verhütung erbkranken Nachwuchses vom 14. Juli 1933', *Zeitschrift für psychische Hygiene* 6, no. 5 (1933): 152–55.
138. Maike Rotzoll et al., *Die nationalsozialistische 'Euthanasie'-Aktion T4 und ihre Opfer: Geschichte und ethische Konsequenzen für die Gegenwart* (Paderborn: Ferdinand Schöningh, 2010).
139. Volker Roelcke, 'Hans Roemer (1878–1948)', *Der Nervenarzt* 84, no. 9 (2013): 1064–68; Hans-Walter Schmuhl, 'Die Genesis der "Euthanasie:" Interpretationsansätze', in *Die nationalsozialistische 'Euthanasie'-Aktion T4 und ihre Opfer: Geschichte und ethische Konsequenzen für die Gegenwart*, ed. Maike Rotzoll et al. (Paderborn: Ferdinand Schöningh, 2010), 67–69.
140. Sommer, 'Organisation', 130.
141. Siemen, *Menschen blieben auf der Strecke*, 119–23.
142. Siemen, 'Reformpsychiatrie', 107.
143. Gerrit Hohendorf, 'Therapieunfähigkeit als Selektionskriterium: Die "Schocktherapieverfahren" und die Organisationszentrale der nationalsozialistischen "Euthanasie" in der Berliner Tiergartenstraße 4, 1939–1945', in '*Heroische Therapien:' Die deutsche Psychiatrie im internationalen Vergleich 1918-1945*, ed. Hans-Walter Schmuhl and Volker Roelcke (Göttingen: Wallstein, 2013), 287–307.
144. Walter, 'Hermann Simon'; Walter, *Psychiatrie und Gesellschaft*, 266–76.
145. Robert Sommer to Gustav Kolb and Hermann Simon, 8 June 1927, Hermann Simon papers, 926/139.
146. Hermann Simon, *Aktivere Krankenbehandlung in der Irrenanstalt* (Berlin and Leipzig: Walter de Gruyter, 1929), 147.
147. Hermann Simon to Hans Roemer, 23 June 1931, Hermann Simon papers, 926/141.
148. Hermann Simon to Hans Roemer, 25 February 1932, Hermann Simon papers, 926/141.

149. Hermann Simon to Robert Sommer, 29 December 1929, Hermann Simon papers, 926/140.
150. Hermann Simon to Hans Roemer, 19 December 1931, Hermann Simon papers, 926/141.
151. Hermann Simon to Robert Sommer, 30 May 1930, Hermann Simon papers, 926/140.
152. Hermann Simon to the board of the DVPH, 10 May 1931, Hermann Simon papers, 926/141.
153. Hermann Simon to the board of the DVPH, 10 May 1931, Hermann Simon papers, 926/141.
154. Hermann Simon to Robert Sommer, 12 July 1933, Hermann Simon papers, 926/142.
155. Hans Roemer to the board of the DVPH, 11 March 1932, Hermann Simon papers, 926/141.
156. Hermann Simon to the board of the DVPH, 8 April 1932, Hermann Simon papers, 926/141.
157. Roemer, 'Die Zweite Tagung'; Hans Roemer, *Bericht über die Zweite Deutsche Tagung für psychische Hygiene in Bonn am 21. Mai 1932* (Berlin and Leipzig: Walter de Gruyter, 1932).
158. Robert Sommer and Hans Roemer, 'Niederschrift über die II. Mitgliederversammlung des Deutschen Verbandes für psychische Hygiene in Bonn im Auditorium maximum der Universität am 20. Mai 1932 17 Uhr', *Zeitschrift für psychische Hygiene* 5 (1932): 179; Roemer, *Bericht über die Zweite Deutsche Tagung*, 7–9.
159. Roemer, 'Die Zweite Tagung', 67.
160. Ibid.
161. Ernst Rüdin, 'Die Ergebnisse der psychiatrischen Erbbiologie für die eugenische Praxis', in *Bericht über die Zweite Deutsche Tagung für psychische Hygiene in Bonn am 21. Mai 1932*, ed. Hans Roemer (Berlin and Leipzig: Walter de Gruyter, 1932), 19–29; Hans Luxenburger, 'Die Sterilisierung aus psychiatrisch-eugenischer Indikation', in *Bericht über die Zweite Deutsche Tagung für psychische Hygiene in Bonn am 21. Mai 1932*, ed. Hans Roemer (Berlin and Leipzig: Walter de Gruyter, 1932), 30–43.
162. Roemer, 'Die Zweite Tagung', 69.
163. Robert Sommer, 'Der natürliche Adel als Ausleseprinzip', in *Bericht über die Zweite Deutsche Tagung für psychische Hygiene in Bonn am 21. Mai 1932*, ed. Hans Roemer (Berlin and Leipzig: Walter de Gruyter, 1932), 132–33.
164. Hans Roemer, ed., 'Merkblatt des Deutschen Verbandes für psychische Hygiene zur Verhütung der erblichen Geistes- und Nervenkrankheiten', in *Bericht über die Zweite Deutsche Tagung für psychische Hygiene in Bonn am 21. Mai 1932* (Berlin and Leipzig: Walter de Gruyter, 1932), 10–18.
165. UAG, Robert Sommer papers, Vol. 13, 19.
166. 'Gesetz zur Verhütung erbkranken Nachwuchses', 152.

167. Schmuhl, *Gesellschaft*, 47–53.
168. Matthias Heinrich Göring and Carl Gustav Jung, 'Geheimrat Sommer zum 70. Geburtstag', *Zentralblatt für Psychotherapie* 7, no. 2 (1934): 314.
169. Hermann Simon to Robert Sommer, 14 March 1933, Hermann Simon papers, 926/142. Walter, 'Hermann Simon'; Walter, *Psychiatrie und Gesellschaft*, 411–14.
170. Robert Sommer, 21 May 1933, Hermann Simon papers, 926/142.
171. Hermann Simon to Robert Sommer, 11 June 1933, Hermann Simon papers, 926/142.
172. Hermann Simon to the Aufklärungsamt für Bevölkerungspolitik und Rassenpflege, 12 June 1933, Hermann Simon papers, 926/142.
173. Hermann Simon to Robert Sommer, 11 June 1933, Hermann Simon papers, 926/142.
174. Hermann Simon to Robert Sommer, 22 June 1933, Hermann Simon papers, 926/142.
175. Hans Roemer to Robert Sommer, 25 June 1933, Hermann Simon papers, 926/142.
176. Hermann Simon to the members of the smaller board of the DVPH, 27 June 1933, Hermann Simon papers, 926/142.
177. Another reason might have been Sommer's age and the poor health of his wife, see Robert Sommer to Matthias Heinrich Göring, 3 October 1933, UAG, Robert Sommer papers, Vol. 68, 1370.
178. Hermann Simon to Hans Roemer and Paul Nitsche, 29 June 1933, Hermann Simon papers, 926/142.
179. Hans Roemer to Wilhelm Weygandt, Hermann Simon, and Paul Nitsche, 6 July 1933, Hermann Simon papers, 926/142.
180. Minutes of the board meeting of the DVPH in Kassel, 16 July 1933, Hermann Simon papers, 926/142.
181. Hermann Simon to Ernst Rüdin, 12 July 1933, Hermann Simon papers, 926/142.
182. Roelcke, 'Psychiatrische Wissenschaft'; Roelcke, 'Ernst Rüdin'.
183. Minutes of the board meeting of the DVPH in Kassel, 16 July 1933, Hermann Simon papers, 926/142. Sheila Faith Weiss, *'The Sword of Our Science' as a Foreign Policy Weapon: The Political Function of German Geneticists in the International Arena During the Third Reich* (Berlin: MPIWG, 2005).
184. Hans Roemer, Die II. Europäische Vereinigung für psychische Hygiene in Rom am 27. und 28. September 1933, 15 October 1933, Hermann Simon papers, 926/142.
185. Roemer had joined the NSDAP on 1 May 1933, Anna Plezko, 'Handlungsspielräume und Zwänge in der Medizin des Nationalsozialismus: Das Leben und Werk des Psychiaters Dr. Hans Roemer (1878–1947)' (MD thesis, University of Gießen, 2011), 17.

186. Guido Cimino and Giovanni Pietro Lombardo, *Sante de Sanctis tra psicologia generale e psicologia applicata* (Milan: Franco Angeli, 2004).
187. Hans Roemer, Die II. Europäische Vereinigung für psychische Hygiene in Rom am 27. und 28. September 1933, 15 October 1933, Hermann Simon papers, 926/142.
188. Ernst Rüdin and Hans Roemer, 'Der Deutsche Verband für psychische Hygiene und Rassenhygiene', *Zeitschrift für psychische Hygiene* 6, no. 5 (1933): 129–30.
189. Hermann F. Hoffmann, 'Der Psychiater und die neue Zeit', *Zeitschrift für psychische Hygiene* 6, no. 6 (1933): 161–67.
190. M. Leonhardt and K. Foerster, 'Hermann F. Hoffmann (1891–1944): Die Tübinger Psychiatrie auf dem Weg in den Nationalsozialismus', *Der Nervenarzt* 67, no. 11 (1996): 947–52.
191. Hoffmann, 'Der Psychiater und die neue Zeit', 161.
192. Ibid., 166.
193. Hans Roemer, 'Die Deutsche Organisation für psychische Hygiene in den Jahren 1930–1936', *Zeitschrift für psychische Hygiene* 10, no. 2 (1937): 37.
194. Ernst Rüdin, *Erblehre und Rassenhygiene im völkischen Staat* (Munich: J. F. Lehmanns, 1934).
195. Hans Roemer, 'Die rassenhygienischen Aufgaben der praktischen Psychiatrie unter besonderer Berücksichtigung der offenen Fürsorge', in *Erblehre und Rassenhygiene im völkischen Staat*, ed. Ernst Rüdin (Munich: J. F. Lehmanns, 1934), 120–35.
196. At the same time, the psychotherapeutic association was undergoing a similar process, leading to a split between an international association and a German General Medical Association for Psychotherapy (*Deutsche Allgemeine Ärztliche Gesellschaft für Psychotherapie*) in September 1933, Carl Gustav Jung, 'Geleitwort', *Zentralblatt für Psychotherapie* 6 (1933): 139–40; 'Mitteilung des Reichsführers der "Deutschen allgemeinen ärztlichen Gesellschaft für Psychotherapie"', *Zentralblatt für Psychotherapie* 6 (1933): 140–41; Regine Lockot, *Erinnern und Durcharbeiten: Zur Geschichte der Psychoanalyse und Psychotherapie im Nationalsozialismus* (Gießen: Psychosozial-Verlag, 2002), 71–74.
197. Minutes of the board meeting of the DVPH in Kassel, 16 July 1933, Hermann Simon papers, 926/142.
198. Ernst Rüdin and Hans Roemer, 'Der Deutsche Ausschuß für psychische Hygiene der Gesellschaft Deutscher Neurologen und Psychiater', *Zeitschrift für psychische Hygiene* 8, no. 4 (1935): 97–99.
199. 'Die Gesellschaft Deutscher Neurologen und Psychiater', *Zeitschrift für psychische Hygiene* 8, no. 1 (1935): 1; Hans-Walter Schmuhl, 'Psychiatrie und Politik: Die Gesellschaft Deutscher Neurologen und Psychiater im Nationalsozialismus', in *Abweichung und Normalität: Psychiatrie in Deutschland*

vom Kaiserreich bis zur Deutschen Einheit, ed. Christine Wolters, Christof Beyer, and Brigitte Lohff (Bielefeld: transcript, 2013), 137–58.
200. Rüdin and Roemer, 'Ausschuß', 98.
201. Schmuhl, 'Psychiatrie und Politik', 138.
202. Rotzoll et al., *Die nationalsozialistische 'Euthanasie'-Aktion T4*.
203. Roelcke, 'Ernst Rüdin'.
204. Ingo Harms, 'Die Gutachter der Meldebogen: Kurzbiografien', in *Die nationalsozialistische 'Euthanasie'-Aktion T4 und ihre Opfer: Geschichte und ethische Konsequenzen für die Gegenwart*, ed. Maike Rotzoll et al. (Paderborn: Ferdinand Schöningh, 2010), 406–7.
205. Ibid., 413–14; Ralf Forsbach, *Die Medizinische Fakultät der Universität Bonn im 'Dritten Reich'* (Munich: Oldenbourg, 2006), 200–13.
206. Hans-Walter Schmuhl, 'Die Patientenmorde', in *Vernichten und Heilen: Der Nürnberger Ärzteprozeß und seine Folgen*, ed. Angelika Ebbinghaus and Klaus Dörner (Berlin: Aufbau Verlag, 2001), 305–6; Hohendorf, 'Therapieunfähigkeit als Selektionskriterium'; Hans-Walter Schmuhl, 'Die Selbstverständlichkeit des Tötens: Psychiater im Nationalsozialismus', *Geschichte und Gesellschaft* 16, no. 4 (1990): 411–39.
207. Hans Aloys Schmitz, 'Der Zweite Internationale Kongreß für Psychische Hygiene in Paris vom 19. bis 25. Juli 1937', *Zeitschrift für psychische Hygiene* 10, nos. 4/5 (1937): 119–25; Russell E. Blaisdell, 'Resume of Papers Presented at the International Congress on Mental Hygiene Held at Paris, July 19–24, 1937', *Psychiatric Quarterly* 12, no. 1 (1938): 26–34.
208. Schmitz, 'Der Zweite Internationale Kongreß', 119.
209. Ernst Rüdin, 'Bedingungen und Rolle der Eugenik in der Prophylaxe der Geistesstörungen', *Zeitschrift für psychische Hygiene* 10, nos. 4/5 (1937): 99–108.
210. Schmitz, 'Der Zweite Internationale Kongreß', 120.
211. Blaisdell, 'Resume of Papers', 27.
212. Forsbach, *Medizinische Fakultät*, 216–20.
213. Schmitz, 'Der Zweite Internationale Kongreß', 120; Blaisdell, 'Resume of Papers', 27.
214. Rüdin, 'Bedingungen und Rolle der Eugenik', 108.
215. Weiss, *The Sword of Our Science*.
216. Ibid., 7–9.
217. Schmitz, 'Der Zweite Internationale Kongreß'; Thomson, 'Mental Hygiene', 286.
218. Blaisdell, 'Resume of Papers', 26.
219. Hans Roemer, 'Die V. Europäische Vereinigung für psychische Hygiene in München vom 22. bis 25. August 1938', *Zeitschrift für psychische Hygiene* 12, no. 1 (1939): 5.
220. Ibid., 6.
221. Ibid., 7.

222. Ibid., 4.
223. Ibid., 6; Ernst Klee, *Das Personenlexikon zum Dritten Reich: Wer war was vor und nach 1945* (Frankfurt am Main: Fischer, 2003), 373.
224. Roemer, 'Die V. Europäische Vereinigung', 6.
225. Walter Morgenthaler, 'Heiratsprophylaxe und psychische Hygiene', *Zeitschrift für psychische Hygiene* 11 (1938): 145–52; Ernst Rüdin, 'Heiratsprophylaxe und psychische Hygiene', *Zeitschrift für psychische Hygiene* 11 (1938): 152–65.
226. Roemer, 'Die V. Europäische Vereinigung', 15.
227. Ibid., 15–26.
228. Kurt Pohlisch and Friedrich Panse, *Schlafmittelmißbrauch* (Leipzig: Thieme, 1934); Ralf Forsbach, 'Friedrich Panse – etabliert in allen Systemen: Psychiater in der Weimarer Republik, im "Dritten Reich" und in der Bundesrepublik', *Der Nervenarzt* 83, no. 3 (2012): 329–36; Forsbach, *Medizinische Fakultät*, 200–16.
229. Roemer, 'Die V. Europäische Vereinigung', 16–17.
230. Maike Rotzoll, 'Rhythmus des Lebens: Arbeit in psychiatrischen Institutionen im Nationalsozialismus zwischen Normalisierung und Selektion', in *Arbeitsrhythmus und Anstaltsalltag: Arbeit in der Psychiatrie vom frühen 19. Jahrhundert bis in die NS-Zeit*, ed. Monika Ankele and Eva Brinkschulte (Stuttgart: Franz Steiner, 2015), 202.
231. Hohendorf, 'Therapieunfähigkeit als Selektionskriterium'.
232. Christine Teller, 'Carl Schneider: Zur Biographie eines deutschen Wissenschaftlers', *Geschichte und Gesellschaft* 16, no. 4 (1990): 464–78; Gerrit Hohendorf, Volker Roelcke, and Maike Rotzoll, 'Innovation und Vernichtung: Psychiatrische Forschung und "Euthanasie" an der Heidelberger Psychiatrischen Klinik 1939–1945', *Der Nervenarzt* 67, no. 11 (1996): 935–46. The 1938 conference was not Schneider's first contact with the mental hygiene movement; in 1930, he had already been involved in the preparations for the section on mental hygiene at the Dresden hygiene exhibition, Carl Schneider, 'Seelische Hygiene', in *Internationale Hygiene-Ausstellung Dresden 1930: Amtlicher Führer* (Dresden: Verlag der Internationalen Hygiene-Ausstellung, 1930), 268–71.
233. Walter, 'Hermann Simon', 1053.
234. Hermann Simon, 'Ergebnisse einer aktiveren Krankenbehandlung in der Heil- und Pflegeanstalt', *Deutsche Medizinische Wochenschrift* 64 (1938): 1224–27; Beddies, 'Aktivere Krankenbehandlung', 272–73.
235. Carl Schneider, *Behandlung und Verhütung der Geisteskrankheiten: Allgemeine Erfahrungen, Grundsätze, Technik, Biologie* (Berlin: J. Springer, 1939).
236. Beddies, 'Aktivere Krankenbehandlung', 279.
237. Schneider, *Behandlung*, 421–82.
238. Ibid., 422.

239. Teller, 'Carl Schneider', 472–73.
240. Ibid., 475–77.
241. Klee, *Personenlexikon zum Dritten Reich*, 98.
242. Petra Stockdreher, 'Heil- und Pflegeanstalt Eglfing-Haar', in *Psychiatrie im Nationalsozialismus: Die Bayerischen Heil- und Pflegeanstalten zwischen 1933 und 1945*, ed. Michael von Cranach and Hans-Ludwig Siemen (Munich: Oldenbourg, 1999), 327–62.
243. Roemer, 'Die V. Europäische Vereinigung', 53.
244. Max Müller, *Erinnerungen: Erlebte Psychiatriegeschichte 1920–1960* (Berlin, Heidelberg, and New York: Springer, 1982), 251.
245. Gabriele Rossi, 'Canevascini, Guglielmo', in *Historisches Lexikon Der Schweiz* (Berne, 2005), http://www.hls-dhs-dss.ch/textes/f/F3499.php.
246. Guglielmo Canevascini, 'Discours d'ouverture', *Gesundheit und Wohlfahrt - Revue Suisse d'Hygiene* 18, nos. 8/9 (1939): 347–48.
247. Repond, 'Die Bewegung für psychische Hygiene in der Schweiz'.
248. J.-D. Zbinden, 'L'organisateur: André Repond (1886–1973)', in *Portraits de psychiatres romands*, ed. Christian Müller (Lausanne: Éditions Payot, 1995), 9–76; Heinz Balmer, 'Walter Morgenthaler 1882–1965', *Verhandlungen der Schweizerischen Naturforschenden Gesellschaft* 146 (1966): 225–46; Vera Koelbing-Waldis, 'Maier, Hans Wolfgang', in *Historisches Lexikon der Schweiz* (Berne, 2008), https://hls-dhs-dss.ch/de/articles/014531/2008-02-27/.
249. André Repond, 'Geistige Hygiene und Politik', *Zeitschrift für psychische Hygiene* 4, no. 6 (1931): 183.
250. Sigmund Freud, *Massenpsychologie und Ich-Analyse* (Leipzig, Vienna, and Zurich: Internationaler Psychoanalytischer Verlag, 1921).
251. Repond, 'Geistige Hygiene', 183–84.
252. Ernst Kretschmer, 'Die konstitutionelle Retardierung und das Problem des sozialen Kontakts', *Gesundheit und Wohlfahrt - Revue Suisse d'Hygiene* 18, no. 8/9 (1939): 372.
253. Hans von Hattingberg, 'Die Bedeutung der polaren psychologischen Typen für die Verständigung', *Gesundheit und Wohlfahrt - Revue Suisse d'Hygiene* 18, nos. 8/9 (1939): 379–87; Carl Gustav Jung, *Psychologische Typen* (Zurich: Rascher, 1921).
254. Jacques Rivière, *L'Allemand: Souvenirs et réflexions d'un prisonnier de guerre* (Paris: Éditions de la Nouvelle Revue Française, 1919).
255. Hattingberg, 'Bedeutung', 387.
256. Bernhard Matz, 'Die Konstitutionstypologie von Ernst Kretschmer: Ein Beitrag zur Geschichte von Psychiatrie und Psychologie des Zwanzigsten Jahrhunderts' (MD thesis, Free University of Berlin, 2000), 4–9; Lockot, *Erinnern und Durcharbeiten*, 74–79.
257. Katharina Eva Keifenheim, 'Hans von Hattingberg between Psychoanalysis and National Socialism', *Luzif Amor* 24, no. 48 (2011): 106–25; Katharina

Eva Keifenheim, 'Hans von Hattingberg (1879–1944): Leben und Werk' (MD thesis, University of Tübingen, 2011); Geoffrey Cocks, *Psychotherapy in the Third Reich: The Göring Institute*, 2nd ed. (New Brunswick and London: Transaction, 1997).

258. Keifenheim, 'Hans von Hattingberg', 2011, 286–93.
259. Matz, 'Konstitutionstypologie', 4–9; Lockot, *Erinnern und Durcharbeiten*, 74–79.
260. Sioli, 'Ausbildung'.
261. Schneider, *Behandlung*, 421–23.
262. Roemer, 'Public Opinion', 284–85.
263. Ibid., 285.
264. Erwin Stransky, 'Richtungen der psychischen Hygiene: Nach einem Vortrag, gehalten am 9. Dezember 1931 in der Jahresversammlung der Gesellschaft für Volksaufartung und Erbkunde', *Wiener Klinische Wochenschrift* 45, no. 2 (1932): 42–46.
265. Thomas Plänkers, 'Hygiene der Seele: Heinrich Meng (1887–1972)', in *Psychoanalyse in Frankfurt am Main: Zerstörte Anfänge, Wiederannäherungen, Entwicklungen*, ed. Thomas Plänkers et al. (Tübingen: edition diskord, 1996), 109–40.
266. Heinrich Meng, *Leben als Begegnung* (Stuttgart: Hippokrates, 1971), 86.
267. Ibid., 25.
268. Ibid., 30–31.
269. Paul Federn and Heinrich Meng, eds., *Das psychoanalytische Volksbuch* (Stuttgart: Hippokrates, 1926).
270. Meng, *Leben als Begegnung*, 86–88.
271. Heinrich Meng, *Seelischer Gesundheitsschutz: Eine Einführung in Diagnostik, Forschung und Nutzanwendung der Psychohygiene* (Basel: Benno Schwabe, 1939); Heinrich Meng, *Praxis der seelischen Hygiene: Erfahrung und Experiment* (Basel: Benno Schwabe, 1943).
272. Meng, *Leben als Begegnung*, 90–91.
273. Ibid., 88.
274. Ibid., 93.
275. Ibid., 91.
276. Heinrich Meng, 'Erziehung zum Verstehen und zur Verständigung', *Gesundheit und Wohlfahrt - Revue Suisse d'Hygiene* 18, nos. 8/9 (1939): 417.
277. Ibid., 421–22.
278. Ibid., 423.
279. Müller, *Erinnerungen*, 251–52.
280. John Carl Flugel, *Proceedings of the International Conference on Mental Hygiene, 11th to 14th August 1948, London* (H. K. Lewis, 1948); Jonathan Toms, 'Political Dimensions of "The Psychosocial": The 1948 International Congress on Mental Health and the Mental Hygiene Movement', *History of the Human Sciences* 25, no. 5 (2012): 91–106.

281. Kenneth Soddy, 'The Mental Hygiene Movement and the Problem of Preventive Mental Health', in *Psychiatrie der Gegenwart: Forschung und Praxis, Vol. III: Soziale und Angewandte Psychiatrie*, ed. Hans W. Gruhle et al. (Berlin, Göttingen, and Heidelberg: Springer, 1961), 36–50.
282. P.-B. Schneider, O. Riggenbach, and R. Egli, 'Au Docteur André Repond, Directeur de la Maison de Santé de Malévoz, Monthey', *Zeitschrift für Präventivmedizin* 1 (1956): 429–31.
283. Hans Hoff, 'Entwicklung der psychischen Hygiene in Österreich', in *Bericht über die 6. Jahresversammlung der Weltvereinigung für Psychische Hygiene, Wien 16.-22. August 1953*, ed. Österreichische Gesellschaft für Psychische Hygiene (Vienna and Bonn: Wilhelm Maudrich, 1956), 21–30.
284. Ernst Brezina and Erwin Stransky, *Psychische Hygiene* (Vienna and Bonn: Wilhelm Maudrich, 1955).
285. Österreichische Gesellschaft für Psychische Hygiene, *Bericht über die 6. Jahresversammlung der Weltvereinigung für Psychische Hygiene, Wien 16.-22. August 1953* (Vienna and Bonn: Wilhelm Maudrich, 1956).
286. Hans Hoff, 'Zum Geleit', *Weltjahr für Geistige Gesundheit: Bulletin der Österreichischen Gesellschaft für Psychische Hygiene* 1 (1960): 1–2.
287. World Federation for Mental Health, 'Mental Health and World Citizenship: A Statement Prepared for the International Congress on Mental Health, London 1948', 1948, 25.

Archival Sources

Institut für Medizingeschichte, Universität Bern

Personennachlässe

Nachlass Walter Morgenthaler

Josephinum, Sammlungen der Medizinischen Universität Wien

Handschriftensammlung

Nachlass Erwin Stransky

LWL-Archivamt für Westfalen, Münster

926, Nachlass Hermann Simon

Österreichische Nationalbibliothek

Handschriften- und Nachlassabteilung

Nachlass Erwin Stransky H11/1980
Teilnachlass Julius Tandler H59/89

D. Freis, *Psycho-Politics between the World Wars*, Mental Health in Historical Perspective, https://doi.org/10.1007/978-3-030-32702-6

Sammelschwerpunkt Paul und Ernst Federn H37/2013

Stadt- und Landesarchiv Wien

1.3.2.119.A32.1939.5695/1939: Verein für angewandte Psychopathologie und Psychologie

1.3.2.119.A32 – Gelöschte Vereine / 1920-1974 ZI 8717/1935 Ärztliche Gesellschaft für Psychotherapie

Universitätsarchiv Gießen

Nachlass Robert Sommer

Universitätsarchiv Wien

Personalakten

PA 251, Kauders, Otto
PA 509, Stransky, Erwin
PA 798, Allers, Rudolf

Rigorosenakten

4783, Roffenstein, Gaston

Senatsakten

S 185.387 Disziplinaruntersuchung Stransky
S 304.924 Pappenheim, Martin

Bibliography

Adams, Andrea. *Psychopathologie und 'Rasse': Verhandlungen 'rassischer' Differenz in der Erforschung psychischer Leiden (1890–1933)*. Bielefeld: transcript, 2013.

Adams, Mark B. *The Wellborn Science: Eugenics in Germany, France, Brazil, and Russia*. New York: Oxford University Press, 1990.

Akavia, Naamah. *Subjectivity in Motion: Life, Art, and Movement in the Work of Hermann Rorschach*. New York and Hove: Routledge, 2013.

Alexander, Jeffrey C. *Trauma: A Social Theory*. Cambridge and Malden: Polity, 2012.

Allers, Rudolf. 'Die internationale Tagung für angewandte Psychopathologie und Psychologie'. *Zentralblatt für Psychotherapie* 3, no. 7 (1930): 389–94.

Alzheimer, Alois. 'Ist die Einrichtung einer psychiatrischen Abteilung im Reichsgesundheitsamt erstrebenswert?' *Zeitschrift für die gesamte Neurologie und Psychiatrie* 6 (1911): 242–46.

Andriopoulos, Stefan. *Possessed: Hypnotic Crimes, Corporate Fiction, and the Invention of Cinema*. Translated by Peter Jansen and Stefan Andriopoulos. Chicago: University of Chicago Press, 2008.

Angetter, Daniela. 'Erwin Stransky: Mitbegründer der modernen Schizophrenielehre', 2012. https://www.oeaw.ac.at/fileadmin/Institute/INZ/Bio_Archiv/bio_2012_01.htm.

Ankele, Monika. 'Arbeitsrhythmus und Anstaltsalltag: Eine Einführung in den Sammelband'. In *Arbeitsrhythmus und Anstaltsalltag: Arbeit in der Psychiatrie vom frühen 19. Jahrhundert bis in die NS-Zeit*, edited by Monika Ankele and Eva Brinkschulte, 9–18. Stuttgart: Franz Steiner, 2015.

Anonymous. 'Massenwahnsinn?' *Die Irrenrechts-Reform* 63 (1919): 181–84.

D. Freis, *Psycho-Politics between the World Wars*, Mental Health in Historical Perspective, https://doi.org/10.1007/978-3-030-32702-6

———. 'Psychiatrisches Ausbreitungsbedürfnis'. *Die Irrenrechts-Reform* 11 (1919): 197–99.

Ash, Mitchell G. 'Wissenschaft und Politik als Ressourcen für einander'. In *Wissenschaften und Wissenschaftspolitik: Bestandsaufnahmen zu Formationen, Brüchen und Kontinuitäten im Deutschland des 20. Jahrhunderts*, edited by Rüdiger vom Bruch and Brigitte Kaderas, 32–51. Stuttgart: Franz Steiner, 2002.

———. 'Wissenschaft(en) und Öffentlichkeit(en) als Ressourcen füreinander: Weiterführende Bemerkungen zur Beziehungsgeschichte'. In *Wissenschaft und Öffentlichkeit als Ressourcen füreinander: Studien zur Wissenschaftsgeschichte im 20. Jahrhundert*, edited by Sybilla Nikolow and Arne Schirrmacher, 349–64. Frankfurt am Main and New York: Campus, 2007.

Ash, Mitchell G., and Thomas Sturm. 'Die Psychologie in praktischen Kontexten: Einleitende Bemerkungen'. *Zeitschrift für Psychologie* 212 (2004): 177–82.

Aubry, Timothy, and Trysh Travis. *Rethinking Therapeutic Culture*. Chicago: Chicago University Press, 2015.

Balmer, Heinz. 'Walter Morgenthaler 1882–1965'. *Verhandlungen der Schweizerischen Naturforschenden Gesellschaft* 146 (1966): 225–46.

Bauer, Kurt. '"Heil Deutschösterreich!" Das deutschnationale Lager zu Beginn der Ersten Republik'. In *… … der Rest ist Österreich: Das Werden der Republik*, edited by Helmut Konrad and Wolfgang Maderthaner, 1:261–80. Vienna: Carl Gerold's Sohn, 2008.

Bauer-Merinsky, Judith. 'Die Auswirkungen der Annexion Österreichs durch das Deutsche Reich auf die medizinische Fakultät der Universität Wien im Jahre 1938: Biographien entlassener Professoren und Dozenten'. PhD Thesis, University of Vienna, 1980.

Beckh-Widmanstetter, H. A. 'Zur Geschichte der Individualpsychologie: Julius Wagner-Jauregg über Alfred Adler'. *Unsere Heimat* 36 (1965): 182–88.

Beddies, Thomas. '"Aktivere Krankenbehandlung" und "Arbeitstherapie:" Anwendungsformen und Begründungszusammenhänge bei Hermann Simon und Carl Schneider'. In *'Heroische Therapien:' Die deutsche Psychiatrie im internationalen Vergleich 1918–1945*, edited by Hans-Walter Schmuhl and Volker Roelcke, 268–86. Göttingen: Wallstein, 2013.

———. '"Generaloberstsachverständiger für alle Lebensformen und Lebensgestaltungen:" Zu gesellschaftlichen Vorstellungen von Ordnung und Normierung "angewandter Psychiatrie" nach dem Ersten Weltkrieg'. In *Norm als Zwang, Pflicht und Traum: Normierende versus individualisierende Bestrebungen in der Medizin*, edited by Eva Brinkschulte and Mariacarla Gadebusch Bondio, 103–34. Frankfurt am Main: Peter Lang, 2015.

Beers, Clifford W. *A Mind That Found Itself: An Autobiography*. New York: Longmans, Green, and Co., 1908.

———. *Eine Seele die sich wiederfand: Autobiographie des Begründers der 'Geistigen Hygiene'*. Translated by Otto Reuter. Basel: Benno Schwabe & Co., 1941.

Benetka, Gerhard. *Psychologie in Wien: Sozial- und Theoriegeschichte des Wiener Psychologischen Instituts 1922–1938*. Vienna: WUV, 1995.

Bergmann, Martin S. *The Hartmann Era*. New York: Other Press, 2000.

Bernays, Edward. *Propaganda: Die Kunst der Public Relations*. Translated by Patrick Schnur. Freiburg: Orange Press, 2007.

Bernfeld, Siegfried. 'Die Psychologie in der Arbeiterbewegung'. In *Antiautoritäre Erziehung und Psychoanalyse: Ausgewählte Schriften*, edited by Lutz von Werder and Reinhart Wolff, 3rd ed., 2:497–506. Frankfurt am Main: März, 1970.

Bessel, Richard. *Germany After the First World War*. Oxford: Clarendon Press, 1993.

Bietak, Wilhelm. 'Feuchtersleben, Ernst Maria Johann Karl von'. In *Neue Deutsche Biographie 5*, 105–8, 1961.

Binding, Karl, and Alfred Hoche. *Die Freigabe der Vernichtung lebensunwerten Lebens: Ihr Maß und ihre Form*. Leipzig: F. Meiner, 1920.

Birnbaum, Karl. *Grundzüge der Kulturpsychopathologie*. Munich: J. Bergmann, 1924.

Blaisdell, Russell E. 'Resume of Papers Presented at the International Congress on Mental Hygiene Held at Paris, July 19–24, 1937'. *Psychiatric Quarterly* 12, no. 1 (1938): 26–34.

Blasius, Dirk. *Einfache Seelenstörung: Geschichte der deutschen Psychiatrie 1800–1945*. Frankfurt am Main: Fischer, 1994.

Bleuler, Eugen. 'Vortrag über Ambivalenz'. *Zentralblatt für Psychoanalyse* 1 (1910): 266–68.

Blumesberger, Susanne, Michael Doppelhofer, Gabriele Mauthe, and Östereichische Nationalbibliothek, eds. *Handbuch österreichischer Autorinnen und Autoren jüdischer Herkunft, 18. bis 20. Jahrhundert*. Munich: Saur, 2002.

Boedeker, Justus Karl Edmund, and Wilhelm Falkenberg. *IV. Internationaler Kongress zur Fürsorge für Geisteskranke, Berlin, Oktober 1910: Offizieller Bericht*. Halle: Carl Marhold, 1911.

Bonhoeffer, Karl. 'Inwieweit sind politische, soziale und kulturelle Zustände einer psychopathologischen Betrachtung zugänglich?' *Klinische Wochenschrift* 2 (1923): 598–601.

Bormuth, Matthias. 'Karl Jaspers the Pathographer'. In *One Century of Karl Jaspers' General Psychopathology*, edited by Giovanni Stanghellini and Thomas Fuchs, 133–49. Oxford: Oxford University Press, 2013.

Br. 'Der Deutschenhaß: Eine Studie von Erwin Stransky'. *Deutsche Revue* 45 (1920): 93.

Brennecke, Hans. 'Debilität, Kriminalität und Revolution'. *Archiv für Psychiatrie und Nervenkrankheiten* 63, no. 1 (1921): 247–60.

———. *Zur Frage der Psychologie und Psychopathologie der Revolution und der Revolutionäre*. Langensalza: Beyer, 1922.

———. 'Zur Frage der Psychopathologie der Revolution und der Revolutionäre'. *Zeitschrift für Kinderforschung* 26, no. 5 (1921): 225–31.

Brezina, Ernst, and Erwin Stransky. *Psychische Hygiene*. Vienna and Bonn: Wilhelm Maudrich, 1955.

Brink, Cornelia. *Grenzen der Anstalt: Psychiatrie und Gesellschaft in Deutschland 1860–1980*. Göttingen: Wallstein, 2010.

———. 'Keine Angst vor dem Psychiater: Psychiatrie, Psychiatriekritik und Öffentlichkeit in der Bundesrepublik Deutschland (1960–1980)'. In *'Moderne' Anstaltspsychiatrie im 19. und 20. Jahrhundert: Legitimation und Kritik*, edited by Heiner Fangerau and Karen Nolte, 341–60. Stuttgart: Steiner, 2006.

Brückweh, Kerstin, Dirk Schumann, Richard F. Wetzell, and Benjamin Ziemann, eds. *Engineering Society: The Role of the Human and Social Sciences in Modern Societies, 1880–1980*. London: Palgrave Macmillan, 2012.

Bruendel, Steffen. *Volksgemeinschaft oder Volksstaat: Die Ideen von 1914 und die Neuordnung Deutschlands im Ersten Weltkrieg*. Berlin: Akademie, 2003.

Budde, Gerhard. 'Die seelische Gesundung unseres Volkes'. *Blätter für Volksgesundheitspflege* 20, no. 1 (1920): 7–10.

Bugmann, Mirjam. *Hypnosepolitik: Der Psychiater August Forel, das Gehirn und die Gesellschaft (1870–1920)*. Vienna, Cologne, and Weimar: Böhlau, 2015.

Bumke, Oswald, Gustav Kolb, Hans Roemer, and Eugen Kahn. *Handwörterbuch der psychischen Hygiene und der psychiatrischen Fürsorge*. Berlin and Leipzig: Walter de Gruyter, 1931.

Burgmair, Wolfgang, Eric J. Engstrom, and Matthias M. Weber. *Emil Kraepelin*. 7 vols. Munich: Belleville, 2000.

Canevascini, Guglielmo. 'Discours d'ouverture'. *Gesundheit und Wohlfahrt - Revue Suisse d'Hygiene* 18, no. 8/9 (1939): 346–48.

Carus, Carl Gustav. *Ueber Geistes-Epidemien der Menschheit*. Leipzig and Meissen: F. W. Goedsche'sche Buchhandlung, 1852.

Caruth, Cathy. *Unclaimed Experience: Trauma, Narrative, and History*. Baltimore: Johns Hopkins University Press, 1996.

Cassata, Francesco. *Building the New Man. Eugenics, Racial Science and Genetics in Twentieth Century Italy*. Budapest, New York: Central European University Press, 2011.

Cimino, Guido, and Giovanni Pietro Lombardo. *Sante de Sanctis tra psicologia generale e psicologia applicata*. Milan: Franco Angeli, 2004.

Clark, Michael, and Catherine Crawford. *Legal History in Medicine*. Cambridge: Cambridge University Press, 1994.

Cocks, Geoffrey. *Psychotherapy in the Third Reich: The Göring Institute*. 2nd ed. New Brunswick and London: Transaction, 1997.

Cohen, Yves. *Le siècle des chefs: Une histoire transnationale du commandement et de l'autorité (1890–1940)*. Paris: Éditions Amsterdam, 2013.

Cowan, Michael. *Cult of the Will: Nervousness and German Modernity*. Pennsylvania: The Pennsylvania State University Press, 2008.

Crouthamel, Jason. *The Great War and German Memory: Society, Politics and Psychological Trauma, 1914–1945*. Exeter: University of Exeter Press, 2009.

Crouthamel, Jason, and Peter Leese, eds. *Psychological Trauma and the Legacies of the First World War*. Basingstoke: Palgrave Macmillan, 2017.

Dain, Norman. *Clifford W. Beers: Advocate of the Insane*. Pittsburgh: University of Pittsburgh Press, 1980.

Dannemann, Adolf. 'Irrenwesen'. In *Handwörterbuch der sozialen Hygiene*, edited by Alfred Grotjahn and Ignaz Kaup, 1:510–23. Leipzig: F.C.W. Vogel, 1912.

Danto, Elizabeth Ann. *Freud's Free Clinics: Psychoanalysis and Social Justice, 1918–1938*. New York: Columbia University Press, 2005.

Decker, Hannah S. *Freud in Germany: Revolution and Reaction in Science, 1893–1907*. New York: International Universities Press, 1977.

'Der II. Internationale Kongreß für psychische Hygiene'. *Zeitschrift für psychische Hygiene* 9, no. 4 (1936): 127–28.

'Die Gesellschaft Deutscher Neurologen und Psychiater'. *Zeitschrift für psychische Hygiene* 8, no. 1 (1935): 1.

'Die Halle 51 der Dresdner Hygieneausstellung'. *Zentralblatt für Psychotherapie* 3, no. 10 (1930): 627–31.

Donath, Julius. 'August Forel†'. *Zeitschrift für die gesamte Neurologie und Psychiatrie* 136 (1931): 642–44.

Dörner, Klaus. *Bürger und Irre: Zur Sozialgeschichte und Wissenschaftssoziologie der Psychiatrie*. Frankfurt am Main: Fischer, 1975.

———. 'Über den Gebrauch klinischer Begriffe in der politischen Diskussion'. In *Die Linke antwortet Jürgen Habermas*, edited by Oskar Negt, 59–69. Frankfurt am Main: Europäische Verlagsanstalt, 1968.

Dowbiggin, Ian Robert. *Keeping America Sane: Psychiatry and Eugenics in the United States and Canada, 1880–1940*. 2nd ed. Ithaca, NY: Cornell University Press, 2003.

Dreikurs, Rudolf. 'Der gegenwärtige Stand der psychischen Hygiene in Wien'. *Volksgesundheit: Zeitschrift für soziale Hygiene* 3, no. 10 (1929): 211–21.

———. 'Die Entwicklung der psychischen Hygiene in Wien: Unter besonderer Berücksichtigung der Alkoholiker- und Psychopathen-(Selbstmörder-)fürsorge'. *Allgemeine Zeitschrift für Psychiatrie und psychisch-gerichtliche Medizin* 88, no. 8 (1928): 469–89.

Dufaud, Grégory. 'Politiser la médecine: La psychiatrie extrahospitalière en Russie soviétique (années 1920 et début des années 1930)'. *Revue d'histoire moderne & contemporaine* 61, no. 3 (2014): 125–48.

Eckart, Wolfgang U. *Medizin und Krieg: Deutschland 1914–1924*. Paderborn: Schöningh, 2014.

Eghigian, Greg. 'A Drifting Concept for an Unruly Menace: A History of Psychopathy in Germany'. *Isis* 106, no. 2 (2015): 283–309.

———. 'Deinstitutionalizing the History of Contemporary Psychiatry'. *History of Psychiatry* 22, no. 2 (2011): 201–14.

Ehrentheil, Otto F. 'The Almost Forgotten Feuchtersleben: Poet, Essayist, Popular Philosopher and Psychiatrist'. *Journal of the History of the Behavioral Sciences* 11, no. 1 (1975): 82–86.

Eissler, Kurt R. *Freud und Wagner-Jauregg vor der Kommission zur Erhebung militärischer Pflichtverletzungen*. 2nd ed. Vienna: Löcker, 2007.

———. 'Julius Wagner-Jaureggs Gutachten über Sigmund Freud und seine Studien zur Psychoanalyse'. *Wiener Klinische Wochenschrift* 70, no. 22 (1958): 401–7.

Eitler, Pascal, Jens Elberfeld, Sabine Maasen, and Maik Tändler. *Das beratene Selbst: Zur Genealogie der Therapeutisierung in den 'langen' Siebzigern*. Bielefeld: transcript, 2011.

Engstrom, Eric J. *Clinical Psychiatry in Imperial Germany*. Ithaca: Cornell University Press, 2003.

———. 'Emil Kraepelin: Psychiatry and Public Affairs in Wilhelmine Germany'. *History of Psychiatry* 2, no. 6 (1991): 111–32.

———. '"On the Question of Degeneration" by Emil Kraepelin (1908)'. *History of Psychiatry* 18, no. 3 (2007): 389–98.

———. 'Organizing Psychiatric Research in Munich (1903–1925): A Psychiatric Zoon Politicon between State Bureaucracy and American Philanthropy'. In *International Relations in Psychiatry: Britain, Germany, and the United States to World War II*, edited by Volker Roelcke, Paul Weindling, and Louise Westwood, 48–66. Rochester: Rochester University Press, 2010.

Engstrom, Eric J., Wolfgang Burgmair, and Matthias M. Weber. 'Psychiatric Governance, Völkisch Corporatism, and the German Research Institute of Psychiatry in Munich (1912–26): Part 1'. *History of Psychiatry* 27 (2016): 38–50.

———. 'Psychiatric Governance, Völkisch Corporatism, and the German Research Institute of Psychiatry in Munich (1912–26), Part 2'. *History of Psychiatry* 27 (2016): 137–52.

Engstrom, Eric J., and Ivan Crozier. 'Race, Alcohol and General Paralysis: Emil Kraepelin's Comparative Psychiatry and His Trips to Java (1904) and North America (1925)'. *History of Psychiatry* 29, no. 3 (2018): 263–81.

Engstrom, Eric J., and Matthias M. Weber. 'Making Kraepelin History: A Great Instauration?' *History of Psychiatry* 18, no. 3 (2007): 267–73.

———. '"On Uprootedness" by Emil Kraepelin (1921)'. *History of Psychiatry* 21, no. 3 (2010): 340–50.

Enke, Ulrike. 'Die ersten Jahre der psychiatrischen Universitätsklinik Gießen unter ihrem Direktor Robert Sommer'. In *Psychiatrie in Gießen: Facetten ihrer Geschichte zwischen Fürsorge und Ausgrenzung, Forschung und Heilung*, edited by

Uta George, Herwig Groß, Michael Putzke, Irmtraud Sahmland, and Christina Vanja, 59–92. Gießen: Psychosozial-Verlag, 2003.

———. 'Ein Liebig-Museum in Gießen: Der Psychiater Robert Sommer, die chemische Hexenküche und das Gießener Liebig-Museum'. *Mitteilungen des oberhessischen Geschichtsvereins* 89 (2004): 63–86.

Etkind, Alexander. *Eros des Unmöglichen: Die Geschichte der Psychoanalyse in Rußland*. Translated by Andreas Tretner. Leipzig: Gustav Kiepenheuer, 1996.

Etzemüller, Thomas. *Die Ordnung der Moderne: Social Engineering im 20. Jahrhundert*. Bielefeld: transcript, 2009.

———. 'Social engineering als Verhaltenslehre des kühlen Kopfes: Eine einleitende Skizze'. In *Die Ordnung der Moderne: Social Engineering im 20. Jahrhundert*, edited by Thomas Etzemüller, 11–40. Bielefeld: transcript, 2009.

Fallend, Karl. 'Marie Frischauf-Pappenheim'. In *Personenlexikon der Sexualforschung*, edited by Volkmar Sigusch, 204–6. Frankfurt am Main: Campus, 2009.

———. *Sonderlinge, Träumer, Sensitive: Psychoanalyse auf dem Weg zur Institution und Profession. Protokolle der Wiener Psychoanalytischen Vereinigung und biographische Studien*. Vienna: Jugend & Volk, 1995.

Federn, Paul. 'Der neurotische Stil'. In *I. Internationale Tagung für angewandte Psychopathologie und Psychologie, Wien, 5.-7. Juni 1930: Referate und Vorträge*, edited by Heinz Hartmann, Martin Pappenheim, and Erwin Stransky, 194–201. Berlin: S. Karger, 1931.

———. 'Schutz vor Nerven- und Geisteskrankheiten'. In *Das psychoanalytische Volksbuch*, edited by Paul Federn and Heinrich Meng, 224–30. Stuttgart: Hippokrates, 1926.

———. *Zur Psychologie der Revolution: Die vaterlose Gesellschaft*. Leipzig and Vienna: Anzengruber, 1919.

Federn, Paul, and Heinrich Meng, eds. *Das psychoanalytische Volksbuch*. Stuttgart: Hippokrates, 1926.

Feichtinger, Johannes. 'Kulturelle Marginalität und wissenschaftliche Kreativität: Jüdische Intellektuelle im Österreich der Zwischenkriegszeit'. In *Das Gewebe der Kultur: Kulturwissenschaftliche Analysen zur Geschichte und Identität Österreichs in der Moderne*, edited by Johannes Feichtinger and Peter Stachel, 311–34. Innsbruck, Vienna, and Munich: Studien Verlag, 2001.

Feldkeller, Paul. *Wörterbuch der Psychopolitik*. Berne and Munich: A. Francke, 1967.

Ferenczi, Sándor. 'Die Psychoanalyse der Kriegsneurosen'. In *Zur Psychoanalyse der Kriegsneurosen: Diskussion gehalten auf dem V. Internationalen Psychoanalytischen Kongress in Budapest, 28. und 29. September 1918*, 9–30. Leipzig and Vienna: Internationaler psychoanalytischer Verlag, 1919.

Feuchtersleben, Ernst von. *Lehrbuch der ärztlichen Seelenkunde*. Vienna: C. Gerold, 1845.

———. *Zur Diätetik der Seele*. Vienna: Carl Armbruster, 1838.

Fink, Angela. *Kunst in der Psychiatrie: Verklärt - Verfolgt - Vermarktet*. Vienna and Berlin: LIT, 2012.
Fischer-Homberger, Esther. *Die traumatische Neurose: Vom somatischen zum sozialen Leiden*. Bern: H. Huber, 1975.
———. *Krankheit Frau: Zur Geschichte der Einbildungen*. Darmstadt: Luchterhand, 1984.
———. *Medizin vor Gericht: Zur Sozialgeschichte der Gerichtsmedizin*. Darmstadt: Luchterhand, 1988.
Flemming, Jens. 'Gegen die intellektualistische Zersetzung der alten moralischen Werte. Die Süddeutschen Monatshefte zwischen Krieg und Nationalsozialismus'. In *Le milieu intellectuel conservateur en Allemagne, sa presse et ses réseaux*, edited by Michel Grunewald, 165–201. Berne: Peter Lang, 2003.
Flugel, John Carl. *Proceedings of the International Conference on Mental Hygiene, 11th to 14th August 1948, London*. H.K. Lewis & Co., 1948.
Föllmer, Moritz. 'Der "kranke Volkskörper": Industrielle, hohe Beamte und der Diskurs der nationalen Regeneration in der Weimarer Republik'. *Geschichte und Gesellschaft* 27 (2001): 41–67.
Föllmer, Moritz, Rüdiger Graf, and Per Leo. 'Die Kultur der Krise in der Weimarer Republik'. In *Die 'Krise' der Weimarer Republik: Zur Kritik eines Deutungsmusters*, edited by Moritz Föllmer and Rüdiger Graf, 9–41. Frankfurt am Main and New York: Campus, 2005.
Forel, Auguste. 'Der Begriff des Monismus'. *Der Monismus* 3, no. 1 (1908): 10–14.
———. *Die Gehirnhygiene der Schüler*. Vienna: Manzsche k.u.k. Hof-Verlags- und Universitätsbuchhandlung, 1908.
———. *Die sexuelle Frage: Eine naturwissenschaftliche, psychologische, hygienische und soziologische Studie für Gebildete*. Munich: Ernst Reinhardt, 1905.
———. *Die Trinksitten, ihre hygienische und sociale Bedeutung und ihre Beziehungen zur akademischen Jugend*. Stuttgart: Ferdinand Enke, 1891.
———. *Die Vereinigten Staaten der Erde: Ein Kulturprogramm*. Berne and Lausanne: Otto Volkart and E. Peytrequin, 1914.
———. *Gehirn und Seele: Ein Vortrag gehalten bei der 66. Versammlung deutscher Naturforscher und Aerzte in Wien am 26. September 1894*. Bonn: Emil Strauss, 1894.
———. *Hygiene der Nerven und des Geistes im gesunden und kranken Zustande*. 4th ed. Stuttgart: Ernst Heinrich Moritz, 1913.
———. *Hygiene of Nerves and Mind in Health and Disease*. Translated by Herbert Austin Aikins. New York and London: G.P. Putnam's Son, 1907.
———. *Malthusianismus oder Eugenik?* Munich: E. Reinhardt, 1911.
———. *Mensch und Ameise: Ein Beitrag zur Frage der Vererbung und Fortschrittsfähigkeit*. Vienna, Berlin, and Leipzig: Rikola, 1922.
———. *Rückblick auf mein Leben*. Zurich: Europa-Verlag, 1935.

Forel, Oscar Louis. 'Walter Morgenthaler als Pionier der Pflegerausbildung'. *Schweizerische Zeitschrift für Psychologie und ihre Anwendungen* 9, no. 1 (1952): 5–10.

Forsbach, Ralf. *Die Medizinische Fakultät der Universität Bonn im 'Dritten Reich'*. Munich: Oldenbourg, 2006.

———. 'Friedrich Panse – etabliert in allen Systemen: Psychiater in der Weimarer Republik, im "Dritten Reich" und in der Bundesrepublik'. *Der Nervenarzt* 83, no. 3 (2012): 329–36.

'Frau Nelly Grosanescu vor den Geschworenen: Heute beginnt der Sensationsprozeß'. *Die Neue Zeitung*, 22 June 1927.

Freimark, Hans. *Die Revolution als psychische Massenerscheinung: Historisch-psychologische Studie*. Munich and Wiesbaden: J. F. Bergmann, 1920.

Freis, David. 'Diagnosing the Kaiser: Psychiatry, Wilhelm II and the Question of German War Guilt'. *Medical History* 62, no. 3 (2018): 273–94.

———. 'Psyche, Trauma und Kollektiv: Der psychiatrische Diskurs über die erschütterten Nerven der Nation'. In *Nerven und Krieg: Psychische Mobilisierungs- und Leidenserfahrungen in Deutschland 1900–1933*, edited by Gundula Gahlen and Oliver Janz. Frankfurt am Main and New York: Campus, forthcoming.

———. '"Subordination, Authority, Psychotherapy:" Psychotherapy and Politics in Inter-War Vienna'. *History of the Human Sciences* 30, no. 2 (2017): 34–53.

———. 'Vertrauen und Subordination: Das psychotherapeutische Ambulatorium der Universität Wien, 1918–1938'. *Schriftenreihe der Deutschen Gesellschaft für Geschichte der Nervenheilkunde* 21 (2015): 557–85.

Freud, Sigmund. *Massenpsychologie und Ich-Analyse*. Leipzig, Vienna, and Zurich: Internationaler Psychoanalytischer Verlag, 1921.

———. 'Zeitgemäßes über Krieg und Tod'. In *Das Unbehagen in der Kultur und andere kulturtheoretische Schriften*, 10th ed., 133–62. Frankfurt am Main: Fischer, 2007.

Frevert, Ute. 'Neue Politikgeschichte: Konzepte und Herausforderungen'. In *Neue Politikgeschichte: Perspektiven einer historischen Politikforschung*, edited by Ute Frevert and Heinz-Gerhard Haupt, 7–26. Frankfurt am Main and New York: Campus, 2005.

Fromm, Erich. 'Forel, August: Rückblick auf mein Leben, 1935'. *Zeitschrift für Sozialforschung* 4, no. 1 (1935): 112–14.

Fussinger, Catherine. '"Therapeutic Community," Psychiatry's Reformers and Antipsychiatrists: Reconsidering Changes in the Field of Psychiatry after World War II'. *History of Psychiatry* 22, no. 2 (2011): 146–63.

Galant, Johann Susmann. 'Robert Sommers Idee der öffentlichen Ruhehallen und ihre Verwirklichung in Sowjet-Rußland'. *Zeitschrift für psychische Hygiene* 1, no. 3 (1928): 91–92.

Galassi, Silviana. *Kriminologie im Deutschen Kaiserreich: Geschichte einer gebrochenen Verwissenschaftlichung*. Stuttgart: Franz Steiner, 2004.

Garscha, Winfried R. 'Euthanasie-Prozesse seit 1945 in Österreich und Deutschland'. In *Medizin im Nationalsozialismus - Wege der Aufarbeitung*, edited by Sonia Horn and Peter Malina, 46–58. Wiener Gespräche zur Sozialgeschichte der Medizin. Vienna: ÖÄK Verlag, 2001.

Gaupp, L. 'Rückblick auf Führungen in der Abteilung des Deutschen Verbandes für psychische Hygiene auf der Internationalen Hygiene-Ausstellung Dresden 1930 und 1931'. *Zeitschrift für psychische Hygiene* 5, no. 6 (1932): 163–67.

Gaupp, Robert. 'Der Arzt als Erzieher seines Volkes'. *Blätter für Volksgesundheitspflege* 19, no. 9/10 (1919): 77–80.

———. 'Der nervöse Zusammenbruch und die Revolution'. *Blätter für Volksgesundheitspflege* 19, no. 5/6 (1919): 43–46.

———. 'Die Unfruchtbarmachung geistig und sittlich Minderwertiger: Erweitertes Referat, erstattet auf der Jahresversammlung des Deutschen Vereins für Psychiatrie am 2. September 1925 in Kassel'. *Zeitschrift für die gesamte Neurologie und Psychiatrie* 100 (1926): 139–81.

———. *Die zukünftige Stellung des Arztes im Volke: Ansprache an die Studierenden der Medizin der Universität Tübingen (23. X. 1919)*. Tübingen: H. Laupp, 1919.

Gay, Peter. *Freud: Eine Biographie für unsere Zeit*. Translated by Joachim A. Frank. 2nd ed. Frankfurt am Main: Fischer, 2006.

Germann, Urs. *Psychiatrie und Strafjustiz: Entstehung, Praxis und Ausdifferenzierung der forensischen Psychiatrie in der deutschsprachigen Schweiz 1850–1950*. Zurich: Chronos, 2004.

Gerwarth, Robert. *The Bismarck Myth: Weimar Germany and the Legacy of the Iron Chancellor*. Oxford: Clarendon Press, 2005.

'Gesetz zur Verhütung erbkranken Nachwuchses vom 14. Juli 1933'. *Zeitschrift für psychische Hygiene* 6, no. 5 (1933): 152–55.

Geuter, Ulfried. 'Polemos panton pater - Militär und Psychologie im Deutschen Reich 1914–1945'. In *Geschichte der deutschen Psychologie im 20. Jahrhundert: Ein Überblick*, edited by Mitchell G. Ash and Ulfried Geuter, 146–71. Opladen: Westdeutscher Verlag, 1985.

Geyer, Martin H. *Verkehrte Welt: Revolution, Inflation und Moderne: München 1914–1924*. Göttingen: Vandenhoeck & Ruprecht, 1998.

Gijswijt-Hofstra, Marijke, and Roy Porter, eds. *Cultures of Neurasthenia from Beard to the First World War*. Amsterdam: Rodopi, 2001.

Ginneken, Jaap van. *Crowds, Psychology and Politics, 1871–1899*. Cambridge: Cambridge University Press, 1992.

Göring, Matthias Heinrich, and Carl Gustav Jung. 'Geheimrat Sommer zum 70. Geburtstag'. *Zentralblatt für Psychotherapie* 7, no. 2 (1934): 313–14.

Goschler, Constantin. 'Wahrheit zwischen Seziersaal und Parlament: Rudolf Virchow und der kulturelle Deutungsanspruch der Naturwissenschaften'. *Geschichte und Gesellschaft* 30, no. 2 (2004): 219–49.

Gottstein, Adolf. 'Soziale Hygiene und Gesundheitsfürsorge'. In *Handwörterbuch der psychischen Hygiene und der psychiatrischen Fürsorge*, edited by Oswald Bumke, Gustav Kolb, Hans Roemer, and Eugen Kahn, 330–40. Berlin and Leipzig: Walter de Gruyter, 1931.

Graf, Rüdiger. 'Optimismus und Pessimismus in der Krise: Der politisch-kulturelle Diskurs in der Weimarer Republik'. In *Ordnungen in der Krise: Zur politischen Kulturgeschichte Deutschlands 1900–1933*, edited by Wolfgang Hardtwig, 115–40. München: Oldenbourg, 2007.

Grigorenko, Elena L., Patricia Ruzgis, and Robert J. Sternberg. *Psychology in Russia: Past, Present, Future.* Commack, NY: Nova Science Publishers, 1997.

Grob, Gerald N. 'The Attack on Psychiatric Legitimacy in the 1960s: Rhetoric and Reality'. *Journal of the History of the Behavioral Sciences* 47, no. 4 (2011): 398–416.

Groddeck, Carl Theodor. *Die demokratische Krankheit, eine neue Wahnsinnsform.* Naumburg: H. Sieling, 1850.

Gröger, Helmut. 'Die Entwicklung der psychischen Hygiene von der Bewegung zur psychiatrischen Disziplin - der österreichische Weg'. *Schriftenreihe der Deutschen Gesellschaft für Geschichte der Nervenheilkunde* 18 (2012): 221–31.

———. 'Josef K. Friedjung'. In *Vertriebene Vernunft II: Emigration und Exil österreichischer Wissenschaft. Internationales Symposium, 19. bis 23. Oktober 1987 in Wien*, edited by Friedrich Stadler, 819–26. Vienna and Munich: Jugend und Volk, 1988.

Groß, Adolf. 'Zeitgemäße Betrachtungen zum wirtschaftlichen Betrieb der Irrenanstalten'. *Allgemeine Zeitschrift für die Psychiatrie und psychisch-gerichtliche Medizin* 76, no. 1 (1923): 60–74.

Gross, Otto. 'Zur Ueberwindung der kulturellen Krise'. *Die Aktion* 3, no. 14 (1913): 384–87.

Grotjahn, Alfred, and Ignaz Kaup. *Handwörterbuch der sozialen Hygiene.* 2 vols. Leipzig: F.C.W. Vogel, 1912.

Groys, Boris. *The Total Art of Stalinism: Avant-Garde, Aesthetic, Dictatorship, and Beyond.* Translated by Charles Rougle. Princeton, NJ: Princeton University Press, 1992.

Gundlach, Horst. 'Reine Psychologie, Angewandte Psychologie und die Institutionalisierung der Psychologie'. *Zeitschrift für Psychologie* 212 (2004): 183–99.

Habermas, Jürgen. 'Die Scheinrevolution und ihre Kinder'. In *Die Linke antwortet Jürgen Habermas*, edited by Oskar Negt, 5–15. Frankfurt am Main: Europäische Verlagsanstalt, 1968.

Hacking, Ian. 'Making Up People'. In *Forms of Desire: Sexual Orientation and the Social Constructionist Controversy*, edited by Edward Stein, 69–88. New York: Routledge, 1992.

Hahnemann, Andy. '"Der Tod jagt durch die Straßen …": Zur Psychopathologisierung der Revolution in Max Glass' Die entfesselte Menschheit (1919)'. In *Friede, Freiheit, Brot! Romane zur deutschen Novemberrevolution*, edited by Ullrich Kittstein and Regine Zeller, 41–58. Amsterdam: Rodopi, 2009.

Hallervorden, Eugen. *Arbeit und Wille: Personenkunde oder klinische Psychologie zur Grundlegung der Psychohygiene*. Würzburg: A. Stuber, 1897.

———. 'Klinische Psychologie, die Vorstufe der Psychohygiene'. *Deutsche Medizinische Wochenschrift* 22, no. 41 (1896): 656–59.

Hamann, Brigitte. *Hitlers Wien: Lehrjahre eines Diktators*. 3rd ed. Munich: Piper, 1996.

Hamdorf, Friedrich Wilhelm. 'Loeb, James'. In *Neue Deutsche Biographie*, 15:18–19, 1987.

Han, Byung-Chul. *Psychopolitik: Neoliberalismus und die neuen Machttechniken*. Frankfurt am Main: S. Fischer, 2014.

Hardtwig, Wolfgang. 'Der Bismarck-Mythos: Gestalt und Funktionen zwischen politischer Öffentlichkeit und Wissenschaft'. In *Politische Kulturgeschichte der Zwischenkriegszeit 1918–1939*, edited by Wolfgang Hardtwig, 61–90. Göttingen: Vandenhoeck & Ruprecht, 2005.

Harms, Ingo. 'Die Gutachter der Meldebogen: Kurzbiografien'. In *Die nationalsozialistische 'Euthanasie'-Aktion T4 und ihre Opfer: Geschichte und ethische Konsequenzen für die Gegenwart*, edited by Maike Rotzoll, Gerrit Hohendorf, Petra Fuchs, Paul Richter, Christoph Mundt, and Wolfgang U. Eckart, 405–20. Paderborn: Ferdinand Schöningh, 2010.

Hartmann, Heinz, Martin Pappenheim, and Erwin Stransky, eds. *I. Internationale Tagung für angewandte Psychopathologie und Psychologie, Wien, 5.-7. Juni 1930: Referate und Vorträge*. Berlin: S. Karger, 1931.

Hattingberg, Hans von. 'Die Bedeutung der polaren psychologischen Typen für die Verständigung'. *Gesundheit und Wohlfahrt - Revue Suisse d'Hygiene* 18, no. 8/9 (1939): 379–87.

Hau, Michael. 'The Humane Expert: The Crisis of Modern Medicine During the Weimar Republic'. In *Experts in Science and Society*, edited by Elke Kurz-Milcke and Gerd Gigerenzer, 105–22. New York: Springer, 2004.

Haymann, Hermann. 'Irrenärztliche Bemerkungen zu Heinrich Mann's neuem Buch'. *Zeitschrift für die gesamte Neurologie und Psychiatrie* 39 (1918): 225–28.

Heinemann, Ulrich. *Die verdrängte Niederlage: Politische Öffentlichkeit und Kriegsschuldfrage in der Weimarer Republik*. Göttingen: Vandenhoeck & Ruprecht, 1983.

Herrn, Rainer. 'Vom Traum zum Trauma: Das Institut für Sexualwissenschaft, 1919–1933'. In *Der Sexualreformer Magnus Hirschfeld: Ein Leben im Spannungsfeld von Wissenschaft, Politik und Gesellschaft*, edited by Elke-Vera Kotowski and Julius Schoeps, 173–200. Berlin: Be.Bra Wissenschaft, 2004.

Hess, Volker, and Benoît Majerus. 'Writing the History of Psychiatry in the 20th Century'. *History of Psychiatry* 22, no. 2 (2011): 139–45.

Hess, Volker, and Heinz-Peter Schmiedebach, eds. *Am Rande des Wahnsinns: Schwellräume einer urbanen Moderne*. Vienna, Cologne, and Weimar: Böhlau, 2012.

Hilberg, Raul. *Die Vernichtung der europäischen Juden: Die Gesamtgeschichte des Holocaust*. Translated by Christian Seeger, Harry Maòr, Walle Bengs, and Wilfried Sczepan. Berlin: Olle & Wolter, 1982.

Hildebrandt, Kurt. 'Forensische Begutachtung eines Spartakisten'. *Allgemeine Zeitschrift für die Psychiatrie und psychisch-gerichtliche Medizin* 76 (1919): 479–518.

Hilken, Susanne, Matthias Bormuth, and Michael Schmidt-Degenhardt. 'Psychiatrische Anfänge der Pathographie'. In *Kunst und Krankheit: Studien zur Pathographie*, edited by Matthias Bormuth, Klaus Podoll, and Carsten Spitzer, 11–26. Göttingen: Wallstein, 2007.

Hippius, Hanns, Hans-Jürgen Möller, Norbert Müller, and Gabriele Neundörfer. *Die Psychiatrische Klinik der Universität München 1904–2004*. Heidelberg: Springer, 2005.

Hirschfeld, Magnus. *Verstaatlichung des Gesundheitswesens*. Berlin: E. Berger, 1919.

Hirschlaff, Leo. 'Zur Psychologie und Hygiene des Denkens'. *Zeitschrift für die gesamte Neurologie und Psychiatrie* 6, no. 1 (1911): 215–41.

Hitschmann, Eduard. 'Prof. Dr. E. Stransky (Wien): Psychopathologie der Ausnahmezustände und Psychopathologie des Alltags'. *Internationale Zeitschrift für Psychoanalyse* 8, no. 2 (1922): 222–23.

———. 'Prof. Erwin Stransky: Psychoanalyse und Kritik'. *Internationale Zeitschrift für Psychoanalyse* 8, no. 2 (1922): 223.

———. 'R. Allers: Über Psychoanalyse'. *Internationale Zeitschrift für Psychoanalyse* 10, no. 4 (1924): 476.

———. 'Zehn Jahre Wiener Psychoanalytisches Ambulatorium: Zur Geschichte des Ambulatoriums'. *Internationale Zeitschrift für Psychoanalyse* 38, no. 2 (1932): 265–71.

Hoeres, Peter. *Krieg der Philosophen: Die deutsche und britische Philosophie im Ersten Weltkrieg*. Paderborn: Schöningh, 2004.

Hofer, Hans-Georg. 'Beyond Freud and Wagner-Jauregg: War, Psychiatry and the Habsburg Army'. In *War, Trauma and Medicine in Germany and Central Europe (1914–1939)*, edited by Hans-Georg Hofer, Cay-Rüdiger Prüll, and Wolfgang U. Eckart, 49–71. Freiburg: Centaurus, 2011.

———. *Nervenschwäche und Krieg: Modernitätskritik und Krisenbewältigung in der österreichischen Psychiatrie (1880–1920)*. Vienna, Cologne, and Weimar: Böhlau, 2004.

Hoff, Hans. 'Entwicklung der psychischen Hygiene in Österreich'. In *Bericht über die 6. Jahresversammlung der Weltvereinigung für Psychische Hygiene, Wien 16.-22. August 1953*, edited by Österreichische Gesellschaft für Psychische Hygiene, 21–30. Vienna and Bonn: Wilhelm Maudrich, 1956.

———. 'In Memoriam: Univ.-Professor Dr. Erwin Stransky'. *Wiener Medizinische Wochenschrift* 112, no. 9 (1962): 181–82.

———. 'Zum Geleit'. *Weltjahr für Geistige Gesundheit: Bulletin der Österreichischen Gesellschaft für Psychische Hygiene* 1 (1960): 1–2.

Hoffmann, Hermann F. 'Der Psychiater und die neue Zeit'. *Zeitschrift für psychische Hygiene* 6, no. 6 (1933): 161–67.

Hohendorf, Gerrit. 'Therapieunfähigkeit als Selektionskriterium: Die "Schocktherapieverfahren" und die Organisationszentrale der nationalsozialistischen "Euthanasie" in der Berliner Tiergartenstraße 4, 1939–1945'. In *'Heroische Therapien:' Die deutsche Psychiatrie im internationalen Vergleich 1918–1945*, edited by Hans-Walter Schmuhl and Volker Roelcke, 287–307. Göttingen: Wallstein, 2013.

Hohendorf, Gerrit, Volker Roelcke, and Maike Rotzoll. 'Innovation und Vernichtung: Psychiatrische Forschung und "Euthanasie" an der Heidelberger Psychiatrischen Klinik 1939–1945'. *Der Nervenarzt* 67, no. 11 (1996): 935–46.

Horley, James. 'The Emergence and Development of Psychopathy'. *History of the Human Sciences* 27, no. 5 (2014): 91–110.

Hubenstorf, Michael. 'Kontinuität und Bruch in der Medizingeschichte'. In *Kontinuität und Bruch 1938 - 1945 - 1955: Beiträge zur österreichischen Kultur- und Wissenschaftsgeschichte*, edited by Friedrich Stadler, 299–334. Münster: LIT, 2004.

———. 'Sozialmedizin, Menschenökonomie, Volksgesundheit'. In *Aufbruch und Untergang: Österreichische Kultur zwischen 1918 und 1938*, edited by Franz Kadrnoska, 247–66. Vienna, Munich, and Zurich: Europaverlag, 1981.

Huber, Wolfgang. *Psychoanalyse in Österreich seit 1933*. Vienna and Salzburg: Geyer-Edition, 1977.

Hüntelmann, Axel C. *Hygiene im Namen des Staates: Das Reichsgesundheitsamt 1876–1933*. Göttingen: Wallstein, 2008.

'Internationale Tagung für angewandte Psychopathologie und Psychologie'. *Wiener Medizinische Wochenschrift* 80, no. 23 (1930): 766–69.

Iso, Isabel Miko, and Bernhard C. Schär. 'Kolonialer Rassismus, eugenisches Denken und Geschlecht: Auguste Forel und Otto Stoll in der Debatte um die "allgemeine Natur des Menschen" um 1900'. In *Gender Scripts: Widerspenstige Aneignungen von Geschlechternormen*, edited by Christa Binswanger, Margaret

Bridges, Brigitte Schnegg, and Doris Wastl-Walter, 61–84. Frankfurt am Main and New York: Campus, 2009.

Jablensky, Assen. 'Living in a Kraepelinian World: Kraepelin's Impact on Modern Psychiatry'. *History of Psychiatry* 18, no. 3 (2007): 381–88.

Jaeger, Siegfried. 'Zur Herausbildung von Praxisfeldern der Psychologie bis 1933'. In *Geschichte der deutschen Psychologie im 20. Jahrhundert: Ein Überblick*, edited by Mitchell G. Ash and Ulfried Geuter, 83–112. Opladen: Westdeutscher Verlag, 1985.

Jaspers, Karl. *Strindberg und Van Gogh: Versuch einer pathographischen Analyse unter vergleichender Heranziehung von Swedenborg und Hölderlin*. Arbeiten zur angewandten Psychiatrie 5. Berne and Leipzig: Bircher, 1922.

Johnston, William M. *The Austrian Mind: An Intellectual and Social History 1848–1938*. Berkeley : University of California Press, 1972.

Jung, Carl Gustav. 'Geleitwort'. *Zentralblatt für Psychotherapie* 6 (1933): 139–40.

———. *Psychologische Typen*. Zurich: Rascher, 1921.

———. 'Zur gegenwärtigen Lage der Psychotherapie'. *Zentralblatt für Psychotherapie* 7, no. 1 (1934): 1–16.

Kaes, Anton. *Shell Shock Cinema: Weimar Culture and the Wounds of War*. Princeton and Oxford: Princeton University Press, 2009.

Kahn, Eugen. 'Psychopathen als revolutionäre Führer'. *Zeitschrift für die gesamte Neurologie und Psychiatrie* 52, no. 1 (1919): 90–106.

———. 'Psychopathie und Revolution'. *Münchener medizinische Wochenschrift* 66, no. 34 (1919): 968–69.

Kanning, Uwe Peter. 'Geschichte der Angewandten und Praktischen Psychologie'. In *Jenseits des Elfenbeinturms: Psychologie als nützliche Wissenschaft*, edited by Uwe Peter Kanning, Lutz von Rosenstiel, and Heinz Schuler, 19–34. Göttingen: Vandenhoeck & Ruprecht, 2010.

Kapner, Gerhardt. 'Der Wiener kommunale Wohnungsbau'. In *Aufbruch und Untergang: Österreichische Kultur zwischen 1918 und 1938*, edited by Franz Kadrnoska, 135–66. Vienna, Munich, and Zurich: Europaverlag, 1981.

Kauders, Anthony D. 'Psychoanalysis Is Good, Synthesis Is Better: The German Reception of Freud, 1930 and 1956'. *Journal of the History of the Behavioral Sciences* 47 (2011): 380–97.

———. 'Truth, Truthfulness, and Psychoanalysis: The Reception of Freud in Wilhelmine Germany'. *German History* 31, no. 1 (2013): 1–22.

Kauders, Otto. 'Geschichte der psychischen Hygiene'. In *Leitfaden der psychischen Hygiene*, edited by Erwin Stransky, 11–15. Vienna: Urban & Schwarzenberg, 1931.

Kaufmann, Doris. 'Science as Cultural Practice: Psychiatry in the First World War and Weimar Germany'. *Journal of Contemporary History* 34, no. 1 (1999): 125–44.

Keifenheim, Katharina Eva. 'Hans von Hattingberg (1879–1944): Leben und Werk'. MD thesis, University of Tübingen, 2011.

———. 'Hans von Hattingberg Between Psychoanalysis and National Socialism'. *Luzif Amor* 24, no. 48 (2011): 106–25.

Kersting, Franz-Werner, and Hans-Walter Schmuhl, eds. 'Minister für Volkswohlfahrt an sämtliche Ober- und Regierungspräsidenten, 2. September 1920, Berlin'. In *Quellen zur Geschichte der Anstaltspsychiatrie in Westfalen*, 2:145–46. Paderborn: Schöningh, 2004.

Kihn, Berthold. 'Die Ausschaltung der Minderwertigen aus der Gesellschaft'. *Allgemeine Zeitschrift für Psychiatrie* 98 (1932): 387–404.

Killen, Andreas. *Berlin Electropolis: Shock, Nerves, and German Modernity*. Berkeley, Los Angeles, and London: University of California Press, 2006.

Kittel, Ingo-Wolf. 'Arthur Kronfeld zur Erinnerung - Schicksal und Werk eines jüdischen Psychiaters in drei deutschen Reichen'. In *Arthur Kronfeld (1886–1941): Ein Pionier der Psychologie, Sexualwissenschaft und Psychotherapie*, edited by Ingo-Wolf Kittel, 7–13. Konstanz: Bibliothek der Universität Konstanz, 1988.

Kittler, Friedrich. *Aufschreibesysteme 1800–1900*. 3rd ed. Munich: Fink, 1995.

———. *Short Cuts*. Frankfurt am Main: Zweitausendeins, 2002.

Klautke, Egbert. *The Mind of the Nation: Völkerpsychologie in Germany, 1851–1955*. New York and Oxford: Berghahn, 2013.

Klee, Ernst. *Das Personenlexikon zum Dritten Reich: Wer war was vor und nach 1945*. Frankfurt am Main: Fischer, 2003.

Kline, Wendy. 'Eugenics in the United States'. In *The Oxford Handbook of the History of Eugenics*, edited by Alison Bashford and Philippa Levine. Oxford: Oxford University Press, 2010.

Knechtle, Eva. 'Walter Morgenthaler (1882–1965) als Pionier der Ausbildung des Psychiatrie-Pflegepersonals in der Schweiz'. MD Thesis, MD thesis, University of Berne, 1992.

Koelbing-Waldis, Vera. 'Forel, Auguste'. *Historisches Lexikon der Schweiz*, 2005.

———. 'Maier, Hans Wolfgang'. In *Historisches Lexikon der Schweiz*. Berne, 2008. https://hls-dhs-dss.ch/de/articles/014531/2008-02-27/.

Kogerer, Heinrich. 'Bericht über die Tätigkeit des Psychotherapeutischen Ambulatoriums an der Psychiatrisch-neurologischen Universitätsklinik in Wien, in den Jahren 1922–1925'. *Wiener Klinische Wochenschrift* 39, no. 12 (1926): 330–33.

———. 'Die Psychotherapie des praktischen Arztes'. *Wiener Klinische Wochenschrift* 41, no. 5 (1928): 167–69.

———. 'I. Jahresbericht Des Psychotherapeutischen Ambulatoriums an Der Psychiatrisch-Neurologischen Universitätsklinik in Wien'. *Wiener Klinische Wochenschrift* 37, no. 11 (1924): 255–57.

———. 'Organisation des Fürsorgewesens in deutschen Ländern'. In *Leitfaden der psychischen Hygiene*, edited by Erwin Stransky, 244–49. Berlin and Vienna: Urban & Schwarzenberg, 1931.

———. 'Psychische Hygiene in Österreich'. *Zeitschrift für psychische Hygiene* 2, no. 4 (1929): 114–18.

———. 'Psychische Hygiene, Neurosenlehre und Psychotherapie'. In *Leitfaden der psychischen Hygiene*, edited by Erwin Stransky, 49–76. Vienna and Berlin: Urban & Schwarzenberg, 1931.

———. *Psychotherapie: Ein Lehrbuch für Studierende und Ärzte*. Vienna: Wilhelm Maudrich, 1934.

———. 'Was leistet die Psychoanalyse für die Psychotherapie?' *Wiener Klinische Wochenschrift* 42, no. 32 (1929): 1068.

Kohlrausch, Martin. *Der Monarch im Skandal: Die Logik der Massenmedien und die Transformation der Wilhelminischen Monarchie*. Berlin: Akademie, 2005.

Kohlrausch, Martin, and Helmuth Trischler. *Building Europe on Expertise: Innovators, Organizers, Networkers*. Houndmills, Basingstoke: Palgrave Macmillan, 2014.

Köhne, Julia Barbara. *Kriegshysteriker: Strategische Bilder und mediale Techniken militärpsychiatrischen Wissens (1914–1920)*. Husum: Matthiessen, 2009.

Kolb, Gustav. 'Inwieweit sind Änderungen im Betriebe der Anstalten geboten?' *Psychiatrisch-Neurologische Wochenschrift*, no. 21/22 (1920): 163–76.

———. 'Inwieweit sind Änderungen im Betriebe der Anstalten geboten?' *Psychiatrisch-Neurologische Wochenschrift*, no. 17/18 (1920): 133–39.

———. 'Reform der Irrenfürsorge'. *Zeitschrift für die gesamte Neurologie und Psychiatrie* 47 (1919): 137–72.

Kollarits, Jenő. 'Die Störung im psychischen Weltgefüge'. *Zeitschrift für die gesamte Neurologie und Psychiatrie* 65 (1921): 331–50.

———. 'Kann die Volksseele aus der Geschichte lernen?' *Deutsche Psychologie* 3 (1920): 177–83.

———. 'Normalzustand und Ausnahmezustand in der Völkerpsyche'. *Zeitschrift für die gesamte Neurologie und Psychiatrie* 66 (1921): 337–42.

Könnemann, Wilhelm. *Über Psychohygiene in Schule und Haus auf Grundlage einer Erörterung über das Verhältnis von Geist und Körper, Seele und Leib*. Posen: Merzbach'sche Buchdruckerei, 1902.

Kracauer, Siegfried. *Von Caligari zu Hitler: Ein Beitrag zur Geschichte des deutschen Films*. Reinbek bei Hamburg: Rowohlt, 1958.

Kraepelin, Emil. 'Das Verbrechen als soziale Krankheit'. *Monatsschrift für Kriminalpsychologie und Strafrechtsreform* 3, no. 1 (1906): 257–79.

———. 'Die Deutsche Forschungsanstalt für Psychiatrie'. *Die Naturwissenschaften* 6, no. 23 (1918): 333–37.

———. *Die psychiatrischen Aufgaben des Staates*. Jena: Gustav Fischer, 1900.

———. 'Die Verfassung der Deutschen Forschungsanstalt für Psychiatrie in München'. *Zeitschrift für die gesamte Neurologie und Psychiatrie* 55 (1920): 310–26.

———. 'Ein Forschungsinstitut für Psychiatrie'. *Zeitschrift für die gesamte Neurologie und Psychiatrie* 32 (1916): 1–38.

———. 'Hundert Jahre Psychiatrie'. *Zeitschrift für die gesamte Neurologie und Psychiatrie* 38 (1918): 161–275.

———. 'On the Question of Degeneration (1908)'. Translated by Eric J. Engstrom. *History of Psychiatry* 18, no. 3 (2007): 399–404.

———. *Psychiatrie: Ein Lehrbuch für Studierende und Ärzte.* 7th ed. Vol. 2. Leipzig: J. A. Barth, 1904.

———. *Psychiatrie: Ein Lehrbuch für Studirende und Aerzte.* 6th ed. 2 vols. Leipzig: Barth, 1899.

———. 'Psychiatrische Randbemerkungen zur Zeitgeschichte'. *Süddeutsche Monatshefte* 16 (1919): 171–83.

———. 'Über die Wachabteilung der Heidelberger Irrenklinik'. *Allgemeine Zeitschrift für Psychiatrie* 51 (1895): 1–21.

———. 'Über Entwurzelung'. *Zeitschrift für die gesamte Neurologie und Psychiatrie* 63 (1921): 1–8.

———. 'Vergleichende Psychiatrie'. *Centralblatt für Nervenheilkunde und Psychiatrie* 27 (1904): 433–37.

———. 'Ziele und Wege der psychiatrischen Forschung'. *Zeitschrift für die gesamte Neurologie und Psychiatrie* 42 (1918): 169–205.

———. 'Zur Entartungsfrage'. *Zentralblatt für Nervenheilkunde und Psychiatrie* 31 (1908): 745–51.

Kraft, Hartmut. *Grenzgänger zwischen Kunst und Psychiatrie.* 3rd ed. Cologne: Deutscher Ärzte-Verlag, 2005.

Kretschmer, Ernst. 'Die konstitutionelle Retardierung und das Problem des sozialen Kontakts'. *Gesundheit und Wohlfahrt - Revue Suisse d'Hygiene* 18, no. 8/9 (1939): 368–72.

Kretschmer, Wolfgang. 'Arthur Kronfeld - ein Vergessener: Zu seinem 100. Geburtstag'. *Der Nervenarzt* 58, no. 12 (1987): 737–42.

Kreuter, Alma. *Deutschsprachige Neurologen und Psychiater: Ein biographisch-bibliographisches Lexikon von den Vorläufern bis zur Mitte des 20. Jahrhunderts.* 3 vols. Munich: K. G. Saur, 1996.

Kronfeld, Arthur. *Das seelisch Abnorme und die Gemeinschaft.* Stuttgart: Julius Püttmann, 1923.

———. *Das Wesen der psychiatrischen Erkenntnis: Beiträge zur allgemeinen Psychiatrie I.* Berlin: Julius Springer, 1920.

———. 'Eine Bedenklichkeit der "angewandten" Psychiatrie'. *Zeitschrift für die gesamte Neurologie und Psychiatrie* 65 (1921): 364–67.

———. 'Rätesystem, Klassenkampf und Ärzte: Eine Entgegnung'. *Rätezeitung* 1, no. 10 (1919): 3.

———. 'Stransky, Erwin (Wien), Psychiatrie und psychologische Methodik'. *Allgemeine ärztliche Zeitschrift für Psychotherapie und psychische Hygiene* 2, no. 12 (1929): 778–79.

———. 'Über die psychologischen Theorien Freuds und verwandte Anschauungen: Systematik und kritische Erörterungen'. *Archiv für die gesamte Psychologie* 22, no. 2/3 (1912): 130–248.

Kuechenhoff, Bernhard. 'The Psychiatrist Auguste Forel and His Attitude to Eugenics'. *History of Psychiatry* 19, no. 2 (2008): 215–23.

Kühl, Stefan. *Die Internationale der Rassisten: Aufstieg und Niedergang der internationalen Bewegung für Eugenik und Rassenhygiene im 20. Jahrhundert.* Frankfurt am Main and New York: Campus, 1997.

———. *Die Internationale der Rassisten: Aufstieg und Niedergang der internationalen eugenischen Bewegung im 20. Jahrhundert.* 2nd ed. Frankfurt am Main and New York: Campus, 2014.

Kumbier, Ekkehardt, and Kathleen Haack. 'Alfred Hauptmann: Schicksal eines deutsch-jüdischen Neurologen'. *Fortschritte der Neurologie, Psychiatrie* 70 (2002): 204–9.

Laak, Dirk van. 'Technokratie im Europa des 20. Jahrhunderts - eine einflussreiche Hintergrundideologie'. In *Theorien und Experimente der Moderne: Europas Gesellschaften im 20. Jahrhundert*, edited by Lutz Raphael, 101–28. Cologne, Vienna and Weimar: Böhlau, 2012.

Labisch, Alfons. *Homo Hygienicus: Gesundheit und Medizin in der Neuzeit.* Frankfurt am Main and New York: Campus, 1992.

Lamb, Susan D. *Pathologist of the Mind: Adolf Meyer and the Origins of American Psychiatry.* Baltimore: Johns Hopkins University Press, 2014.

———. 'Pathologist of the Mind: Adolf Meyer, Psychobiology and the Phipps Psychiatric Clinic at the Johns Hopkins Hospital, 1908–1917'. PhD thesis, Johns Hopkins University, 2010.

Lamiell, James T. *William Stern (1871–1938): A Brief Introduction to His Life and Works.* Lengerich and Berlin: Pabst Science Publishers, 2010.

Latour, Bruno. *Science in Action: How to Follow Scientists and Engineers Through Society.* Cambridge, MA: Harvard University Press, 1987.

Lebeau, Vicky. 'Psychopolitics: Frantz Fanon's Black Skin, White Masks'. In *Psycho-Politics and Cultural Desires*, edited by Jan Campbell and Janet Harbord, 113–23. London and Bristol, PA: UCL Press, 1998.

Leist, Anton, ed. *Auguste Forel: Eugenik und Erinnerungskultur.* Zurich: vdf Hochschulverlag, 2006.

Lemke, Thomas. *Biopolitics: An Advanced Introduction.* Translated by Eric Frederick Trump. New York and London: New York University Press, 2011.

Lengwiler, Martin. 'Im Zeichen der Degeneration: Psychiatrie und internationale Abstinenzbewegung im ausgehenden 19. Jahrhundert'. In *Biopolitik und Sittlichkeitsreform: Kampagnen gegen Alkohol, Drogen und Prostitution 1880–1950*, edited by Judith Große, Francesco Spöring, and Jana Tschurenev, 85–110. Frankfurt am Main: Campus, 2014.

Leonhardt, M., and K. Foerster. 'Hermann F. Hoffmann (1891–1944): Die Tübinger Psychiatrie auf dem Weg in den Nationalsozialismus'. *Der Nervenarzt* 67, no. 11 (1996): 947–52.

Lerner, Paul. *Hysterical Men: War, Psychiatry, and the Politics of Trauma in Germany, 1890–1930*. Ithaca: Cornell University Press, 2003.

Leser, Norbert. *Skurille Begegnungen: Mosaike zur österreichischen Geistesgeschichte*. Vienna: Böhlau, 2011.

Levelt, Willem J. M. *A History of Psycholinguistics: The Pre-Chomskyan Era*. Oxford: Oxford University Press, 2013.

Lévy, Alfred. 'Rudolf Allers - ein katholischer Individualpsychologe'. In *Gestalten um Alfred Adler: Pioniere der Individualpsychologie*, edited by Alfred Lévy and Gerald Mackenthun, 27–36. Würzburg: Königshausen & Neumann, 2002.

Ley, Astrid. 'Psychiatriekritik durch Psychiater: Sozialreformerische und professionspolitische Ziele des Erlanger Anstaltsdirektors Gustav Kolb (1870–1938)'. In *'Moderne' Anstaltspsychiatrie im 19. und 20. Jahrhundert: Legitimation und Kritik*, edited by Heiner Fangerau and Karen Nolte, 195–220. Stuttgart: Franz Steiner, 2006.

Lockot, Regine. *Erinnern und Durcharbeiten: Zur Geschichte der Psychoanalyse und Psychotherapie im Nationalsozialismus*. Gießen: Psychosozial-Verlag, 2002.

Löscher, Monika. 'Zur Popularisierung von Eugenik und Rassenhygiene in Wien'. In *Wissenschaft, Politik und Öffentlichkeit: Von der Wiener Moderne bis zur Gegenwart*, edited by Mitchell G. Ash and Christian H. Stifer, 233–66. Vienna: WUV, 2002.

———. 'Zur Umsetzung und Verbreitung von eugenischem/rassenhygienischen Gedankengut in Österreich bis 1934 unter besonderer Berücksichtigung Wiens'. In *Medizin im Nationalsozialismus - Wege der Aufarbeitung*, edited by Sonia Horn and Peter Malina, 99–127. Wiener Gespräche zur Sozialgeschichte der Medizin. Vienna: ÖÄK Verlag, 2001.

Luchsinger, Katrin. *Die Vergessenskurve: Werke aus psychiatrischen Kliniken in der Schweiz um 1900: eine kulturanalytische Studie*. Zurich: Chronos, 2016.

Luxenburger, Hans. 'Die Sterilisierung aus psychiatrisch-eugenischer Indikation'. In *Bericht über die Zweite Deutsche Tagung für psychische Hygiene in Bonn am 21. Mai 1932*, edited by Hans Roemer, 30–43. Berlin and Leipzig: Walter de Gruyter & Co., 1932.

———. 'Psychopathologie und Erblichkeit'. In *I. Internationale Tagung für angewandte Psychopathologie und Psychologie, Wien, 5.-7. Juni 1930: Referate und*

Vorträge, edited by Heinz Hartmann, Martin Pappenheim, and Erwin Stransky, 77–93. Berlin: S. Karger, 1931.

Maderthaner, Wolfgang. 'Die eigenartige Größe der Beschränkung: Österreichs Revolution im mitteleuropäischen Spannungsfeld'. In *… … der Rest ist Österreich: Das Werden der Republik*, edited by Helmut Konrad and Wolfgang Maderthaner, 1:187–206. Vienna: Carl Gerold's Sohn, 2008.

Maier, Hans W. 'Zum gegenwärtigen Stand der Frage der Kastration und Sterilisation aus psychiatrischer Indikation'. *Zeitschrift für die gesamte Neurologie und Psychiatrie* 98 (1925): 200–219.

Mann, Thomas. *Betrachtungen eines Unpolitischen.* Berlin: S. Fischer, 1918.

Mapother, Henry. 'Emil Kraepelin'. *British Journal of Psychiatry* 73, no. 303 (1927): 509–15.

Marcuse, Julian. 'Nervenkraft als Grundlage des Wiederaufbaus'. *Blätter für Volksgesundheitspflege* 21, no. 10–12 (1921): 117–18.

Marx, Hugo. 'Aerztliche Gedanken zur Revolution'. *Berliner Klinische Wochenschrift* 12 (1919): 279.

Marx, Karl. *Das Kapital: Kritik der Politischen Ökonomie.* Vol. 1. MEW 23. Berlin: Dietz, 1962.

Matz, Bernhard. 'Die Konstitutionstypologie von Ernst Kretschmer: Ein Beitrag zur Geschichte von Psychiatrie und Psychologie des Zwanzigsten Jahrhunderts'. MD thesis, Free University of Berlin, 2000.

Mayer, Thomas. '"…dasz die eigentliche österreichische Rassenhygiene in der Hauptsache das Werk Reichels ist:" Der (Rassen-)Hygieniker Heinrich Reichel (1876–1943) und seine Bedeutung für die eugenische Bewegung in Österreich'. In *Vorreiter der Vernichtung? Eugenik, Rassenhygiene und Euthanasie in der österreichischen Diskussion vor 1938*, edited by Heinz Eberhard Gabriel and Wolfgang Neugebauer, 65–98. Vienna, Cologne, and Weimar: Böhlau, 2005.

McGuire, William, ed. *The Freud/Jung Letters: The Correspondence Between Sigmund Freud and C. G. Jung.* Translated by Ralph Manheim and R. F. C. Hull. London: The Hogarth Press and Routledge & Kegan Paul, 1977.

Meier, Rolf. *August Forel, 1848–1931: Arzt, Naturforscher, Sozialreformer.* Zurich: Universität Zürich, 1986.

Meier, Ulrich, Martin Papenheim, and Willibald Steinmetz, eds. *Semantiken des Politischen: Vom Mittelalter bis ins 20. Jahrhundert.* Göttingen: Wallstein, 2012.

Meißel, Theodor. 'Freud und die österreichische Psychiatrie seiner Zeit'. In *Psychoanalyse und Psychiatrie*, edited by Heinz Böker, 54–69. Heidelberg: Springer, 2006.

Meng, Heinrich. 'Erziehung zum Verstehen und zur Verständigung'. *Gesundheit und Wohlfahrt - Revue Suisse d'Hygiene* 18, no. 8/9 (1939): 416–23.

———. *Leben als Begegnung.* Stuttgart: Hippokrates, 1971.

———. *Praxis der seelischen Hygiene: Erfahrung und Experiment.* Basel: Benno Schwabe, 1943.

———. *Seelischer Gesundheitsschutz: Eine Einführung in Diagnostik, Forschung und Nutzanwendung der Psychohygiene.* Basel: Benno Schwabe & Co., 1939.

Meng, Heinrich, and André Repond. 'Vorwort'. In *Eine Seele die sich wiederfand: Autobiographie des Begründers der 'Geistigen Hygiene'*, edited Clifford W. Beers. Basel: Benno Schwabe & Co., 1941.

Mergel, Thomas. 'Führer, Volksgemeinschaft und Maschine: Politische Erwartungsstrukturen in der Weimarer Republik und dem Nationalsozialismus 1918–1936'. In *Politische Kulturgeschichte der Zwischenkriegszeit 1918–1939*, edited by Wolfgang Hardtwig, 91–128. Göttingen: Vandenhoeck & Ruprecht, 2005.

Meyer zum Wischen, Michael. *'Der Seele Tiefen zu ergründen…' Robert Sommer (1864–1937) und das Konzept einer ganzheitlichen, erweiterten Psychiatrie.* Gießen: Wilhelm Schmitz, 1988.

Micale, Mark S. 'The Ten Most Important Changes in Psychiatry Since World War II'. *History of Psychiatry* 25, no. 4 (2014): 485–91.

Micale, Mark S., and Paul Lerner, eds. *Traumatic Pasts: History, Psychiatry, and Trauma in the Modern Age, 1870–1930.* Cambridge: Cambridge University Press, 2001.

Mills, China. *Decolonizing Global Mental Health: The Psychiatrization of the Majority World.* London and New York: Routledge, 2014.

'Mitteilung des Reichsführers der "Deutschen allgemeinen ärztlichen Gesellschaft für Psychotherapie"'. *Zentralblatt für Psychotherapie* 6 (1933): 140–41.

Morgenthaler, Walter. 'Der Kampf um das Erscheinen der Psychodiagnostik: Hermann Rorschach zum 70. Geburtstag (8. November 1954)'. *Rorschachiana* 2, no. 3 (1954): 255–62.

———. *Der Mensch Karl Marx.* Berne: Schweizerisches Ost-Institut, 1962.

———. *Ein Geisteskranker als Künstler.* Arbeiten zur angewandten Psychiatrie 1. Berne and Leipzig: Bircher, 1921.

———. 'Heiratsprophylaxe und psychische Hygiene'. *Zeitschrift für psychische Hygiene* 11 (1938): 145–52.

———. 'Neurologie, Psychiatrie, Psychotherapie'. *Zentralblatt für Psychotherapie* 9, no. 1 (1935): 25–36.

———. *Persönliche Neutralität und Geistige Wehrkraft.* Berne: Hans Huber, 1941.

———. 'Psychotherapie und Politik'. In *I. Internationale Tagung für angewandte Psychopathologie und Psychologie, Wien, 5.-7. Juni 1930: Referate und Vorträge*, edited by Heinz Hartmann, Martin Pappenheim, and Erwin Stransky, 229–35. Berlin: S. Karger, 1931.

———. 'Über seelische Hygiene'. In *Seelische Hygiene*, 37–59. Berne: Stämpfli & Cie., 1931.

———. 'Zur Psychologie der Orientierung nach unten'. *Sozialärztliche Rundschau* 2 (1930).

———. 'Zur Psychologie des Zeitgeschehens: Über Hitler und Mussolini'. *Schweizerische Zeitschrift für Psychologie und ihre Anwendungen* 4, no. 2 (1945): 137–48.

Moser, Gabriele. '"Die Zukunft gehört der prophylaktischen Medizin:" Sozialhygiene, medizinisches Präventionsverständnis und Gesundheitsbegriff Ende der 1920er Jahre'. In *Sozialmedizin, Sozialhygiene und Public Health: Konzepte und Visionen zum Verhältnis von Medizin und Gesellschaft in historischer Perspektive*, edited by Udo Schagen and Sabine Schleiermacher, 15–20. Berlin: Forschungsstelle Zeitgeschichte im Institut für Geschichte der Medizin, 2002.

Mosse, George L. 'Shell-Shock as a Social Disease'. *Journal of Contemporary History* 35, no. 1 (2000): 101–8.

Mühlberger, Kurt. *Vertriebene Intelligenz 1938: Der Verlust geistiger und menschlicher Potenz an der Universität Wien von 1938 bis 1945*. 2. Vienna: Archiv der Universität Wien, 1993.

Mühlleitner, Elke. *Biographisches Lexikon der Psychoanalyse: Die Mitglieder der Psychoanalytischen Mittwoch-Gesellschaft und der Wiener Psychoanalytischen Vereinigung 1902–1938*. Tübingen: edition diskord, 1992.

———. *Medizinische Psychologie und Psychotherapie in Österreich 1900–1950*. 2 vols. Klagenfurt: Institut für Psychologie der Universität Klagenfurt, 1994.

Müller, Christian. 'Morgenthaler, Walter'. *Historisches Lexikon Der Schweiz*, 2008.

———. *Verbrechensbekämpfung im Anstaltsstaat: Psychiatrie, Kriminologie und Strafrechtsreform in Deutschland 1871–1933*. Göttingen: Vandenhoeck & Ruprecht, 2004.

Müller, Max. *Erinnerungen: Erlebte Psychiatriegeschichte 1920–1960*. Berlin, Heidelberg, and New York: Springer, 1982.

Münsterberg, Hugo. *Grundzüge der Psychotechnik*. Leipzig: J.A. Barth, 1914.

Neuner, Stephanie. *Politik und Psychiatrie: Die staatliche Versorgung psychisch Kriegsbeschädigter in Deutschland 1920–1939*. Göttingen: Vandenhoeck & Ruprecht, 2011.

Neve, Michael. 'A Commentary on the History of Social Psychiatry and Psychotherapy in Twentieth-Century Germany, Holland and Great Britain'. *Medical History* 48, no. 4 (2004): 407–12.

Nitzschke, Bernd. '"Ich muss mich dagegen wehren, still kaltgestellt zu werden." Voraussetzungen, Begleitumstände und Folgen des Ausschlusses Wilhelm Reichs aus der DGP/IPV in den Jahren 1933/34'. In *Der 'Fall' Wilhelm Reich: Beiträge zum Verhältnis von Psychoanalyse und Politik*, edited by Karl Fallend and Bernd Nitzschke, 83–133. Gießen: Psychosozial-Verlag, 2002.

Nolan, James L. *The Therapeutic State: Justifying Government at Century's End*. New York: New York University Press, 1998.

Nolte, Karen. *Gelebte Hysterie: Erfahrung, Eigensinn und psychiatrische Diskurse im Anstaltsalltag um 1900*. Frankfurt am Main: Campus, 2003.

Nordau, Max. *Entartung*. Vol. 1. Berlin: C. Duncker, 1892.

Oosterhuis, Harry. 'Outpatient Psychiatry and Mental Health Care in the Twentieth Century: International Perspectives'. In *Psychiatric Cultures Compared: Psychiatry and Mental Health Care in the Twentieth Century. Comparisons and Approaches*, edited by Marijke Gijswijt-Hofstra, Harry Oosterhuis, Joost Vijselaar, and Hugh Freeman, 248–76. Amsterdam: Amsterdam University Press, 2005.

Oppenheim, Hermann. 'Seelenstörung und Volksbewegung'. *Berliner Tageblatt*, 16 April 1919.

Österreichische Gesellschaft für Psychische Hygiene. *Bericht über die 6. Jahresversammlung der Weltvereinigung für Psychische Hygiene, Wien 16.-22. August 1953.* Vienna and Bonn: Wilhelm Maudrich, 1956.

Pappenheim, Else. *Hölderlin, Feuchtersleben, Freud: Beiträge zur Geschichte der Psychoanalyse, der Psychiatrie und Neurologie.* Translated by Wilfried Prantner, Else Pappenheim, and Stephen Frishauf. Graz and Vienna: Nausner & Nausner, 2004.

———. 'Politik und Psychoanalyse in Wien vor 1939'. *Psyche* 43, no. 2 (1989): 120–41.

———. 'Zeitzeugin'. In *Vertriebene Vernunft II: Emigration und Exil österreichischer Wissenschaft. Internationales Symposium, 19. bis 23. Oktober 1987 in Wien*, edited by Friedrich Stadler, 221–29. Vienna and Munich: Jugend und Volk, 1988.

Pappenheim, Martin. 'Eröffnungsansprache'. In *I. Internationale Tagung für angewandte Psychopathologie und Psychologie, Wien, 5.-7. Juni 1930: Referate und Vorträge*, edited by Heinz Hartmann, Martin Pappenheim, and Erwin Stransky, 1–4. Berlin: S. Karger, 1931.

———. 'Medizinisches und Aerztliches aus Sowjetrußland'. *Wiener Klinische Wochenschrift* 35, no. 8 (1922): 185–87.

———. '[Report from Soviet Russia]'. *Internationale Zeitschrift für Psychoanalyse* 7, no. 3 (1921): 387–88.

Pappenheim, Martin, Erwin Stransky, and Heinz Hartmann. 'Zum Geleit'. In *I. Internationale Tagung für angewandte Psychopathologie und Psychologie, Wien, 5.-7. Juni 1930: Referate und Vorträge*, edited by Heinz Hartmann, Martin Pappenheim, and Erwin Stransky, III–IV. Berlin: S. Karger, 1931.

Parenžanin, Ratko. *Gavrilo Princips Bekenntnisse: Ein geschichtlicher Beitrag zur Vorgeschichte des Attentats von Sarajevo.* Vienna: Rudolf Lechner & Sohn, 1926.

Paskauskas, R. Andrew. *The Complete Correspondence of Sigmund Freud and Ernest Jones, 1908–1939.* Cambridge, MA: Harvard University Press, 1993.

Patzel-Mattern, Katja. '"Dispositionen des Individuums" im Produktionsprozess: Die industrielle Psychotechnik der Weimarer Republik zwischen Selbstbehauptung, Unternehmererwartungen und Arbeiterinteressen'. In *Das Selbst zwischen Anpassung und Befreiung: Psychowissen und Politik im 20. Jahrhundert*, edited by Maik Tändler and Uffa Jensen, 60–84. Göttingen: Wallstein, 2012.

Peukert, Detlev J. K. *Die Weimarer Republik: Krisenjahre der Klassischen Moderne.* Frankfurt am Main: Suhrkamp, 1987.

Pick, Daniel. *Faces of Degeneration: A European Disorder, c. 1848–c. 1918.* Cambridge: Cambridge University Press, 1989.

Pisa, Karl. *Ernst Freiherr von Feuchtersleben: Pionier der Psychosomatik.* Vienna, Cologne, and Weimar: Böhlau, 1998.

Plänkers, Thomas. 'Hygiene der Seele: Heinrich Meng (1887–1972)'. In *Psychoanalyse in Frankfurt am Main: Zerstörte Anfänge, Wiederannäherungen, Entwicklungen*, edited by Thomas Plänkers, Michael Laier, Hans-Heinrich Otto, Hans-Joachim Rothe, and Helmut Siefert, 109–40. Tübingen: edition diskord, 1996.

Plezko, Anna. 'Handlungsspielräume und Zwänge in der Medizin des Nationalsozialismus: Das Leben und Werk des Psychiaters Dr. Hans Roemer (1878–1947)'. MD thesis, University of Gießen, 2011.

Pohlisch, Kurt, and Friedrich Panse. *Schlafmittelmißbrauch.* Leipzig: Thieme, 1934.

Pollak, Gustav. *The Hygiene of the Soul: The Memoir of a Physician and Philosopher.* New York: Dodd, Mead and Co., 1910.

Pols, Hans. '"Beyond the Clinical Frontiers:" The American Mental Hygiene Movement, 1910–1945'. In *International Relations in Psychiatry: Britain, Germany, and the United States to World War II*, edited by Volker Roelcke, Paul Weindling, and Louise Westwood, 111–33. Rochester: University of Rochester Press, 2010.

———. 'Managing the Mind: The Culture of American Mental Hygiene, 1910–1950'. PhD thesis, University of Pennsylvania, 1997.

Pongratz, Ludwig J., ed. 'Rudolf Dreikurs'. In *Psychotherapie in Selbstdarstellungen*, 107–28. Berne, Stuttgart, and Vienna: Hans Huber, 1973.

Porter, Roy. 'The Patient's View: Doing Medical History from Below'. *Theory and Society* 14, no. 2 (1985): 175–98.

Porter, Roy, and David Wright. *The Confinement of the Insane: International Perspectives 1800–1965.* Cambridge: Cambridge University Press, 2003.

Prinzhorn, Hans. *Bildnerei der Geisteskranken: Ein Beitrag zur Psychologie und Psychologie der Gestaltung.* Berlin: Julius Springer, 1922.

Proctor, Hannah. 'Lost Minds: Sedgwick, Laing and the Politics of Mental Illness'. *Radical Philosophy* 197, no. 5/6 (2016): 36–48.

Prüll, Cay-Rüdiger. 'The Exhausted Nation—Psychiatry and Medicine on the Home Front (1914–1918): The Case of Robert Sommer and the City of Giessen'. In *War, Trauma and Medicine in Germany and Central Europe (1914–1939)*, edited by Hans-Georg Hofer, Cay-Rüdiger Prüll, and Wolfgang U. Eckart, 30–48. Freiburg: Centaurus, 2011.

Radkau, Joachim. *Das Zeitalter der Nervosität: Deutschland zwischen Bismarck und Hitler.* Munich: Hanser, 1998.

Raggam-Blesch, Michaela. '"Mischlinge" und "Geltungsjuden." Alltag und Verfolgungserfahrungen von Männern und Frauen halbjüdischer Herkunft in Wien 1938–1945'. In *Alltag im Holocaust: Jüdisches Leben im Großdeutschen Reich 1941–1945*, edited by Andrea Löw, Doris L. Bergen, and Anna Hájková, 81–98. Munich: Oldenbourg, 2013.

Raphael, Lutz. 'Die Verwissenschaftlichung des Sozialen als methodische und konzeptionelle Herausforderung für eine Sozialgeschichte des 20. Jahrhunderts'. *Geschichte und Gesellschaft* 22, no. 2 (1996): 165–93.

———. 'Embedding the Human and Social Sciences in Western Societies, 1880–1980: Reflections on Trends and Methods of Current Research'. In *Engineering Society: The Role of the Human and Social Sciences in Modern Societies, 1880–1980*, edited by Kerstin Brückweh, Dirk Schumann, Richard F. Wetzell, and Benjamin Ziemann, 41–58. London: Palgrave Macmillan, 2012.

Rathkolb, Oliver, Peter Autengruber, Birgit Nemec, and Florian Wenninger. 'Forschungsprojektendbericht: Straßennamen Wiens seit 1860 als "Politische Erinnerungsorte"'. Vienna: Kulturabteilung der Stadt Wien (MA 7), 9 July 2013.

Reich, Eduard. *Die Geschichte der Seele, die Hygieine des Geisteslebens und die Civilisation*. Minden: J.C.C. Bruns, 1884.

———. *Studien über die Volksseele aus dem Gesichtspunkte der Physiologie und Hygieine*. 2nd ed. Jena: Hermann Costenoble, 1879.

Reichmayr, Johannes, and Elke Mühlleitner. 'Psychoanalysis in Austria After 1933–34: History and Historiography'. *International Forum of Psychoanalysis* 12, no. 2/3 (2003): 118–29.

Reichmayr, Johannes, and Elisabeth Wiesbauer. 'Das Verhältnis von Sozialdemokratie und Psychoanalyse in Österreich zwischen 1900 und 1938'. In *Beiträge zur Geschichte der Psychoanalyse in Österreich*, edited by Wolfgang Huber, 25–60. Vienna and Salzburg: Geyer-Edition, 1978.

Repond, André. 'Die Bewegung für psychische Hygiene in der Schweiz'. *Zeitschrift für psychische Hygiene* 1, no. 6 (1928): 187–91.

———. 'Geistige Hygiene und Politik'. *Zeitschrift für psychische Hygiene* 4, no. 6 (1931): 183–84.

'Revolution Im Irrenwesen'. *Die Irrenrechts-Reform* 62 (1919): 160–61.

Richter, A. 'Über die Ernährungsverhältnisse in der Irrenanstalt Buch während des Krieges 1914/1918 und deren Folgen'. *Allgemeine Zeitschrift für Psychiatrie und psychisch-gerichtliche Medizin* 75 (1919): 407–23.

Riedesser, Peter, and Axel Verderber. *Maschinengewehre hinter der Front: Zur Geschichte der deutschen Militärpsychiatrie*. Frankfurt am Main: Fischer, 1996.

Rieff, Philip. *The Triumph of the Therapeutic*. New York: Harper & Row, 1966.

Ritter, Hans Jakob. *Psychiatrie und Eugenik: Zur Ausprägung eugenischer Denk- und Handlungsmuster in der schweizerischen Psychiatrie 1850–1950*. Zurich: Chronos, 2009.

Rivière, Jacques. *L'Allemand: Souvenirs et réflexions d'un prisonnier de guerre*. Paris: Éditions de la Nouvelle Revue Française, 1919.

Roelcke, Volker. 'Biologizing Social Facts: An Early 20th Century Debate on Kraepelin's Concepts of Culture, Neurasthenia, and Degeneration'. *Culture, Medicine, and Psychiatry* 21, no. 4 (1997): 383–403.

———. 'Continuities or Ruptures? Concepts, Institutions and Contexts of Twentieth-Century German Psychiatry and Mental Health Care'. In *Psychiatric Cultures Compared: Psychiatry and Mental Health Care in the Twentieth Century: Comparisons and Approaches*, edited by Marijke Gijswijt-Hofstra, Harry Oosterhuis, Joost Vijselaar, and Hugh Freeman, 162–83. Amsterdam: Amsterdam University Press, 2005.

———. 'Die Entwicklung der Psychiatrie zwischen 1880 und 1932: Theoriebildung, Institutionen, Interaktionen mit zeitgenössischer Wissenschafts- und Sozialpolitik'. In *Wissenschaften und Wissenschaftspolitik: Bestandsaufnahmen zu Formationen, Brüchen und Kontinuitäten im Deutschland des 20. Jahrhunderts*, edited by Rüdiger vom Bruch and Brigitte Kaderas, 109–24. Stuttgart: Franz Steiner, 2002.

———. 'Ernst Rüdin: Renommierter Wissenschaftler, radikaler Rassenhygieniker'. *Der Nervenarzt* 83, no. 3 (2012): 303–10.

———. 'Hans Roemer (1878–1948)'. *Der Nervenarzt* 84, no. 9 (2013): 1064–68.

———. *Krankheit und Kulturkritik: Psychiatrische Gesellschaftsdeutungen im bürgerlichen Zeitalter (1790–1914)*. Frankfurt am Main: Campus, 1999.

———. 'Prävention in Hygiene und Psychiatrie zu Beginn des 20. Jahrhunderts: Krankheit, Gesellschaft, Vererbung und Eugenik bei Robert Sommer und Emil Gotschlich'. In *Die Medizinische Fakultät der Universität Gießen: Institutionen, Akteure und Ereignisse von der Gründung 1607 bis ins 20. Jahrhundert*, edited by Ulrike Enke, 395–416. Stuttgart: Franz Steiner, 2007.

———. 'Psychiatrische Wissenschaft im Kontext nationalsozialistischer Politik und Euthanasie: Zur Rolle Ernst Rüdins und der Deutschen Forschungsanstalt für Psychiatrie/Kaiser-Wilhelm-Institut'. In *Geschichte der Kaiser-Wilhelm-Gesellschaft im Nationalsozialismus: Bestandsaufnahme und Perspektiven der Forschung*, edited by Doris Kaufmann, 1:112–50. Göttingen: Wallstein, 2000.

———. 'Psychiatry in Munich and Yale, ca. 1920–1935: Mutual Perceptions and Relations, and the Case of Eugen Kahn (1887–1973)'. In *International Relations in Psychiatry: Britain, Germany, and the United States to World War II*, edited by Volker Roelcke, Paul Weindling, and Louise Westwood, 156–78. Rochester: University of Rochester Press, 2010.

———. 'Unterwegs zur Psychiatrie als Wissenschaft: Das Projekt einer Irrenstatistik und Emil Kraepelins Neuformulierung der psychiatrischen Klassifikation'. In *Psychiatrie im 19. Jahrhundert: Forschungen zur Geschichte von psychiatrischen Institutionen, Debatten und Praktiken im deutschen Sprachraum*, edited by Eric J. Engstrom and Volker Roelcke, 189–218. Basel: Schwabe, 2003.

Roemer, Hans, ed. *Bericht über die Erste Deutsche Tagung für Psychische Hygiene in Hamburg am 20. September 1928*. Berlin and Leipzig: Walter de Gruyter, 1929.

———. *Bericht über die Zweite Deutsche Tagung für psychische Hygiene in Bonn am 21. Mai 1932*. Berlin and Leipzig: Walter de Gruyter & Co., 1932.

———. 'Die Deutsche Organisation für psychische Hygiene in den Jahren 1930–1936'. *Zeitschrift für psychische Hygiene* 10, no. 2 (1937): 33–39.

———. 'Die rassenhygienischen Aufgaben der praktischen Psychiatrie unter besonderer Berücksichtigung der offenen Fürsorge'. In *Erblehre und Rassenhygiene im völkischen Staat*, edited by Ernst Rüdin, 120–35. Munich: J. F. Lehmanns, 1934.

———. 'Die V. Europäische Vereinigung für psychische Hygiene in München vom 22. bis 25. August 1938'. *Zeitschrift für psychische Hygiene* 12, no. 1 (1939): 2–54.

———. 'Die Zweite Tagung für psychische Hygiene in Bonn am 21. Mai 1932'. *Zeitschrift für psychische Hygiene* 5, no. 3/4 (1932): 65–80.

———. 'Eine humanitäre Bewegung: Der Erste Weltkongreß für psychische Hygiene'. *Frankfurter Zeitung*, 20 July 1930.

———, ed. 'Merkblatt des Deutschen Verbandes für psychische Hygiene zur Verhütung der erblichen Geistes- und Nervenkrankheiten'. In *Bericht über die Zweite Deutsche Tagung für psychische Hygiene in Bonn am 21. Mai 1932*, 10–18. Berlin and Leipzig: Walter de Gruyter & Co., 1932.

———. 'Psychische Hygiene'. In *Handwörterbuch der psychischen Hygiene und der psychiatrischen Fürsorge*, edited by Oswald Bumke, Gustav Kolb, Hans Roemer, and Eugen Kahn, 296–312. Berlin and Leipzig: Walter de Gruyter, 1931.

———. 'To What Extent Does Public Opinion Help, and to What Extent Does It Impair the Work of Mental Hygiene?' In *Proceedings of the First International Congress on Mental Hygiene, Held at Washington, D.C., U.S.A. May 5th to 10th, 1930*, edited by Frankwood E. Williams, 1:266–93. New York: The International Committee for Mental Hygiene, 1932.

———. 'Was will die internationale Bewegung für geistige Hygiene?' *Zeitschrift für psychische Hygiene* 1, no. 2 (1928): 33–38.

Roffenstein, Gaston. 'Das Problem der Ideologie in der materialistischen Geschichtsauffassung und das moderne Parteiwesen'. In *Partei und Klasse im Lebensprozeß der Gesellschaft*, edited by Richard Thurnwald, 1–46. Leipzig: C. L. Hirschfeld, 1926.

———. *Das Problem des psychologischen Verstehens: Ein Versuch über die Grundlagen von Psychologie, Psychoanalyse und Individualpsychologie*. Stuttgart: Julius Püttmann, 1926.

———. *Das Problem des Unbewußten*. Stuttgart: Julius Püttmann, 1923.

———. 'Einige grundsätzliche Bemerkungen zum Problem Psychopathologie und Gesellschaft'. *Zeitschrift für die gesamte Neurologie und Psychiatrie* 109 (1927): 151–58.

———. *Zur Psychologie und Psychopathologie der Gegenwartsgeschichte*. Arbeiten zur angewandten Psychiatrie 4. Berne and Leipzig: Bircher, 1921.

Rogge, Heinrich. 'Psychopolitik und Führerproblem'. *Zeitschrift für Menschenkunde* 1, no. 1 (1925): 18–24.

Rolnik, Eran. *Freud auf Hebräisch: Geschichte der Psychoanalyse im jüdischen Palästina*. Translated by David Ajchenrand. Göttingen: Vandenhoeck & Ruprecht, 2013.

Rorschach, Hermann. *Psychodiagnostik: Methodik und Ergebnisse eines wahrnehmungsdiagnostischen Experiments (Deutenlassen von Zufallsformen)*. Arbeiten zur angewandten Psychiatrie 2. Berne and Leipzig: Bircher, 1921.

Rose, Nikolas. *Inventing Our Selves: Psychology, Power, and Personhood*. Cambridge: Cambridge University Press, 1996.

———. *The Psychological Complex: Psychology, Politics, and Society in England, 1869–1939*. London and Boston: Routledge & Kegan Paul, 1985.

Rosenstein, Gaston. 'Eine Kritik'. *Jahrbuch für psychoanalytische und psychopathologische Forschungen* 4, no. 2 (1912): 741–99.

Rossi, Gabriele. 'Canevascini, Guglielmo'. In *Historisches Lexikon Der Schweiz*. Berne, 2005. http://www.hls-dhs-dss.ch/textes/f/F3499.php.

Roth, Gottfried, and Ruth Koblizek. 'Die Geschichte der Nervenheilanstalt Rosenhügel'. In *50 Jahre Schlaganfallzentrum Rosenhügel - 90 Jahre Nathaniel Freiherr von Rothschild'sche Stiftung für Nervenkranke in Wien*, edited by Ruth Koblizek and Gernot Schnaberth, 27–36. Vienna: Eigenverlag Verein MEMO, 2002.

Rotzoll, Maike. 'Rhythmus des Lebens: Arbeit in psychiatrischen Institutionen im Nationalsozialismus zwischen Normalisierung und Selektion'. In *Arbeitsrhythmus und Anstaltsalltag: Arbeit in der Psychiatrie vom frühen 19. Jahrhundert bis in die NS-Zeit*, edited by Monika Ankele and Eva Brinkschulte, 189–214. Stuttgart: Franz Steiner, 2015.

Rotzoll, Maike, Gerrit Hohendorf, Petra Fuchs, Paul Richter, Christoph Mundt, and Wolfgang U. Eckart. *Die nationalsozialistische 'Euthanasie'-Aktion T4 und ihre Opfer: Geschichte und ethische Konsequenzen für die Gegenwart*. Paderborn: Ferdinand Schöningh, 2010.

Roudinesco, Elisabeth, and Michel Plon. *Wörterbuch der Psychoanalyse: Namen, Länder, Werke, Begriffe*. Translated by Christoph Eissing-Christophersen, Marion Müllerburg, Renate Nentwig, Michel Ramaharomanana, Franziska Roelcke, and Michael Wiesmüller. Vienna and New York: Springer, 2004.

'Rückblick auf die I. Internationale Tagung für angewandte Psychopathologie und Psychologie in Wien, 5.-7. Juni 1930'. *Wiener Medizinische Wochenschrift* 80, no. 31 (1930): 1036–37.

Rüdin, Ernst. 'Bedingungen und Rolle der Eugenik in der Prophylaxe der Geistesstörungen'. *Zeitschrift für psychische Hygiene* 10, no. 4/5 (1937): 99–108.

———. 'Die Ergebnisse der psychiatrischen Erbbiologie für die eugenische Praxis'. In *Bericht über die Zweite Deutsche Tagung für psychische Hygiene in Bonn am 21. Mai 1932*, edited by Hans Roemer, 19–29. Berlin and Leipzig: Walter de Gruyter & Co., 1932.

———. 'Emil Kraepelin, Zur Entartungsfrage'. *Archiv Für Rassen- Und Gesellschaftsbiologie* 6, no. 2 (1909): 254–57.

———. 'Erbbiologisch-psychiatrische Streitfragen'. *Zeitschrift für die gesamte Neurologie und Psychiatrie* 108 (1927): 247–97.

———. *Erblehre und Rassenhygiene im völkischen Staat*. Munich: J. F. Lehmanns, 1934.

———. 'Heiratsprophylaxe und psychische Hygiene'. *Zeitschrift für psychische Hygiene* 11 (1938): 152–65.

———. 'The Significance of Eugenics and Genetics for Mental Hygiene'. In *Proceedings of the First International Congress on Mental Hygiene, Held at Washington, D.C., U.S.A. May 5th to 10th, 1930*, edited by Frankwood E. Williams, 1:471–95. New York: The International Committee for Mental Hygiene, 1932.

Rüdin, Ernst, and Hans Roemer. 'Der Deutsche Ausschuß für psychische Hygiene der Gesellschaft Deutscher Neurologen und Psychiater'. *Zeitschrift für psychische Hygiene* 8, no. 4 (1935): 97–99.

———. 'Der Deutsche Verband für psychische Hygiene und Rassenhygiene'. *Zeitschrift für psychische Hygiene* 6, no. 5 (1933): 129–30.

———. 'Robert Sommer†'. *Zeitschrift für psychische Hygiene* 10, no. 1 (1937): 1–2.

Russel, William L. 'A Brief Account of the Life and Work of Dr. Salmon'. In *Proceedings of the First International Congress on Mental Hygiene, Held at Washington,D.C., U.S.A. May 5th to 10th, 1930*, edited by Frankwood E. Williams, 1:515–23. New York: The International Committee for Mental Hygiene, 1932.

Sablik, Karl. *Julius Tandler: Mediziner und Sozialreformer*. Frankfurt am Main: Peter Lang, 2010.

Sack, A. *Die geistigen Typen der Juden und die Revolutionsbewegung*. Heidelberg: Wolff, 1920.

Sack, Martin. *Von der Neuropathologie zur Phänomenologie: Alfred Prinz Auersperg und die Geschichte der Heidelberger Schule*. Würzburg: Königshausen & Neumann, 2005.

Sarasin, Philipp. 'Das obszöne Genießen der Wissenschaft: Über Populärwissenschaft und mad scientists'. In *Geschichtswissenschaft und Diskursanalyse*, 231–57. Frankfurt am Main: Suhrkamp, 2003.

———. 'Kampf ums Dasein'. In *Evolution: Ein interdisziplinäres Handbuch*, edited by Philipp Sarasin and Marianne Sommer, 33–36. Stuttgart and Weimar: J. B. Metzler, 2010.

'Satzungen des Deutschen Verbands für psychische Hygiene'. *Zeitschrift für psychische Hygiene* 1, no. 5 (1928): 137–40.

Schäfer, Armin. 'Die Archivfunktion der Psychiatrie (Kraepelin, Jaspers)'. In *Gewalt der Archive: Studien zur Kulturgeschichte der Wissensspeicherung*, edited by Thomas Weitin and Burkhardt Wolf, 235–54. Konstanz: Konstanz University Press, 2012.

Schelenz, Hermann. 'Jean Paul Marat'. *Münchener medizinische Wochenschrift* 66, no. 27 (1919): 752–53.

Scheler, Max. *Die Ursachen des Deutschenhasses: Eine nationalpädagogische Erörterung*. Leipzig: K. Wolff, 1917.

Schmiedebach, Heinz-Peter. 'Eine "antipsychiatrische Bewegung" um die Jahrhundertwende'. In *Medizinkritische Bewegungen im Deutschen Reich (ca. 1870–ca. 1933)*, edited by Martin Dinges, 127–60. Stuttgart: Steiner, 1996.

———, ed. *Entgrenzungen des Wahnsinns: Psychopathie und Psychopathologisierungen um 1900*. Berlin and Boston: Walter de Gruyter, 2016.

Schmiedebach, Heinz-Peter, and Stefan Priebe. 'Social Psychiatry in Germany in the Twentieth Century: Ideas and Models'. *Medical History* 48, no. 4 (2004): 449–72.

Schmitz, Hans Aloys. 'Der Zweite Internationale Kongreß für Psychische Hygiene in Paris vom 19. bis 25. Juli 1937'. *Zeitschrift für psychische Hygiene* 10, no. 4/5 (1937): 119–25.

Schmuhl, Hans-Walter. 'Die Genesis der "Euthanasie:" Interpretationsansätze'. In *Die nationalsozialistische 'Euthanasie'-Aktion T4 und ihre Opfer: Geschichte und ethische Konsequenzen für die Gegenwart*, edited by Maike Rotzoll, Gerrit Hohendorf, Petra Fuchs, Paul Richter, Christoph Mundt, and Wolfgang U. Eckart, 66–76. Paderborn: Ferdinand Schöningh, 2010.

———. *Die Gesellschaft Deutscher Neurologen und Psychiater im Nationalsozialismus*. Berlin: Springer, 2016.

———. 'Die Patientenmorde'. In *Vernichten und Heilen: Der Nürnberger Ärzteprozeß und seine Folgen*, edited by Angelika Ebbinghaus and Klaus Dörner, 295–329. Berlin: Aufbau Verlag, 2001.

———. 'Die Selbstverständlichkeit des Tötens: Psychiater im Nationalsozialismus'. *Geschichte und Gesellschaft* 16, no. 4 (1990): 411–39.

———. 'Psychiatrie und Politik: Die Gesellschaft Deutscher Neurologen und Psychiater im Nationalsozialismus'. In *Abweichung und Normalität: Psychiatrie in Deutschland vom Kaiserreich bis zur Deutschen Einheit*, edited by Christine Wolters, Christof Beyer, and Brigitte Lohff, 137–58. Bielefeld: transcript, 2013.

———. *Rassenhygiene, Nationalsozialismus, Euthanasie: Von der Verhütung zur Vernichtung 'lebensunwerten Lebens,' 1890–1945*. Göttingen: Vandenhoeck & Ruprecht, 1987.

Schmuhl, Hans-Walter, and Volker Roelcke, eds. *'Heroische Therapien:' Die deutsche Psychiatrie im internationalen Vergleich 1918–1945*. Göttingen: Wallstein, 2013.

Schnaberth, Gernot. 'Das neurologische Krankenhaus Rosenhügel seit dem Ende des Zweiten Weltkriegs'. In *50 Jahre Schlaganfallzentrum Rosenhügel - 90 Jahre*

Nathaniel Freiherr von Rothschild'sche Stiftung für Nervenkranke in Wien, edited by Ruth Koblizek and Gernot Schnaberth, 58–69. Vienna: Eigenverlag Verein MEMO, 2002.

Schneider, Carl. *Behandlung und Verhütung der Geisteskrankheiten: Allgemeine Erfahrungen, Grundsätze, Technik, Biologie*. Berlin: J. Springer, 1939.

———. 'Seelische Hygiene'. In *Internationale Hygiene-Ausstellung Dresden 1930: Amtlicher Führer*, 268–71. Dresden: Verlag der Internationalen Hygiene-Ausstellung, 1930.

Schneider, Ernst. 'Schutz durch Beratung in Lebensfragen'. In *Das psychoanalytische Volksbuch*, edited by Paul Federn and Heinrich Meng, 278–87. Stuttgart: Hippokrates, 1926.

Schneider, P.-B., O. Riggenbach, and R. Egli. 'Au Docteur André Repond, Directeur de la Maison de Santé de Malévoz, Monthey'. *Zeitschrift für Präventivmedizin* 1 (1956): 429–31.

Schorske, Carl E. *Fin-de-Siècle Vienna: Politics and Culture*. New York: Vintage Books, 1981.

Schreber, Daniel Paul. *Denkwürdigkeiten eines Nervenkranken*. Frankfurt am Main: Syndikat, 1985.

Schröder, Christina. *Der Fachstreit um das Seelenheil: Psychotherapiegeschichte zwischen 1880 und 1932*. Frankfurt am Main: Peter Lang, 1995.

Scull, Andrew. 'A Failure to Communicate? On the Reception of Foucault's Histoire de La Folie by Anglo-American Historians'. In *The Insanity of Place/The Place of Insanity: Essays on the History of Psychiatry*, 30–37. London and New York: Routledge, 2006.

———. 'Some Reflections on Madness and Culture in the Post-War World'. *History of Psychiatry* 25 (2014): 395–403.

Searls, Damion. *The Inkblots: Hermann Rorschach, His Iconic Test, and the Power of Seeing*. New York: Crown, 2017.

Sedgwick, Peter. *Psychopolitics: Laing, Foucault, Goffman, Szasz, and the Future of Mass Psychiatry*. New York: Harper & Row, 1982.

Shamdasani, Sonu. 'Psychotherapy: The Invention of a Word'. *History of the Human Sciences* 18, no. 1 (2005): 1–22.

Shepherd, Michael. 'Two Faces of Emil Kraepelin'. *British Journal of Psychiatry* 167, no. 2 (1995): 174–83.

Shillady, John R. 'The Story of the Congress'. In *Proceedings of the First International Congress on Mental Hygiene, Held at Washington, D.C., U.S.A. May 5th to 10th, 1930*, edited by Frankwood E. Williams, 1:1–31. New York: The International Committee for Mental Hygiene, 1932.

Shorter, Edward. *A History of Psychiatry: From the Era of the Asylum to the Age of Prozac*. New York: Wiley, 1997.

Shorvon, Simon D., Giselle Weiss, and Howard P. Goodkin. 'Notes on the Origins of Epilepsia and the International League Against Epilepsy'. *Epilepsia* 50, no. 3 (2009): 368–76.

Showalter, Elaine. *The Female Malady: Women, Madness and English Culture, 1830–1980*. New York: Pantheon Books, 1985.

Siemen, Hans Ludwig. 'Die Reformpsychiatrie der Weimarer Republik: Subjektive Ansprüche und die Macht des Faktischen'. In *Nach Hadamar: Zum Verhältnis von Psychiatrie und Politik im 20. Jahrhundert*, edited by Franz-Werner Kersting, Karl Teppe, and Bernd Walter, 98–108. Paderborn: Ferdinand Schöningh, 1993.

———. *Menschen blieben auf der Strecke …: Psychiatrie zwischen Reform und Nationalsozialismus*. Gütersloh: Jakob von Hoddis, 1987.

———. 'Reform und Radikalisierung: Veränderungen der Psychiatrie in der Weltwirtschaftskrise'. In *Medizin und Gesundheitspolitik in der NS-Zeit*, edited by Norbert Frei, 191–200. München: Oldenbourg, 1991.

Simon, Hermann. *Aktivere Krankenbehandlung in der Irrenanstalt*. Berlin and Leipzig: Walter de Gruyter, 1929.

———. 'Ergebnisse einer aktiveren Krankenbehandlung in der Heil- und Pflegeanstalt'. *Deutsche Medizinische Wochenschrift* 64 (1938): 1224–27.

———. 'Krankenbehandlung in der Heilanstalt, insbesondere Beschäftigung, in ihren Beziehungen zur psychischen Hygiene'. In *Bericht über die Erste Deutsche Tagung für psychische Hygiene in Hamburg am 20. Dezember 1928*, edited by Hans Roemer, 19–24. Berlin and Leipzig: Walter de Gruyter, 1929.

Sioli, Franz. 'Ausbildung der mit psychischer Hygiene befaßten Personenkreise'. In *Handwörterbuch der psychischen Hygiene und der psychiatrischen Fürsorge*, edited by Oswald Bumke, Gustav Kolb, Hans Roemer, and Eugen Kahn, 31–34. Berlin and Leipzig: Walter de Gruyter, 1931.

Smith, R. Percy. 'The International Committee for the Study of the Causes and Prophylaxis of Mental Disease'. *British Journal of Psychiatry* 56, no. 234 (1910): 389–405.

Soddy, Kenneth. 'The Mental Hygiene Movement and the Problem of Preventive Mental Health'. In *Psychiatrie der Gegenwart: Forschung und Praxis, Vol. III: Soziale und Angewandte Psychiatrie*, edited by Hans W. Gruhle, R. Jung, W. Mayer-Gross, and Max Müller, 36–50. Berlin, Göttingen, and Heidelberg: Springer, 1961.

Sommer, Robert. *Aerztlicher Notruf zum Ende des Jahres 1918*. n.p.: self-published, 1918.

———. *Bericht über den II. Kurs mit Kongress für Familienforschung, Vererbungs- und Regenerationslehre in Gießen vom 9. bis 13. April 1912*. Halle: Carl Marhold, 1912.

———. 'Beseitigung funktioneller Taubheit, besonders bei Soldaten, durch eine experimental-psychologische Methode'. *Archiv für Psychiatrie und Nervenkrankheiten* 57 (1917): 574–75.

———. 'Clifford Whittingham Beers, A mind that found itself (Eine Seele, die sich fand)'. *Zeitschrift für psychische Hygiene* 1, no. 1 (1928): 5–9.

———. 'Der natürliche Adel als Ausleseprinzip'. In *Bericht über die Zweite Deutsche Tagung für psychische Hygiene in Bonn am 21. Mai 1932*, edited by Hans Roemer, 132–33. Berlin and Leipzig: Walter de Gruyter & Co., 1932.

———. *Diagnostik der Geisteskrankheiten für praktische Ärzte und Studierende.* Berlin and Vienna: Urban & Schwarzenberg, 1901.

———. 'Die Einrichtung von öffentlichen Schlaf- und Ruhehallen'. *Die Krankenpflege* 2 (1902): 528–30.

———. *Die Goldmacher: Eine Komödie.* Giessen: von Münchow'sche Univ.-Druckerei, 1921.

———. 'Die I. Tagung des Deutschen Verbands für Psychische Hygiene in Hamburg-Friedrichsberg vom 19.-21. Sept. 1928'. *Allgemeine ärztliche Zeitschrift für Psychotherapie und psychische Hygiene* 1 (1928): 619–22.

———. 'Die körperliche Erziehung der deutschen Studentenschaft'. *Zeitschrift für Schulgesundheitspflege* 29, no. 9 (1916): 393–409.

———. 'Die nationale und internationale Organisation der psychischen Hygiene'. *Allgemeine Zeitschrift für die Psychiatrie und psychisch-gerichtliche Medizin* 83, no. 5/6 (1926): 391–94.

———. 'Die nationale und internationale Organisation der psychischen Hygiene'. *Deutsches Ärzteblatt* 59, no. 11 (1930): 130–31.

———. 'Die öffentlichen Schlaf- und Ruhehallen bei der Internationalen Hygiene-Ausstellung in Dresden'. *Psychiatrisch-Neurologische Wochenschrift* 13 (1911): 202–5.

———. 'Die psychische Hygiene der Arbeit und Erholung'. In *Bericht über die Erste Deutsche Tagung für psychische Hygiene in Hamburg am 20. Dezember 1928*, edited by Hans Roemer, 94. Berlin and Leipzig: Walter de Gruyter, 1929.

———. 'Die psychische Hygiene des Lärms'. *Allgemeine ärztliche Zeitschrift für Psychotherapie und psychische Hygiene* 2, no. 1 (1929): 33–34.

———. 'Die psychische Hygiene und die Leibesübungen'. In *Bericht über die Erste Deutsche Tagung für psychische Hygiene in Hamburg am 20. Dezember 1928*, edited by Hans Roemer, 95. Berlin and Leipzig: Walter de Gruyter, 1929.

———. 'Die weitere Entwicklung der öffentlichen Ruhehallen'. *Klinik für psychische und nervöse Krankheiten* 6 (1911): 368–79.

———. *Die Werk-Währung.* Giessen: Druck der Oberhessischen Volkszeitung, 1931.

———. 'Eine psychiatrische Abteilung des Reichsgesundheitsamts'. *Psychiatrisch-Neurologische Wochenschrift* 12, no. 12 (1910): 295–98.

———. *Familienforschung und Vererbungslehre.* 1st ed. Leipzig: Johann Ambrosius Barth, 1907.

———. *Familienforschung und Vererbungslehre.* 2nd ed. Leipzig: Johann Ambrosius Barth, 1922.

———. *Familienforschung, Vererbungs- und Rassenlehre*. 3rd ed. Leipzig: Johann Ambrosius Barth, 1927.

———. 'Krieg und Seelenleben'. *Wiener Medizinische Wochenschrift* 65, no. 39 (1915): 1441–48.

———. *Krieg und Seelenleben*. Leipzig: Otto Nemnich, 1916.

———. 'Organisation und Aufgaben eines Reichsinstituts für Familienforschung und Vererbungslehre'. *Deutsche Medizinische Wochenschrift*, no. 14 (1914): 708–11.

———. 'Psychiatrische Erblichkeitsforschung und psychische Hygiene'. In *Bericht über die Erste Deutsche Tagung für psychische Hygiene in Hamburg am 20. Dezember 1928*, edited by Hans Roemer, 96–100. Berlin and Leipzig: Walter de Gruyter, 1929.

———. 'Psychotherapie und psychische Hygiene'. *Allgemeine ärztliche Zeitschrift für Psychotherapie und psychische Hygiene* 1, no. 1 (1928): 6–10.

———. 'Psychotherapie und psychische Hygiene'. *Allgemeine ärztliche Zeitschrift für Psychotherapie und psychische Hygiene* 1, no. 2 (1928): 129–34.

———. 'Schlusswort'. In *Bericht über die Erste Deutsche Tagung für psychische Hygiene in Hamburg am 20. Dezember 1928*, edited by Hans Roemer, 136. Berlin and Leipzig: Walter de Gruyter, 1929.

———. 'The Meaning of Recreation and Avocation in Mental Hygiene'. In *Proceedings of the First International Congress on Mental Hygiene, Held at Washington, D.C., U.S.A. May 5th to 10th, 1930*, edited by Frankwood E. Williams, 2:550–64. New York: The International Committee for Mental Hygiene, 1932.

———. 'Zu dem internationalen Kongress für psychische Hygiene'. *Wiener Medizinische Wochenschrift* 75, no. 18 (1925): 1060–61.

———. 'Zur Frage einer psychiatrischen Abteilung des Reichsgesundheitsamts'. *Psychiatrisch-Neurologische Wochenschrift* 13 (1911): 31–34.

Sommer, Robert, and Hans Roemer. 'Niederschrift über die erste Mitgliederversammlung des Deutschen Verbandes für psychische Hygiene in Hamburg in der Staatskrankenanstalt Friedrichsberg am 19. September 1928'. *Zeitschrift für psychische Hygiene* 1, no. 5 (1928): 134–37.

———. 'Niederschrift über die II. Mitgliederversammlung des Deutschen Verbandes für psychische Hygiene in Bonn im Auditorium maximum der Universität am 20. Mai 1932 17 Uhr'. *Zeitschrift für psychische Hygiene* 5 (1932): 179–83.

Sommer, Robert, Wilhelm Weygandt, Hans Roemer, Gustav Kolb, and Hermann Simon. 'Zum Ersten Internationalen Kongreß für psychische Hygiene'. *Zeitschrift für psychische Hygiene* 3, no. 2 (1930): 33–35.

Spaulding, Ernest Wilder. *The Quiet Invaders: The Story of the Austrian Impact upon America*. Vienna: Österreichischer Bundesverlag, 1968.

Spoerri, Elka. *Adolf Wölfli: Draftsman, Writer, Poet, Composer*. Ithaca: Cornell University Press, 1997.

Spöring, Francesco. '"Du musst Apostel der Wahrheit werden:" Auguste Forel und der sozialhygienische Antialkoholdiskurs, 1886–1931'. In *Biopolitik und Sittlichkeitsreform: Kampagnen gegen Alkohol, Drogen und Prostitution 1880–1950*, edited by Judith Große, Francesco Spöring, and Jana Tschurenev, 111–44. Frankfurt am Main: Campus, 2014.

Spreng, Hanns. 'Zum Geleit'. *Schweizerische Zeitschrift für Psychologie und ihre Anwendungen* 9, no. 1 (1952): 1–2.

Springer, Alfred. 'Die Verwirklichung der "geeinten deutschen Seelenkunde" im Nationalsozialistischen Österreich: Ideengeschichtliche Aspekte'. In *Gründe der Seele: Die Wiener Psychiatrie im 20. Jahrhundert*, edited by Brigitta Keintzel, 90–135. Vienna: Picus, 1999.

Stanghelleni, Giovanni, and Thomas Fuchs, eds. *One Century of Karl Jaspers' General Psychopathology*. Oxford: Oxford University Press, 2013.

Staudacher, Anna L. *'... meldet den Austritt aus dem mosaischen Glauben:' 18.000 Austritte aus dem Judentum in Wien, 1868–1914: Namen - Quellen - Daten*. Frankfurt am Main: Peter Lang, 2009.

Steger, Heinrich. *Verteidigungsrede im Prozesse gegen Frau Nelly Grosavescu wegen Verbrechens des Gattenmordes, gehalten am 25. Juni 1927 vor dem Wiener Schwurgerichtshofe*. Vienna and Leipzig: Moritz Perles, 1927.

Steinberg, Holger. *Kraepelin in Leipzig: Eine Begegnung von Psychiatrie und Psychologie*. Bonn: Psychiatrie-Verlag, 2001.

Steinberg, Holger, and Matthias C. Angermeyer. 'Emil Kraepelin's Years at Dorpat as Professor of Psychiatry in Nineteenth-Century Russia'. *History of Psychiatry* 12, no. 47 (2001): 297–327.

Steinmetz, Willibald, and Heinz-Gerhard Haupt. 'The Political as Communicative Space in History: The Bielefeld Approach'. In *Writing Political History Today*, edited by Willibald Steinmetz, Ingrid Gilcher-Holtey, and Heinz-Gerhard Haupt, 11–36. Frankfurt am Main and New York: Campus, 2013.

Stelzner, Helenefriderike. 'Psychopathologisches in der Revolution'. *Zeitschrift für die gesamte Neurologie und Psychiatrie* 49 (1919): 393–408.

Stern, William. 'Angewandte Psychologie'. *Beiträge zur Psychologie der Aussage* 1 (1903): 4–45.

Stiegler, Bernard. *Prendre soin: De la jeunesse et des générations*. Paris: Flammarion, 2008.

Still, Arthur, and Irving Velody. *Rewriting the History of Madness: Studies in Foucault's Histoire de La Folie*. London: Routledge, 1992.

Stockdreher, Petra. 'Heil- und Pflegeanstalt Eglfing-Haar'. In *Psychiatrie im Nationalsozialismus: Die Bayerischen Heil- und Pflegeanstalten zwischen 1933 und 1945*, edited by Michael von Cranach and Hans-Ludwig Siemen, 327–62. Munich: Oldenbourg, 1999.

Stokes, Aldwyn. 'In Memoriam: Clarence B. Farrar (1874–1970)'. *American Journal of Psychiatry* 127 (1970): 387–88.

Stransky, Erwin. 'Angewandte Psychiatrie: Motive und Elemente zu einem Programmentwurf'. *Allgemeine Zeitschrift für Psychiatrie und psychisch-gerichtliche Medizin* 74, no. 1–3 (1918): 22–53.

———. 'Angewandte Psychopathologie und Gegenwartszivilisation'. In *I. Internationale Tagung für angewandte Psychopathologie und Psychologie, Wien, 5.-7. Juni 1930: Referate und Vorträge*, edited by Heinz Hartmann, Martin Pappenheim, and Erwin Stransky, 146–61. Berlin: S. Karger, 1931.

———. 'Angewandte Psychopathologie: Vortrag gehalten im Akademischen Verein für medizinische Psychologie in Wien am 10. Dezember 1931'. *Psychiatrisch-Neurologische Wochenschrift* 16 (1932): 195–98.

———. 'Aus einem Gelehrtenleben um die Zeitenwende: Rückschau, Ausblick, Gedanken', n.d. Josephinum Wien, Autographensammlung, no. 2065.

———. 'Auswirkungen der Psychopathologie auf das Gegenwartsdenken'. *Wissenschaft und Weltbild* 15 (1962): 1–18.

———. 'Behandlungs- und Beratungsstellen für Psychisch-Nervöse'. *Wiener Medizinische Wochenschrift* 69, no. 9 (1919): 435–38.

———. 'Curriculum Vitae', n.d. Autographensammlung, Josephinum Wien, no. 2064.

———. *Der Deutschenhaß*. Vienna and Leipzig: Franz Deuticke, 1919.

———. 'Der Fachärzteverband und die Kliniker'. *Wiener Klinische Wochenschrift* 38, no. 46 (1925): 1241–43.

———. 'Der seelische Wiederaufbau des deutschen Volkes und die Aufgaben der Psychiatrie: Erweiterter Vortrag, gehalten auf der Deutschen Psychiaterversammlung in Hamburg, am 27./28. Mai 1920'. *Zeitschrift für die gesamte Neurologie und Psychiatrie* 60, no. 1 (1920): 271–80.

———. 'Der Tagung für angewandte Psychopathologie und Psychologie zum Gruße'. *Wiener Klinische Wochenschrift* 80, no. 23 (1930): 766.

———. 'Die Verhandlung gegen Hofrat Professor Dr. Wagner-Jauregg und Genossen. Oder: Dank vom Hause Österreich. Ein Nachruf'. *Wiener Medizinische Wochenschrift* 70, no. 45 (1920): 1901–2.

———. 'Gaston Roffenstein'. *Wiener Medizinische Wochenschrift* 77, no. 39 (1927): 1330–31.

———. 'Großdeutschland und die Ärzteschaft'. *Wiener Medizinische Wochenschrift* 69, no. 2 (1919): 117–25.

———. 'Keine Bedenklichkeit der angewandten Psychiatrie'. *Zeitschrift für die gesamte Neurologie und Psychiatrie* 69 (1921): 327–31.

———. *Krieg und Geistesstörung: Feststellungen und Erwägungen zu diesem Thema vom Standpunkte der angewandten Psychiatrie*. Wiesbaden: J. F. Bergmann, 1918.

———. 'Kriegspsychiatrie und Kriegsgerichtsbarkeit'. *Wiener Medizinische Wochenschrift* 69, no. 28 (1919): 1361–68.

———. 'Kriegspsychiatrie und Kriegsgerichtsbarkeit'. *Wiener Medizinische Wochenschrift* 69, no. 29 (1919): 1425–30.

———. *Lehrbuch der allgemeinen und speziellen Psychiatrie*. Vol. 2. Leipzig: F. C. W. Vogel, 1919.

———, ed. *Leitfaden der psychischen Hygiene*. Vienna: Urban & Schwarzenberg, 1931.

———. 'Menschenbehandlung und Menschenführung aus ärztlicher Schau'. In *Menschenführung im Blickfeld der Pädagogik und Psychohygiene*, edited by Ludwig Hänsel, Karl Dienelt, and Erwin Stransky, 94–140. Vienna and Munich: Österreichischer Bundesverlag für Unterricht, Wissenschaft und Kunst, 1960.

———. 'Modeströmungen und Kurzschlüsse in der Psychiatrie'. *Zeitschrift für die gesamte Neurologie und Psychiatrie* 101 (1926): 770–85.

———. 'Psychiatrie und psychologische Methodik'. *Wiener Medizinische Wochenschrift* 79, no. 21 (1929): 671–76.

———. 'Psychoanalyse und Kritik'. *Wiener Medizinische Wochenschrift* 71, no. 16 (1921): 716–18.

———. *Psychopathie und Staatsführung*. Vienna and Innsbruck: Urban & Schwarzenberg, 1952.

———. *Psychopathologie der Ausnahmezustände und Psychopathologie des Alltags*. Arbeiten zur angewandten Psychiatrie 3. Berne and Leipzig: Bircher, 1921.

———. 'Rasse und Psychotherapie'. *Zentralblatt für Psychotherapie* 10 (1937): 9–28.

———. 'Remarks Concerning the Development of Applied Psychopathology'. *American Journal of Psychiatry* 92 (1936): 1043–49.

———. 'Richtungen der psychischen Hygiene: Nach einem Vortrag, gehalten am 9. Dezember 1931 in der Jahresversammlung der Gesellschaft für Volksaufartung und Erbkunde'. *Wiener Klinische Wochenschrift* 45, no. 2 (1932): 42–46.

———. *Subordination, Autorität, Psychotherapie: Eine Studie vom Standpunkt des klinischen Empirikers*. Vienna: Julius Springer, 1928.

———. *Über die Dementia Praecox: Streifzüge durch Klinik und Psychopathologie*. Wiesbaden: Bergmann, 1909.

———. 'Vorträge für Abiturienten über psychische Hygiene in Wien'. *Zeitschrift für psychische Hygiene* 5, no. 6 (1932): 184–85.

———. 'Wesen und Programmatik der psychischen Hygiene'. In *Leitfaden der psychischen Hygiene*, edited by Erwin Stransky, 1–10. Vienna: Urban & Schwarzenberg, 1931.

———. 'Zur nervösen und psychischen Morbität der städtischen Hausgehilfinnen'. *Wiener Klinische Wochenschrift* 44, no. 47 (1931): 1460–64.

Stransky, Erwin, and Bernard Dattner. *Über Psychoanalyse: Einleitender Vortrag von Rudolf Allers in Wien, mit daranschließender Aussprache im Verein für angewandte Psychopathologie und Psychologie in Wien (S.-S. 1920)*. Berlin: S. Karger, 1922.

Szasz, Thomas. *The Myth of Mental Illness: Foundations of a Theory of Personal Conduct*. New York: Harper & Row, 1961.

———. *The Therapeutic State: Psychiatry in the Mirror of Current Events*. Buffalo, N.Y.: Prometheus Books, 1984.

Tandler, Julius. 'Gefahren Der Minderwertigkeit'. *Das Wiener Jugendhilfswerk: Jahrbuch*, 1928, 3–22.

Tanner, Jakob. 'Auguste Forel als Ikone der Wissenschaft: Ein Plädoyer für historische Forschung'. In *Auguste Forel: Eugenik und Erinnerungskultur*, edited by Anton Leist, 81–106. Zurich: vdf Hochschulverlag, 2006.

'Tätigkeitsbericht der Österr. Gesellschaft für Volksgesundheit über das 5. Vereinsjahr. (Mitte November 1929 bis Mitte November 1930)'. *Volksgesundheit: Zeitschrift für soziale Hygiene* 4, no. 10/11 (1930): 207–17.

Teller, Christine. 'Carl Schneider: Zur Biographie eines deutschen Wissenschaftlers'. *Geschichte und Gesellschaft* 16, no. 4 (1990): 464–78.

Thomson, Mathew. 'Mental Hygiene as an International Movement'. In *International Health Organisations and Movements, 1918–1939*, edited by Paul Weindling, 283–304. Cambridge: Cambridge University Press, 1995.

———. 'Mental Hygiene in Britain during the First Half of the Twentieth Century: The Limits of International Influence'. In *International Relations in Psychiatry: Britain, Germany, and the United States to World War II*, edited by Volker Roelcke, Paul Weindling, and Louise Westwood, 134–55. Rochester: University of Rochester Press, 2010.

———. 'The Psychological Sciences and the Scientization and Engineering of Society in Twentieth-Century Britain'. In *Engineering Society: The Role of the Human and Social Sciences in Modern Societies, 1880–1980*, edited by Kerstin Brückweh, Dirk Schumann, Richard F. Wetzell, and Benjamin Ziemann, 141–58. London: Palgrave Macmillan, 2012.

Toller, Ernst. *Eine Jugend in Deutschland*. Reinbek: Rowohlt, 1963.

Toms, Jonathan. 'Political Dimensions of "the Psychosocial": The 1948 International Congress on Mental Health and the Mental Hygiene Movement'. *History of the Human Sciences* 25, no. 5 (2012): 91–106.

Triarhou, Lazaros C. 'Erwin Stransky (1877–1962)'. *Journal of Neurology* 259, no. 9 (2012): 2012–13.

Tyndel, Milo. 'In Memoriam: Erwin Stransky, M.D. 1878–1962'. *The American Journal of Psychiatry* 119 (1962): 287–88.

Uekötter, Frank. *Umweltgeschichte im 19. und 20. Jahrhundert*. Munich: Oldenbourg, 2007.

'Verein für angewandte Psychopathologie und Psychologie'. *Wiener Medizinische Wochenschrift* 85, no. 37 (1935): 999–1002.

'Verein für angewandte Psychopathologie und Psychologie in Wien'. *Wiener Medizinische Wochenschrift* 84, no. 22 (1934): 621.

'Verein für angewandte Psychopathologie und Psychologie in Wien'. *Wiener Medizinische Wochenschrift* 87, no. 32 (1937): 854–56.

'Verein für angewandte Psychopathologie und Psychologie in Wien: Bericht über die Tätigkeit im Wintersemester 1920'. *Wiener Medizinische Wochenschrift* 70, no. 47 (1920): 1981–84.

'Verein für angewandte Psychopathologie und Psychologie: Sitzung vom 20. Juni 1927'. *Wiener Medizinische Wochenschrift* 77, no. 47 (1927): 1602.

Verhey, Jeffrey. *The Spirit of 1914: Militarism, Myth and Mobilization in Germany.* New York: Cambridge University Press, 2000.

Virchow, Rudolf. 'Der Armenarzt'. *Die medicinische Reform*, no. 18 (1848).

Vogel, Martin. 'Aufklärung, hygienische und Volksaufklärung: Allgemeines, Grundsätzliches und Geschichtliches'. In *Handwörterbuch der psychischen Hygiene und der psychiatrischen Fürsorge*, edited by Oswald Bumke, Gustav Kolb, Hans Roemer, and Eugen Kahn, 23–30. Berlin and Leipzig: Walter de Gruyter, 1930.

'Vorträge über psychische Hygiene, veranstaltet vom österreichischen Unterausschuss für psychische Hygiene in Wien'. *Zentralblatt für Psychotherapie* 5, no. 4 (1932): 193.

Wagner-Jauregg, Julius. *Lebenserinnerungen.* Vienna: Springer, 1950.

———. 'Über Eugenik'. *Wiener Klinische Wochenschrift* 44 (1931): 1–6.

Walter, Bernd. 'Hermann Simon: Psychiatriereformer, Sozialdarwinist, Nationalsozialist?' *Der Nervenarzt* 73, no. 11 (2002): 1047–54.

———. *Psychiatrie und Gesellschaft in der Moderne: Geisteskrankenfürsorge in der Provinz Westfalen zwischen Kaiserreich und NS-Regime.* Paderborn: Ferdinand Schöningh, 1996.

Watson, Alexander. *Enduring the Great War: Combat, Morale and Collapse in the German and British Armies, 1914–1918.* Cambridge: Cambridge University Press, 2009.

Weber, Matthias M. 'Psychiatric Research and Science Policy in Germany: The History of the Deutsche Forschungsanstalt Für Psychiatrie (German Institute for Psychiatric Research) in Munich from 1917 to 1945'. *History of Psychiatry* 11, no. 43 (2000): 235–58.

———. 'Rassenhygienische und genetische Forschungen an der Deutschen Forschungsanstalt für Psychiatrie/Kaiser-Wilhelm-Institut in München vor und nach 1933'. In *Geschichte der Kaiser-Wilhelm-Gesellschaft im Nationalsozialismus: Bestandsaufnahme und Perspektiven der Forschung*, edited by Doris Kaufmann, 1:95–111. Göttingen: Wallstein, 2000.

Weber, Matthias M., Wolfgang Burgmair, and Eric J. Engstrom. 'Emil Kraepelin: Zwischen klinischen Krankheitsbildern und "psychischer Volkshygiene"'. *Deutsches Ärzteblatt* 103, no. 41 (2006): 2685–90.

Weidner, Tobias. *Die unpolitische Profession. Deutsche Mediziner im langen 19. Jahrhundert.* Frankfurt am Main: Campus, 2012.

Weihsmann, Helmut. *Das Rote Wien: Sozialdemokratische Architektur und Kommunalpolitik 1919–1934*. Vienna: Promedia, 2002.

Weindling, Paul. *Health, Race and German Politics Between National Unification and Nazism, 1870–1945*. Cambridge: Cambridge University Press, 1989.

———. 'Public Health in Germany'. In *The History of Public Health and the Modern State*, edited by Dorothy Porter, 119–32. Amsterdam and Atlanta: Editions Rodopi, 1994.

———. 'The Sonderweg of German Eugenics: Nationalism and Scientific Internationalism'. *The British Journal for the History of Science* 22, no. 3 (1989): 321–33.

Weingart, Peter, Jürgen Kroll, and Kurt Bayertz. *Rasse, Blut und Gene: Geschichte der Eugenik und Rassenhygiene in Deutschland*. Frankfurt am Main: Suhrkamp, 1992.

Weinländer, Georg. 'Stranskys Deutschenhaß'. *Wiener Medizinische Wochenschrift* 70 (1920): 1017–18.

Weiss, Sheila Faith. *'The Sword of Our Science' as a Foreign Policy Weapon: The Political Function of German Geneticists in the International Arena During the Third Reich*. Berlin: MPIWG, 2005.

Wettley, Annemarie. 'Forel, August'. In *Neue Deutsche Biographie*, 5:298–99, 1961.

Wetzell, Richard F. 'Die Rolle medizinischer Experten in Strafjustiz und Strafrechtsreformbewegung: Eine Medikalisierung des Strafrechts?' In *Experten und Expertenwissen in der Strafjustiz von der Frühen Neuzeit bis zur Moderne*, edited by Alexander Kästner and Sylvia Kesper-Biermann, 57–72. Leipzig: Meine, 2008.

———. *Inventing the Criminal: A History of German Criminology, 1880–1945*. Chapel Hill and London: University of North Carolina Press, 2000.

Weygandt, Wilhelm. 'Das Leben und Wirken von Robert Sommer'. *Zeitschrift für psychische Hygiene* 10, no. 3 (1937): 65–82.

———. 'Psychohygienische Tagung und Ausstellung in der Schweiz'. *Zeitschrift für psychische Hygiene* 4, no. 6 (1931): 182–83.

———. 'Über die Aufgaben des deutschen Verbandes für psychische Hygiene und die erste deutsche Tagung'. In *Bericht über die Erste Deutsche Tagung für psychische Hygiene in Hamburg am 20. Dezember 1928*, edited by Hans Roemer, 8–12. Berlin and Leipzig: Walter de Gruyter, 1929.

White, William A. 'The Origin, Growth, and Significance of the Mental-Hygiene Movement'. In *Proceedings of the First International Congress on Mental Hygiene, Held at Washington, D.C., U.S.A. May 5th to 10th, 1930*, edited by Frankwood E. Williams, 1:523–33. New York: The International Committee for Mental Hygiene, 1932.

Whitrow, Magda. *Julius Wagner-Jauregg (1857–1940)*. London: Smith-Gordon, 1993.

Williams, Frankwood E. *Proceedings of the First International Congress on Mental Hygiene, Held at Washington, D.C., U.S.A. May 5th to 10th, 1930*. 2 vols. New York: The International Committee for Mental Hygiene, 1932.

———, ed. 'The Founding of the International Committee for Mental Hygiene'. In *Proceedings of the First International Congress on Mental Hygiene, Held at Washington, D.C., U.S.A. May 5th to 10th, 1930*, 1:32–49. New York: The International Committee for Mental Hygiene, 1932.

———, ed. 'World View of Mental Hygiene'. In *Proceedings of the First International Congress on Mental Hygiene, Held at Washington, D.C., U.S.A. May 5th to 10th, 1930*, 1:86–139. New York: The International Committee for Mental Hygiene, 1932.

Winter, Jay. 'Shell-Shock and the Cultural History of the Great War'. *Journal of Contemporary History* 35, no. 1 (2000): 7–11.

Wolters, Christine, Christof Beyer, and Brigitte Lohff. *Abweichung und Normalität: Psychiatrie in Deutschland vom Kaiserreich bis zur Deutschen Einheit*. Bielefeld: transcript, 2013.

World Federation for Mental Health. 'Mental Health and World Citizenship: A Statement Prepared for the International Congress on Mental Health, London 1948', 1948.

Zalashik, Rakafet. *Das unselige Erbe: Die Geschichte der Psychiatrie in Palästina und Israel*. Translated by David Ajchenrand. Frankfurt am Main: Campus, 2012.

Zaretsky, Eli. *Secrets of the Soul: A Social and Cultural History of Psychoanalysis*. New York: Vintage, 2005.

Zbinden, J.-D. 'L'organisateur: André Repond (1886–1973)'. In *Portraits de psychiatres romands*, edited by Christian Müller, 9–76. Lausanne: Éditions Payot, 1995.

Zeller, Uwe. *Psychotherapie in der Weimarer Zeit: Die Gründung der 'Allgemeinen Ärztlichen Gesellschaft für Psychotherapie' (AÄGP)*. Tübingen: Köhler, 2001.

Zulliger, Hans. *Einführung in den Behn-Rorschach-Test*. 2 vols. Arbeiten zur angewandten Psychiatrie 6. Berne: Huber, 1941.

'Zum Geleit'. *Allgemeine ärztliche Zeitschrift für Psychotherapie und psychische Hygiene* 1, no. 1 (1928): 1–6.

'Zur Einführung'. *Zeitschrift für angewandte Anatomie und Konstitutionslehre* 1, no. 1 (1913): 1–3.

'Zur Frage der Arbeitstherapie in den Heil- und Pflegeanstalten'. *Zeitschrift für psychische Hygiene* 2, no. 2 (1929): 50–61.

Zweig, Stefan. *Die Welt von Gestern: Erinnerungen eines Europäers*. Stockholm: Bermann-Fischer, 1941.

'Zweiter Bericht über die Deutsche Forschungsanstalt für Psychiatrie in München zur Stiftungsratssitzung am 30. April 1921'. *Zeitschrift für die gesamte Neurologie und Psychiatrie* 70, no. 1 (1921): 342–59.

Index

D. Freis, *Psycho-Politics between the World Wars*, Mental Health in Historical Perspective, https://doi.org/10.1007/978-3-030-32702-6

FSC
www.fsc.org
MIX
Papier | Fördert
gute Waldnutzung
FSC® C083411

Kolibri 360 GmbH
Ferdinand-Jühlke-Straße 7
99095 Erfurt, Deutschland
produktsicherheit@kolibri360.de